DEDICATION

To Mom and Dad...I shall always lift you up!

To my sons, Adam and Dylan...Life will never be the same.
And without you, I would not have known life as completely.

To my soul mate, Candice...
"As soon as I saw you, I knew an adventure was going to happen..." (A. A. Milne)
And, the adventures continue to grow through each one of you.

To my Lord God...Thank you for giving your Son.

DSB

TABLE OF CONTENTS

INTRODUCTION

Having trained an average of 50 clients per week for 9 years, I understand the struggle that you, the personal trainer, face with a limited number of hours each day. Personal training, any way you size it up, is labor intensive. One of my biggest frustrations while training was the effort of trying to interpret volumes of complex, scientific information, and at the same time give 110% effort, service and follow-up to 10 clients on any given day.

I wanted to write a book that would be of great use to personal trainers in the "trenches." Those trainers who train one-on-one every day and/or supervise other staff simply have very little time available for professional growth and personal priorities. I hope that *Program Design for Personal Trainers* helps ease your time crunch.

This book is for trainers who need practical information supported by science and current research. *Program Design* is partially a physiology text, and partially a guide to applying those complex theories to everyday program design for a variety of settings and clients. This is what I call "bridging theory into application." If you can not apply new information and research to your everyday situation, I ask, "Of what practical use is it?"

This book is written so chapters stand on their own. To this end, some information is repeated, but often from a new and different perspective. I think the best learning experience will be gained by reading the book from cover to cover. But, *Program Design* is also an excellent source to use as a quick reference to identify the information you need for a particular program-design challenge. Whether it is exercise physiology, strength training, fat loss, special populations or other concerns, I think you will find the answer here. And, maybe best of all, you will be able to use your limited time efficiently because all the resources you need to develop effective programming are available in one place.

Douglas Brooks

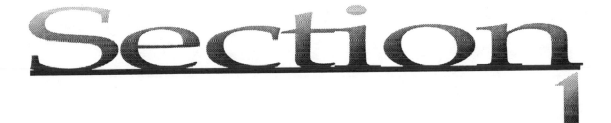

Section 1

Foundations of Effective Program Design

"Being above average is not all that difficult. To put it bluntly, the average person has settled for less, has accepted mediocrity. The goal in life is not to be an average human being but to be the best you can possibly be. This attitude is a matter of making the most out of what you were born with. It follows from acknowledging an obligation to excellence."

George Sheehan, MD, 1986

CHAPTER 1

TEN STEPS TO PROGRAM DESIGN

"You mean you planned this *for me*!?" exclaimed one of my first clients when we began introducing variety into her workout by changing exercises and intensity of effort. As a new trainer I had wrongly assumed that clients understood my professional dedication and the time I invested in planning and periodizing their programs. In that moment I realized that many trainers do little to progress individual training programs. Her emphasis on "for me" magnified the importance of the words "individual," "personal," "commitment" and "service," which are the essence of personal training.

Whether or not you are an experienced personal trainer, you probably have questions about program design. It does not take long to realize that a one-size-fits-all program design does not work. Every individual has unique needs, interests and responses to various activities and protocols. Although an understanding of exercise physiology and movement sciences is a prerequisite to creative exercise programming, personal trainers armed with only this information may still be puzzled about the practical solutions to their clients' individual needs.

I understand that challenge—the need to build a bridge between the science and the individual. After training an average of 40 to 50 clients a week for 9 years, I learned to blend the usable and practical aspect of theory into the reality of day-to-day personal training. How? By planning quality programs using a step-by-step process. Many personal trainers—and their clients—do not understand the necessity and importance of a plan of action. Many clients assume (too often, correctly) that a personal training session has little forethought attached to its implementation.

If you are retelling the same story day in and day out, not only will your clients fail to progress, but you will fail to create a sense of value regarding the services you provide to your clients on a long-term basis. Personal training must evolve beyond a "flurry of unplanned activity." We need to create programs that change the perception of the consumer that the only way to progress or add variety is to move to another personal trainer.

By moving through each of these 10 steps with each client, I had a format to follow that ensured each training program was built on a solid foundation of science while being customized to each client's individual needs. That way, the clients were able to maintain their motivation and trust in my skills, and I was confident that the program was safe, effective and sufficiently multidimensional to keep them interested. You can use them, too, to get your clients results.

Table 1. Ten Steps for Effective Program Design	
Step 1: Information Gathering	Step 6: Active Rest
Step 2: Balanced Physical Programming	Step 7: Cross Training
Step 3: Cardiorespiratory Conditioning	Step 8: Special Needs for Healthy Populations
Step 4: Muscle Strength and Endurance	Step 9: Success and Adherence
Step 5: Flexibility Training	Step 10: The Reality Factor

Step 1: Information Gathering

The information-gathering process involves 3 steps:

1. medical history/health questionnaire

2. client interview

3. fitness testing (optional)

The **medical history/health questionnaire** asks questions that elicit information you need to help identify medical concerns, your clients' personal understanding of basic fitness concepts, current and past fitness activities, goals and interests, and eating habits. An additional lifestyle profile includes such things as job type and personality traits.

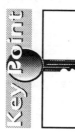

> Your questionnaire should ask only for information that you understand and can interpret to determine your client's course of action.

The **client interview** will become an ongoing dialogue that takes your medical history/health questionnaire to the next, more personal level. For the program to be effective you must consider the goals and preferences of your clients, understand how you can best communicate with them, and encourage feedback at every opportunity. It is important to create a motivational environment where communication comes first and program compliance is high. How you interact with your clients greatly influences how they feel about themselves and how they feel about you.

Fitness testing is an *optional* motivational tool that many trainers use to define a starting point and to excite their clients about changes in their fitness over time. (In no way is it a diagnostic tool that assesses the diseased, or non-diseased, status of an individual.) Fitness testing *can* be highly motivational to certain individuals.

Typically personal trainers test submaximal cardiorespiratory fitness, muscle strength and endurance, and flexibility. The results serve as a benchmark from which further improvements in these components of fitness may be objectively measured. To do so, the exact procedure used in the initial test must be replicated in the retest.

For example, a positive adaptation to cardiorespiratory training could be a lower heart rate. Heart rate is an example of a tangible and objective measure of improvement—or lack of improvement—in fitness over a specific time period. For the test to be a valid measure of the client's progress, you could use a stationary bicycle with indicators that allow you to measure the overload and the rpm (speed) so you can duplicate the test later.

All of the current models for testing have both strengths and weaknesses in their abilities to assess improvements in the different areas of fitness. Most of the concern lies in appropriateness (safety and needs) to the individual and the ability of the tests (especially muscle strength and endurance, and flexibility) to reflect balanced fitness.

Quick Index:

Chapter 2, health history and fitness tests
Chapter 3, interpreting lab reports, learning about medically related conditions

Step 2: Balanced Physical Programming

Once the stage has been set and the client's goals are well understood, physical programming for the majority of the population includes cardiorespiratory conditioning, muscular strength and endurance conditioning, and flexibility training. All of these key components of fitness must be addressed correctly to ensure that a balanced approach to your client's health and fitness has been taken.

Within each component, you likewise balance fitness. For example, within the muscular strength and endurance component, all agonist and antagonist muscle pairs, such as the biceps and triceps, need to be challenged.

Balanced physical programming walks a fine line between *listening* to what your client is telling you that she *wants*, and incorporating these interests into a program that also contains what she *needs* from a total wellness perspective. Don't neglect to explain to your client the importance of including all the components.

Quick Index:

Chapter 6, monitoring intensity levels
Chapter 10, integrating program variables such as progression, overload, specificity and rest
Chapter 11, appropriate maintenance levels

Step 3: Cardiorespiratory Conditioning

Cardiorespiratory conditioning consists of activity that involves large-muscle, rhythmic, continuous movement that simultaneously increases heart rate and blood flow back to the heart. This type of conditioning can decrease the risk factors associated with heart disease, increase endurance and personal vitality, and help with weight maintenance or loss. Use a variety of cardiorespiratory activities (walking, running, biking, swimming) to challenge the heart and lungs, and to avoid an increased risk of overuse injury that is associated with unrelenting and repetitive motions.

Quick Index:

Chapters 4 and 12, the interrelationship among energy systems and fat burning
Chapter 5, physiology and methods for cardiorespiratory conditioning

Step 4: Muscular Strength and Endurance Conditioning

Most of your clients should engage in strength training. Proper strength training can boost metabolism, help decrease fat mass or maintain ideal weight, decrease the risk for osteoporosis, increase self-esteem, preserve personal physical independence and increase strength.

Effective muscular strength and endurance conditioning is dependent on a progressive increase in resistance over time that challenges all of the movements that muscles contribute to. Be sure to include all of the body's paired agonist/antagonist muscular relationships.

Quick Index:

Chapter 4, interrelationship among energy systems
Chapter 7, the physiology of muscles
Chapter 14, manipulating numbers of reps and sets and weight loads
Chapter 15, evaluating resistance training exercises

Step 5: Flexibility Training

Flexibility is most simply defined as range of motion (ROM) available to a joint or joints. Active range of motion (AROM) and functional range of motion (FROM) expand this limited view. Healthy, or desired, flexibility is a capacity to move freely in every *intended direction*. The movement should be confined to the joint's FROM or intended movement capabilities. This is different from the joint's *normal* ROM because normal is not always healthy, or adequate for individual movement pattern needs. The development of functional or usable flexibility entails challenging range of motion in a manner that closely mimics daily or functional movement.

An active stretch (AROM) occurs when an agonist muscle(s) moves a body part through the farthest possible range of motion without outside assistance. For example, if the knee is extended, the contracting (agonist) quadriceps actively stretch the opposing (antagonist) hamstring musculature.

Adapting the concept of FROM and utilizing AROM technique in your flexibility programming may allow your client to participate more effectively in daily domestic activities and recreational pursuits, with less potential of injury. Since flexibility is specific to each joint's musculature, design a program that stretches areas of the body that are often lacking in adequate flexibility.

Quick Index:

Chapter 8, physiology of flexibility
Chapter 17, flexibility training techniques

Step 6: Active Rest

Regardless of fitness level, thread the concept of active rest throughout the fitness routines. The active rest concept sequences exercises to structure a workout that optimizes workout time and accommodates the fitness level of the individual. Typically, a large amount of time in traditional fitness programs involves recovery from work performed. There are several ways to minimize wasted recovery time or to eliminate it.

1. Use perceived exertion and intervals (work, recovery) to keep your client in motion during cardiorespiratory conditioning.

2. Sequence resistance training exercises so that they alternate from muscle group to muscle group, or from upper to lower body to the trunk.

3. If a muscle group is targeted for consecutive multiple sets, the recovery phase(s) can be utilized for flexibility training.

For your clients who are looking for maximum results with minimum time investment, this is an excellent way to optimize the finite time you have available.

Quick Index:

Chapter 10, integrating program variables such as progression, overload, specificity and rest
Chapter 12, interval training philosophy and application
Chapter 14, ways to challenge the musculoskeletal system

Step 7: Cross Training

Now that your base approach is set, the fun continues as you change the program with cross training. By understanding the concept of specific overloads and their effects on the body's energy systems and the 3 components of fitness, the world of programming choices becomes less confusing. Overload definitions reveal exactly what effect a certain intensity, duration, frequency and type of activity will have on any component of fitness. This leads to productive and time-efficient activity that fulfills your client's program goals.

A client may cross train within a component of fitness, such as cardiorespiratory fitness (running, walking, stepping, etc.), or between components of fitness (circuit with muscular endurance and cardiorespiratory fitness emphasized). Utilizing cross training within your program gives you big advantages, such as:

- variety and change
- new physiological stimulation (new fitness gains)
- motivation
- compliance ("sticking with it")

Some clients like change and some do not. Continued communication (the ongoing "interview") and feedback from your clients is essential before and after you initiate any program changes. Changing for the sake of variety, or because you (the trainer) need a change, are the wrong reasons. Change is best implemented when your client is ready physiologically and psychologically.

Quick Index:

Step 8: Special Needs for Healthy Populations

All of your clients have special concerns. You already have the tools to balance fitness among cardiorespiratory, muscular strength and endurance, and flexibility components. Now, you will need to consider issues such as exercise for performance versus fitness versus health; safe weight maintenance and loss; and strength plateaus or pregnancy. You may also need to address nutritional concerns, motivational and psychological needs. You will need to determine what style of communication will work best with your client. Taking all these into account will help you design the perfect, customized program.

Quick Index:

Step 9: Success and Adherence

Encouraging the client's perception that she is successful is one—if not the most—important aspect of program design. Four factors ensure exercise adherence and a successful business.

- Time—keep most workouts around one hour; 2-3 times per week.

- Variety—use cross training when appropriate.

- Intrinsic motivation—both you and your client should know

  why she wants to exercise (ask her!).

- Lifestyle changes—people must like what they are doing to incorporate

  the new behavior into their lifelong habits.

Success in program design means a healthy, happy client, as well as a thriving business.

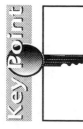

Many people do not want to exercise "hard." Most exercise to feel better and have more energy for daily living. We, as trainers, need to step away from our own preferences and walk into the lives of our clients. Most of our clients would not plan their exercise programs like we plan our own. Consider this thought seriously and you're on your way to effective and safe program design!

Step 10: The Reality Factor

I have worked with clients in a personal training situation for 11 years, and counting. I don't work out 50 clients per week anymore, but the "reality factor" is as evident today as it was years ago when I was working with clients from early in the morning to late at night. Many clients still do not perform perfect exercise technique. Some do not have all of the ideal components of a balanced fitness program comfortably inserted into their daily schedule. Others have never linked their cardiorespiratory interval segments into a continual effort. Most will never experience proprioceptive neuromuscular facilitation (PNF) stretching in its true and intense form.

Though the majority of clients are not the perfect models of textbook programming, their individual improvement is great. Their lives are better. Rather than create a program that your peers would approve, attempt to optimize your client's involvement in fitness for a lifetime, with whatever techniques it takes.

Don't be a robotic trainer who uses one recipe/program for every client. Fitness programming is not a clear-cut issue. More often than not, an effective program and business offers a smorgasbord of options that change as your client does.

Case Study: Designing for Individual Need

Bob was evaluated as clinically obese and had the approval of his primary health care professional to begin an exercise program. His overfat state and my conversations with his doctor indicated that his cardiorespiratory conditioning was low, and there were orthopedic concerns related to his knees, hips and low back. Yet Bob was extremely strong and agile at 6 feet 4 inches and 350-plus pounds.

After gathering information on Bob, I felt it was imperative to focus on *his* goals and psychological makeup. (At a later date, I would let him know fitness testing was an option he could choose.) One of his long-term goals was to be able to run 10K distances. Was it going to be possible? I didn't know.

Since his diagnostic stress test indicated no limitations with regard to exercising heart rate, the immediate concern was orthopedic. Bob was excited to begin his journey toward the 10K goal, so we started to develop baseline fitness by walking, walking inclines, recumbent stationary biking, stair and machine stepping, participating in a balanced strength program, and flexibility training. We did not initially focus on a host of "negative" issues such as diet or weight loss (Bob had been there, done that). Still, I made no promises.

My concerns as a trainer were the obvious goals of strengthening the joints and joint musculature and improving Bob's cardiorespiratory system. To these I attached a host of health-related issues, such as fat loss, decreased risk of heart disease, decreased blood pressure, improved lipid profile, decreased risk of orthopedic injury, decreased risk for adult onset diabetes (NIDDM), and an increased awareness on Bob's part regarding his physical self.

Bob, on the other hand, simply wanted to run.

Over a period of months we "shuffled" our way to a walk/jog. Bob soon complained of discomfort in the lower leg and foot. We immediately backed off. One day as we exited my studio to take a fast stride, I grabbed a small football. Bob fancied himself as a strong, fleet-footed athlete. My plan was to institute a form of interval conditioning by tossing the football back and forth. Bob would walk/shuffle/run a pass pattern, make the spectacular catch and recover as I ran my requisite pattern.

The result: Bob's perceived exertion a 10; perceived fun a 10; and no resultant orthopedic problems. He accomplished more total work during his time slot, became more fit and burned more calories (see Chapter 12 on interval training). This is certainly not your textbook program (and following the "rules" by the book would not have worked with Bob), but it worked because Bob seeks fun and variety as his number-one requirement for fitness activities.

From day to day we utilize various cardiovascular options. Excellent choices have included the recumbent stationary bike, stepping, treadmill, cross-country ski simulator, water fitness and of course, tossing the football as our personal favorite. We utilize recovery phases or steady-state (rate) work loads to discuss his current health concerns and further optimize the training session.

Bob never did run a 10K, or even a continuous 5K. But, in his pursuit of the 10K he discovered something of more value—*fun!* Bob told me that he felt "fun and success are direct derivatives from a program that works with, instead of against, your body." That is what training smart is all about! The pearls of wisdom that I derived from Bob, and continue to use with every one of my clients, include:

- Listen to your client. It merits repeating: Listen!
- Pay attention to what your client wants, while simultaneously formulating a program that also encompasses his needs.
- Have your client listen closely to what his body is telling him.
- Encourage your client to communicate to you how he feels.
- Act on your client's personal feelings and perceptions.
- Lead your client to understand why he exercises by asking him to express his emotions and needs, and to identify the activities that meet them.

The point, of course, is to flow with your client. My first reaction to Bob's request was that Bob would never run injury-free, which would have slammed the door shut on Bob's personal, self-generated motivation. It was more effective to use that motivation and work toward *his* goal. Much of the success of a personal trainer is borne in technical competency. However, equally as important are people skills and interpreting, by listening, what the needs of your client are.

Effective Advisors for Effective Programs

Where do you get help for a client who has a special problem? How do you locate health professionals you can refer to? Part of the success of your program design and of your business depends on the expertise you can access. An advisory board is an important step in the right direction. When thoughtfully selected, your advisory board members can become a professional referral system and a management team.

Include a diverse representation from business people and licensed health professionals (such as a registered dietitian, physical therapist, physician, osteopathic doctor, chiropractor or massage therapist) to other qualified fitness professionals. I like to include at least one other personal trainer who owns her own business, as well as another trainer who works for a club.

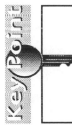

If a particular client's needs cannot be met by your organization in a safe and competent manner, a responsible referral must be made to the appropriate specialist. This is both ethical and a professional courtesy to clients. Here is the warning: take time to interview these professionals, and check their references so you are confident about the referral. Since you are recommending them, their services are a direct reflection on you.

Utilization of an advisory board can keep you from becoming myopic, stagnant and complacent in your approach to running your business and in your program design. Representation from the business community and the health and fitness sector gives you direct communication to the pulse of the "real world." This can help you solve your business and programming challenges in a time-efficient and effective manner, and keeps you fresh and challenged by a constant introduction to "cutting edge" ideas.

The smart leaders of today surround themselves with excellence. They absorb personality qualities and information from knowledgeable sources by observing behavior, listening and asking questions. An openness to learn and a desire to exude their personal best propels their services and businesses to the top.

Fitness Programming That Fails to Deliver

Fitness programming that fails to deliver results is often a direct consequence of a poor understanding of applied physiology and biomechanics. We have to understand how the human body works and attain a high level of technical competence.

Programming that fails is also a result of program design that is driven by consumer demands, fads, exercise trends based on little scientific substance or traditional approaches that have never been questioned. More often than not, little importance is given to the scientific backing, for example, of a particular strength training movement or utilization of a particular piece of exercise equipment. Variety for the sake of variety becomes the fashion and the form.

To choose a programming philosophy that uses this approach will compromise your integrity, effectiveness and—most importantly—your client's program. Short-lived variety and current "fitness fashion" can lead to client injury, disillusionment, dropout and, needless to say, a decline in your business. Consumer/client interests must be satisfied, but they can be done in an entertaining, reputable and effective way.

Effective programming maintains a close interaction between science, yourself and the client's needs. And, it goes beyond activity. To create programming that delivers, keep these 5 points in mind:

1. Programming that meets the ongoing and changing needs of your clients is a dynamic process of personal interaction and versatile program choices.

2. Keep the client and his or her needs as the center of focus.

3. Continue to educate yourself and constantly ask, "Why?"

4. Implement programming ideas when you fully understand the concept and can communicate it to your client.

5. Always keep and encourage open communication.

Program design is certainly a dynamic and ever-changing process. Armed with a solid physiological and philosophical basis for your decision making, you are on the road to creating the best exercise programming for your clients.

The Bridge

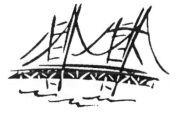

Using these 10 steps to create a comprehensive, individualized plan for each client is the "secret" to excellent fitness programming. Your ability to apply these steps relies as much on your knowledge of each client's needs and goals as on your knowledge of science. As trainers our job is to focus on the client—not reproduce the exercise program that we personally prefer. These 10 steps provide the structure to make professional recommendations.

Step-by-Step Program Design

Step One: Information Gathering

___1. Did I obtain a complete medical history/health questionnaire?

Medical concerns such as blood pressure, smoking, blood lipid profile, orthopedic and cardiovascular history, allergies, medications, last physical examinations and family histories.

___2. Did I determine relevant information, such as personal understanding of fitness concepts and past fitness experiences?

___3. Did I determine individual goals and interests?

___4. Did I have a thorough initial client interview, and am I prepared to encourage ongoing communication?

___5. Did I provide optional, appropriate fitness testing?

Step Two: Balanced Physical Programming

___6. Did I explain the primary components of physical fitness? This includes cardiorespiratory and muscular strength and endurance conditioning, and flexibility training.

___7. Am I prepared to differentiate between training for athletic performance and creating fitness/health improvements?

Step Three: Cardiorespiratory Conditioning

___8. Did I plan exercises that provide rhythmic, continuous, large-muscle activity that promotes a simultaneous increase in heart rate and return of blood to the heart?

___9. Did I generally recommend cardiorespiratory exercise 3-5 times per week, at 40-85% of my client's max VO_2 (this compares to 55-90% of maximum heart rate), for 20-60 minutes?

___10. Did I consider the option of planning unstructured activities that will positively impact my client's health?

___11. Am I sure I did not create a workout that is too hard?

Step Four: Muscle Strength and Endurance Conditioning

___12. Did I plan exercises that offer a progressive increase in resistance over time and challenge all of the movements the muscles make?

___13. Did I generally recommend 8-12 repetitions, 3-5 times per week, for each muscle group (8-10 exercises)?

___14. Was I careful to err on the side of conservatism, recognizing that intensity is relative to the individual?

___15. Did I include exercise for balanced muscle strength between all of the paired agonist/antagonist muscles of the body (for example, biceps/triceps)?

___16. Did I design a program that will maintain the client's interest and produce results?

Step Five: Flexibility Training

__17. Did I plan static (no bouncing), sustained (10-60 seconds) stretches held to the point of mild tension, 3-5 times a week?

__18. Did I plan stretching for *functional* flexibility, rather than extreme ranges of motion?

__19. Did I plan stretching for areas of the body that are often lacking adequate flexibility (chest, anterior shoulder, hamstrings, hip flexors, gastrocnemius/soleus muscle groups of the lower leg)?

Step Six: Active Rest

__20. For time-crunched clients, did I optimize time availability and accommodate the fitness level of the individual using various active-rest techniques?

Step Seven: Cross Training

__21. Did I apply the definitions of overload for each component of fitness to all cross training activities?

__22. Did I utilize cross training for variety and change, new physiological stimulation (new fitness gains), motivation and compliance ("sticking with it")?

__23. Did I find what level of change and variety the client needs or wants?

Step Eight: Special Needs for Healthy Populations

__24. Did I plan for the client's special interest, such as performance vs. fitness vs. health, safe weight control, strength plateaus and health issues such as pregnancy?

Step Nine: Success and Adherence

__25. Am I prepared to provide continuing feedback to encourage the client's perception that she is successful?

__26. If it is a beginner workout, did I keep it around one hour, 2-3 times a week?

__27. Did I understand and incorporate the client's intrinsic motivation to exercise?

__28. Did I consider my client's enjoyment of exercises so she can incorporate fitness into a lifestyle change?

__29. Did I keep in mind that most people do not want to exercise "hard?" Many clients simply want to feel better and have more energy for daily living.

Step Ten: The Reality Factor

__30. Did I keep in mind my ultimate goal of improving my client's quality of life?

__31. Did I remember and emphasize the goal of progress, not perfection?

CHAPTER 2

GATHERING INFORMATION

Jerry was referred to me by a cardiologist. Six months earlier Jerry had undergone a second, successful heart bypass surgery. I quickly realized that Jerry's perception of his health status was very different from his doctor's perception. On his medical history questionnaire he treated his heart disease as though it was no more serious than a mild cold. He told me the doctor said, "You can do anything; everything is perfect with your health." During a conversation with his doctor, however, I received explicit limitations and guidelines regarding cardiorespiratory exercise type and intensity. The doctor was very specific about heart rate and blood pressure monitoring and resistance training exercises.

I realized Jerry's written responses revealed that he truly believed surgery could correct any health problems he might have. His doctor vehemently denounced this, and added that "my goal is to get Jerry to the 'wake-up call' before he's run out of second chances." Jerry was in denial about the seriousness of his heart disease because of fear and his desire to go on with life in his usual, unrestricted manner.

Jerry felt that he knew best and he wanted to control the direction of his workouts, whether or not it was beneficial to his health. He made it clear that he despised cardiorespiratory activity and did not like to perspire. He liked lifting heavy weights. If I was to successfully work with Jerry, I had to create an environment that would work with his personality rather than fight against it. If our relationship became a battle of "right" versus "wrong," Jerry would win, but ultimately both of us would be losers.

The physical programming challenge was solved by introducing Jerry to a circuit-training design that emphasized cardiorespiratory conditioning. I told him that the "cardio" stations were just rest stations so that he could perform his "strength" workout more effectively. His high repetition overload (20-25 reps per set) "strength" stations were established by "doctor's orders." Yes, it was manipulation. But as far as Jerry was concerned, he was lifting weights, in control, doing what he wanted, and he forgot that he did not like sweat!

Obviously, if I had relied on Jerry as my only source of information, I may have put my client at risk of serious complication or even death. Also, I would have never developed an effective support network for optimizing Jerry's health. Jerry presented a new challenge to me every time we got together. I learned many of my approaches from Jerry's wife and his attending physician, because both had much more experience at dealing with his disposition. Because we all had at the top of our list his well-being, my team had expanded to client, wife and doctor.

After 4 years, Jerry was a changed and much healthier man. He has made numerous lifestyle changes, insists that his denial and anxiety about his health have decreased, and that the quality of his life has improved.

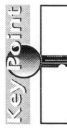

> The only way you can build a bridge between your knowledge of exercise science and a program that will meet each client's specific needs is by gathering information. Even when you are designing exercise programs for healthy, asymptomatic people, there are many considerations you must uncover in addition to your client's current health status.

The information-gathering process includes:

- medical history/health questionnaire—get it in writing!
- client interview—get it by talking!
- fitness testing (optional)

Proper written and verbal (interview) screening—along with the development of key liaisons with appropriate medical professionals—takes the burden off your shoulders. Use your advisory board. Do not be caught in the predicament of having to make decisions completely on your own. Failing to consult with or refer to the proper professional is a mistake that can totally undermine your personal training business. The liability implications are obvious. The risk for a successful lawsuit against you increases when (1) you accept a client when you do not have the capacity to render appropriate services, and (2) you pretend to have competence in a particular area.

Even if you are not sued, the client may lose confidence in your integrity and ability to deliver competent service. This can certainly affect client referrals and is a very short-sighted way to look at the "big picture" of growing your business. Take the pressure off. Ask the right questions and take the time for the appropriate pre-exercise groundwork.

If you have *any* questions or hesitations concerning the safety of proceeding with an individual's program, check with your client's physician or qualified health care provider. Establishing a relationship with your client's health care provider is very important, particularly when working with higher risk clients. In addition, this kind of attention also will allow you to create your own opportunities in the health care industry.

Health management organizations (HMOs) often prefer to focus on prevention and early detection of disease. For example, you may discover high blood pressure in a client and refer the person to a medical doctor. You will have decreased the potential long-term costs to the individual and insurance company and demonstrated your ability to a physician. A process like this can open up many doors of opportunity. And, it all begins with a simple screening process that has your client's well-being at the center of attention.

The Medical History/Health Questionnaire

The medical history/health questionnaire asks questions about medical concerns and other useful personal information, such as activities and lifestyle behaviors. This questionnaire, as well as informed consent and consent/release forms, is your means of identifying clients who may need medical clearance before participating in an exercise program. These forms also document that you have acted in a legally responsible manner, in accordance with industry standards and guidelines.

The questionnaire should ask *only for information that you understand and can interpret* to determine your client's course of action. The profile may include questions to learn more about:

- blood pressure, smoking and blood-lipid profiles (cholesterol ratio, HDL and LDL)
- personal and family cardiovascular history, chest pain, angina, heart attacks and strokes
- breathing or lung disorders
- personal and family history of diabetes
- allergies, medications, last physical examination, current family health and general histories
- orthopedic problems that include back pain, recent surgery, muscle or joint pains and any other related condition that is considered chronic
- pregnancy. Is the client pregnant, or has she given birth within the previous 6 weeks to several months?
- chronic illnesses such as osteoporosis, arthritis, epilepsy, multiple sclerosis and Parkinson's disease
- the client's personal level of understanding of basic fitness concepts. This includes cardiovascular fitness, muscular strength and endurance, flexibility training and safe weight loss
- current and past involvement with fitness activities
- personal goals and interests
- personal dietary practices. Include questions that help reveal information about eating habits and nutritional knowledge.
- personal lifestyle and stress profile
- job type and personality traits

The **short-form medical history/health questionnaire** (see sample at the end of this chapter) is appropriate for apparently low-risk clients, or short-term clients requesting only a consultation or program design. It also makes sense if you are not comfortable using an involved medical history questionnaire, or if a client resists a longer form. A properly designed short-form certainly is not a compromise for information gathering, but simply a matter of appropriateness to your situation.

The **long-form medical/health history** (see sample at the end of this chapter) is designed to be repetitive with regard to the questions asked. I have found that asking relatively similar questions in different ways and in different sections of the form is more likely to elicit the information that I need. If the first version of the question does not alert me to a consideration, then the second or third approach may. For example, a client may not indicate risk factors for heart disease, but may give the information in a different form when answering questions about relatives, blood pressure and blood lipids. While some of my clients have observed that the form is repetitive and are curious as to why, the majority see no connection, and often their answers reflect this.

The **informed and release consent forms** (see samples at the end of this chapter) explain the exercise test(s) or procedure(s) your client is going to be part of, discusses possible risks or discomforts and answers your client's questions. The release/consent form acknowledges that your client is participating voluntarily and retains the right to deny consent or stop the procedures at any point during the testing/evaluation. Forms like these can help protect you from a liability standpoint, and informs your clients as to exactly what they will be experiencing.

"Red Flags"

When something on the medical/health history questionnaire appears out of the ordinary, I term this a "red flag." Red flags generally need some kind of attention or follow-up that may be beyond your expertise. A few examples of red flags include: age of the individual, history of heart disease, orthopedic concerns, high blood pressure, pregnancy and diabetes.

If your client informs you about any of these medical concerns and you are not confident you have the expertise to safely and effectively work with this individual or particular situation, refer him to a physician or other medical expert for evaluation and clearance before he begins exercising. This is where your advisory board can be of invaluable assistance if you do not know the best direction to take.

A red flag can also signify an area where you simply need more information before you can begin to create the best, and safest, program for your client. For example, your new client Susan appears for an initial consultation holding her new baby. She is only 2 weeks postpartum and anxious to "whip her body back into shape, starting today."

Though you may not be an expert in working with perinatal clients, you are concerned with the possibility of postpartum bleeding that often occurs if new moms start exercising too soon. In addition, you have read that the hormone relaxin, secreted during pregnancy, maintains its effect on joint laxity for about 4-6 weeks, or longer, after child birth. You explain to Susan some of your concerns regarding her recent pregnancy and the importance of your pre-screening process.

She is impressed by your professionalism, knowledge and concern, and is eager to introduce you to her obstetrician. She now understands the necessity for you to gather invaluable information about her. "I can't believe this. Other trainers that I have worked with started me on a program as soon as they could schedule me in. I think I'm beginning to understand what a professional personal trainer is really like. I'll fax this medical form back to you as soon as possible and I'll call my ob/gyn tomorrow to introduce you. By the way, my mom has diabetes and my dad struggles with high blood pressure and arthritis. Could you help them with their exercise and health?"

Physician-Directed Diagnostic Testing

When should you proceed with this step? The purpose of a **diagnostic health evaluation** is to detect the presence of disease. Conducted by a physician, it may include a coronary risk factor analysis, physical examination and laboratory tests (Heyward, 1991). Based on the results, individuals are classified as apparently healthy, at higher risk, or with disease.

The American College of Sports Medicine (ACSM, 1991) *recommends* a physical examination and medical clearance from a physician for new exercisers who meet the following criteria:

- men over 40 years of age

- women over 50 years of age

- individuals at higher-risk who have one or more coronary risk factors or symptoms of cardiopulmonary or metabolic disease

- known cardiovascular, pulmonary or metabolic disorders

It may be in the best interests of individuals who fall into one or more of the categories listed above to have a **diagnostic stress test** administered with medical supervision. Your advisory board can help you identify clients who may benefit from this type of testing. These tests are administered with physician supervision and conducted by exercise technicians who are well trained and experienced in monitoring exercise tests and emergencies.

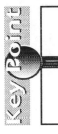

If you have questions about beginning an exercise program with any client, contact the client's health care provider and/or enlist the assistance of your advisory board.

ACSM recommends a diagnostic exercise stress test for healthy older men (over 40 years) and women (over 50 years) before beginning a *vigorous* (greater than 60% of functional aerobic capacity) exercise program.

Moderate exercise (exercise intensity at 40-60% of max VO2) may be appropriate for any aged clientele *without* maximal stress testing. Moderate exercise is an intensity level well within the individual's current capacity that can be comfortably sustained for a prolonged period of time and is generally noncompetitive.

Quick Index:

The Client Interview

The client interview is a dialogue that really never ends. Initially, it allows you to gather facts regarding your client's interests, needs and understanding of fitness in relationship to health. This conversation expands upon the information you receive from the written medical history questionnaire.

> The interview helps you to find out what the *client* wants to accomplish. By acknowledging the client's perspective of what direction the program should take, you encourage your client to feel ownership and responsibility for the program content. This intrinsic motivation will go a long way in exciting your client to be compliant. And it's easy to incorporate any interests of his into a program where you also cover his health and fitness needs.

For example, Jani was a busy mom with 2 young children. She loved to play tennis and was concerned about her overall health and fitness program. She told me, "Even though I live for improving my tennis skills, I'm concerned about other areas of fitness I may be ignoring, like flexibility and strength. How do I fit it all in?"

The balanced physical programming solution was a total conditioning program that took place entirely on court. We created a program that spent 15 minutes on tennis-specific aerobic conditioning, agility and skill drills. Eight minutes of tennis-specific flexibility training followed this cardiorespiratory segment. This served as a perfect preparation for her match. Next, she would play her match. After the match, she completed 15 minutes of upper-body strength work using elastic resistance attached to a court-side net standard. During her competitive season, Jani plays tennis 3 times per week and enters tournaments on weekends. Since she completed her sport-specific workout 3 times per week on her own during tennis season, we added 2 workouts per week with me to concentrate on lower-body and trunk strength. We also integrate some upper-body strength exercises and include flexibility training.

Your clients must always remain a part of the *process*. Their input and sense of personal involvement are important components in directing your program design. This type of interactive communication continues throughout successful personal trainer/client relationships. And, if you have done a thorough job of gathering information, you should understand the inner workings of your client and know what makes him tick.

An excellent tool you can use to gain better knowledge and understanding of yourself and your clients is *The Personal Fitness System: Interactive Wellness© (PFS)*. After completing the 10-minute PFS questionnaire, computer software is available that creates a behavior profile based on the responses. You can use this information to:

1. Gain commitment for improving compliance to programs.
2. Gain commitment for improving fitness and wellness.
3. Accelerate client achievement.
4. Give constructive feedback and criticism.
5. Avoid misunderstanding between client and professional.
6. Get new clients off to a fast and productive start.

7. Build a strong client-professional relationship from the beginning.

8. Discover what makes your client feel comfortable and at ease during a session.

By having a handle on these 8 powerful and crucial issues, you will enhance your effectiveness and your client's success. Also the PFS process, or one that you design by yourself, creates another difference between you and the trainer next door. It loudly proclaims your interest in identifying each client's motivation, as well as your desire to communicate effectively.

Fitness Testing—An Optional Motivational Tool

Fitness testing (as opposed to diagnostic fitness assessment) is an optional motivation tool that many trainers use to excite their clients about improvement in their fitness over time. By recording measurements over specific time periods, such as every 4-6 weeks, clients can see their physical changes. Measurable physical changes include:

- heart-rate responses to cardiorespiratory effort
- resistance being lifted a specific number of times or the amount of resistance being
  lifted, which represents muscular endurance and strength
- changes in range of motion (flexibility) or posture

Fitness testing is *not* a diagnostic tool that assesses the diseased, or nondiseased, status of an individual. Nor is it a tool to determine your client's readiness to engage in activity. A properly designed medical history/health questionnaire, verbal client interviews and a relationship with your client's health care professional(s) determine your client's readiness to participate safely.

Fitness testing is never an absolute necessity. Does the test put your client in a high-risk performance situation inappropriate for his current fitness and health status? For example, can you see the absurdity of maximally testing an individual who is just beginning a strength program to determine his starting weights? Additionally, does the test have the potential to be an embarrassment to the client? If so, don't use it. For example, if you are working with an extremely overfat, sedentary individual, is it really necessary to administer tests to establish that the person is overfat, has a low cardiorespiratory status and has flexibility/postural imbalances? A visual check, proper health screening and conversation will detail all of this.

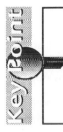

> Administer tests only when they have the potential to have an effect as positive feedback. It is not very motivating for an obese individual to be told that the jaws of the skinfold caliper will not open wide enough to allow a measurement. Stay sensitive to your clients!

At best, the world of fitness testing and assessment is confusing. This topic demands a book in itself to catalog the array of testing methods. Regardless, some of my favorite sources are listed at the end of this chapter.

There are 2 approaches to fitness assessment. One is to compare assessment results to the results (or norms) of other people who have taken the tests. The second is to compare the client's own assessment results to determine the percentage of improvement from test-to-test. Which approach you use depends on the needs of the client. His medical history questionnaire, current level of fitness and health, psychological profile, understanding of the assessment process and client interview will help influence appropriate assessment procedures.

Using Norms. With this method, the client's results are compared to age-adjusted norms. A norm is a standard pattern of response that is regarded as typical for a specific group of people being tested. By comparing your client's results with norms, you are able to *somewhat* quantify your client's effort using a percentile or a rating scale that ranges, for example, from excellent to very poor. When your client tests at the 90th percentile on a particular evaluation, this means that approximately 89% of the people who take this test score *lower*. On the other hand, if your client tests at the 11th percentile, about 89% of the testees score *higher*.

If you are comparing testing results to norms, the exact procedures (protocols) used to establish the norms must be followed. For example, if the test calls for a specific cadence and step height, this must be replicated.

I often call norms the "judgment" scale. Norms are a double-edged sword that can motivate or demotivate, depending on how the scale rates your client's performance. Moreover, comparison to norms may or may not be relevant to your client's current situation. Any improvement, regardless of absolute starting point, is positive. And, even after significant improvement, norm ratings may still leave your client in the lowest category. When I have a client who I anticipate will perform very well, I exploit norms and/or percentiles. Occasionally a "negative," or low rating, could motivate a client in a positive direction. However, be careful with this approach as it could prevent him from continuing his program.

Using Percent Improvement. In my opinion, the better approach for most clients is to show improvement relative to the client's starting point. This enables you to track improvements in fitness that are specific to the individual client. I have had clients who would find it very disheartening to be compared to a standard of excellence that, at this time in their health and fitness journey, seems impossible to achieve.

Also, you can develop your own testing protocols when using percent improvement. By modifying existing tests, creating your own tests and introducing postural assessment techniques, the needs of your clients will be more effectively and safely met.

As part of the screening/fitness testing process, I encourage personal trainers to administer skinfold, circumference measurements (Brittingham, Golding, Heyward, Jackson, Lohman, McArdle), and resting blood-pressure measurements (Golding, Heyward). All 3 procedures are simple skills to learn and safe to administer. An excellent way to attain the ability to accurately learn these assessment skills is to attend educational conferences that offer hands-on learning experiences. Depending on client readiness, these assessments should occur early in the screening process and continue on a fairly regular basis throughout the relationship.

Quick Index:

Case Study: Norms or Percent Improvement?

Let's look at how 3 clients could (and did!) react to fitness assessment. The information you choose to emphasize from your testing and assessment can obviously have very different impacts.

John's initial cardiorespiratory assessment put him near a zero percentile ranking, a level rated as "very poor." I did not share this information with John, as it was obvious it would not have been much of a motivator. John was excited to have simply, as he put it, "... finished in one piece and still breathing." I explained to him that we would refer to this starting point (his heart rate response) of fitness to objectively establish some of the improvements that he would be certain to achieve over a fairly short time period.

After training with Sue for several weeks, she told me that she wanted to have a percentage body-fat assessment performed with skinfold calipers. I had previously discussed an array of possible assessment approaches and had given her several options, which included body composition assessment. After recording the measurements, I entered the data into a popular generalized equation.

Sue's body fat was 48%. It was obvious that it would be very negative to inform her that her percent fat rated at the zero percentile in the "very, very poor category" and that she was, technically, clinically obese. Since she did not ask, I did not offer to disclose. Instead, I said, "Now, we've got your site-specific measurements (see Table 3) that we can refer to as you start to lose fat weight and change your body composition and shape."

About 6 weeks later, at their urging, I retested both John and Sue. John's exercise/recovery heart rate dropped 16% (from 168 to 142) for the same exercise test protocol we had used weeks earlier (see Table 2). Although I knew he only moved to the 5th percentile and was still rated "very poor" when compared to norms, the test "felt easier" and John was ecstatic. As an investment banker, he said, "I'd take a 16% return on my money anytime!"

Sue's body-fat percentage, upon retesting, dropped from 48% to 44%. This is an 8% improvement. I had to chuckle when Sue, who manages a large mutual fund said, "I wish I could get that return on all of my investments." You would have liked her comment when I told her that her sum of skinfolds, which had gone down from 232 to 160, was a 31% improvement (see Table 3). However, when compared to norms, this significant improvement only moved Sue toward the 10th percentile, and she was still categorically rated "very, very poor." She certainly did not need this type of information. Needless to say, she left my studio with the light step of a new person, filled with hope.

Also, in terms of my personal worth to both John and Sue, I had attained a new level. After all, I had just gotten them a 16% and 31% return on their investments. Not bad for a Wall Street rookie!

Sally, on the other hand, is an age-group triathlete champion. Testing is perceived by her as simply another competitive event that she will do very well at, or probably even "win." Her first 2 questions were, "What performance standards do I have to attain to beat the highest scores and what percentage of body fat puts me at levels that compare with world-class triathletes?"

It is obvious that her competitive nature and self-esteem will benefit with norm comparison because she is always rated by the "judgment" scale as excellent and she is usually in the 99th percentile based on her results. Obviously, fitness testing and assessment for Sally is fun since it is not a question of her doing well, but instead, how well will she test?

Table 2. Calculating Percentage Improvement

Percent improvement is easily calculated by subtracting the most recent test result/data from the previous test. This difference is then divided by the previous test result. For the percentage improvement to have any validity related to previous efforts, the testing protocol must be identical. The following chart uses John's raw cardiorespiratory testing data.

A. Initial or previous test result/data	B. Retest #1 or most recent test result/data	C. Difference between previous and most recent test result/data (A minus B)	D. Difference divided by initial or previous test result/data (C divided by A)
168 heart rate	142 heart rate	26 beats per minute	26 divided by 168 equals .1547 or about 16% improvement

Initial and Follow-up Fitness Assessments

Timing of the initial fitness assessment depends primarily on the needs and fitness history of your client. For many of your clients, it is prudent to create a foundation of conditioning before testing, especially if you choose to assess your clients with tests that require physical activity.

Retesting coincides nicely with the phases of (1) initial conditioning, (2) improvement and (3) maintenance described by the American College of Sports Medicine (ACSM, 1991). The greatest gains in conditioning will be in the first 4-6 weeks in a properly designed program. Maintenance conditioning, for the average participant, can begin around 6 months if your client has taken part in steady and progressive training.

Retesting 6-8 weeks after the initial test makes sense from a standpoint of physiological adaptation. You are also likely to motivate your clients with the probable "before and after" improvements. Testing again at 6 months, one year and once a year thereafter is a reasonable plan to follow, based on documented adaptations to a progressive training program.

Evaluating and Improvising Fitness Tests

Personal trainers typically test submaximal cardiorespiratory fitness, muscle strength and endurance, and flexibility. Examples and descriptions of traditional testing and assessment models can be found in the list of resources at the end of this chapter. Many of the current models have both strengths and weaknesses in their abilities to assess improvements in your client's different areas of fitness. In fact, some tests not only may have very little relevance to a client's current situation, they may even put him at risk. To the unsuspecting trainer, the inadequacies may not be easily identified for a specific client's unique needs.

Have you, for example, ever looked closely at the progression of overload for submaximal bicycle ergometer, treadmill and step tests when measuring cardiorespiratory fitness? Is the steady-rate building phase long enough to ensure a safe test? Is the incremental increase in heart rate or functional capacity (VO2) that is required to perform the cardiorespiratory test within a safe limit of effort for your client?

Here's another example. A standard cardiorespiratory test protocol calls for the use of a step height of 12 inches and cadence of 96 beats per minute. A step height of 12 inches may quickly elicit a maximal heart rate from your client, *and* the step height might add orthopedic stress to his knee because it is too high in relation to the client's unique anatomic considerations. Is that really safe?

Though maximal strength tests are not "bad," they are often inappropriately administered because the client is not physically or psychologically ready. Furthermore, most muscular strength and endurance tests *fail* to measure balanced muscular strength and endurance. If balanced muscular fitness is the goal, we would need to assess all of the major muscle groups in the body. Yet testing of all the paired agonist and antagonist (for example, quadriceps and hamstrings) muscle relationships is rarely performed. Many of these tests use traditional protocols that often test only maximal muscular strength and/or use exercises that are biomechanically unsafe or have little relevance to your client's daily movement and exercise patterns.

You may have to create your own exercise and test standards to test muscular balance, strength and endurance. A simple way to do this is to select a number of exercises, perform them at a specific cadence and select an overload that tests both muscular strength and endurance. The test ends when the controlled lifting cadence cannot be maintained. Then, calculate percentage of improvement after the second testing date.

And finally, assessing only "flexibility" is not adequate. See the section on "Flexibility and Postural Assessment" to find out why.

While I would need an entire book to completely discuss the pros and cons of fitness assessment procedures and describe proper procedures, I hope these thoughts will encourage you to question and investigate the appropriateness of traditional fitness assessment "recipes." Too often, a series of evaluations is used again and again, regardless of the unique needs of individual clients and limitations of the tests.

Before choosing any tests, ask yourself the following questions from the "Any Assessment Drill." This drill will help you identify tests that are appropriate, safe and useful for motivating your client toward success in a goal-oriented, individualized program.

Any Assessment Drill

1. Why am I administering these tests? What am I measuring, and how will I use these measurements to motivate my client toward his goals and to aid exercise compliance?

2. Are the tests safe in relation to my client's current level of fitness?

3. Are the tests appropriate to my client's personal health and fitness needs?

4. Do the tests reflect balanced fitness by measuring and assessing all of the major components of fitness?

5. Do the tests accurately measure what they are intended to measure, and if so, is it a useful criterion by which to motivate and measure client improvement? (For example, if you choose to administer a hand dynamometer test to measure static strength and endurance of grip-squeezing muscles of the hand, the answer to this question will not reveal whether this is a "good" or "bad" test, but rather its usefulness to the client.)

If you are not sure of the answer to any of these 5 questions, and especially if you question whether the procedure has any relevance or potential risk to your client, do not use it!

You can easily create your own testing protocol by borrowing ideas from traditional tests. For example, I often modify step tests by using a 2- to 4-inch step platform versus 10, 12 or 18 inches, and often decrease the commonly recommended cadence of 96 beats per minute to a lesser number. By doing this, the norms of the standard test no longer apply, and I must replicate this exact procedure on the retest if I am going to effectively use percentage of improvement. However, the results are relevant to my client's current situation and the previous test. As a result, I feel I have the best world of options and, most important, can better fulfill the testing and assessment necessities of individual clients.

Skinfold Measurements

Skinfold measurements may be used to predict a percentage of body fat or to show improvements in body composition. Body composition measurements are motivational because they can demonstrate safe and progressive fat loss and reinforce the effectiveness of the training program.

I prefer using the process illustrated in Table 3, *How to Practically Use Fat Fold Measurements*, because all of the changes are specific to the individual client. On the other hand, predicting a percentage of body fat or referring to norms compares the client to others. For people who are lean and fit, or otherwise mentally prepared, this can be an exciting motivator. For overfat individuals, this can be a powerful form of negative feedback and another slap in the face to their motivation to become fit.

In Joyce's example in Table 3, I calculated her overall body fat percentage difference from test one to test 2 and it only changed 2.5%. While this is significant to a scientist, it is difficult to convince many clients that this percentage improvement was worth their last 4-6 weeks of effort. I chose not to disclose this calculation to Joyce. However, it was easy and fun for both of us to identify where Joyce was losing body fat, based on her genetic profile, what the site-specific measurements revealed and how her clothes were fitting her.

During previous months she had lost significant fat in the scapulae and triceps area. Joyce was initially frustrated and questioned why she could not selectively "spot reduce" the areas of the body that she viewed as problem regions. I had explained, with patience and consistency, that by "doing the right things" her program would come full circle and allow her to finally lose fat in other areas of the body. She understood and accepted that this was her genetic profile for fat distribution and loss, and its pattern could not be altered. Because of this, Joyce was quite excited to see her consistent effort pay off with a huge percentage of improvement (28% and 31.9% respectively) in 2 site-specific measurements of the abdominal and hip (iliac crest) regions. And overall, her relative degree of fatness (sum of fat fold measures) decreased 12.8%.

Joyce was ecstatic and ready to progress to her next goal of healthy weight loss. I never told her about my 2.5% "secret," yet I think this was the right professional choice because today she is maintaining a healthy and fit 17% body fat.

Blood Pressure

High blood pressure (BP) or hypertension is often a symptomless disease that influences the progression of various vascular diseases, including coronary heart disease (CHD). Early detection of hypertension and consistent monitoring of blood pressure may help your client avoid symptomatic vascular disease, such as heart attack, stroke, intermittent claudication or pain in the lower extremities in later life.

Working with your client's physician to help interpret the blood pressure values you obtain can be an invaluable service to the client. This holds particularly true if your client does not receive regular medical checkups. In this case, you become a vital "health information link" to your client's health care experts.

Table 3. How to Practically Use Fat Fold Measurements
(without predicting percent body fat)

There are 3 ways to use fat fold measurements without predicting a percentage of body fat. The **sum of the measurements** of all fat (skin) fold measurement sites can be used to estimate a relative degree of fatness for comparison over time. However, it is not necessary to label this degree of fatness. It is simply a number.

Second, body fat distribution that is **specific to each site measured** ("site-specific") can be documented and changes noted at each retest. From this information, a genetically determined profile of where fat is lost and gained can be observed. This type of information is useful in counseling clients who are frustrated by the pattern of fat loss that is determined by genetics and cannot be altered.

The third way to use fat fold measurements is as a "before and after" **percentage of change**. Before and after percentage of change can be used with both individual site-specific measures and the sum of measurements. In Table 3, percentage of change is calculated by (1) dividing the change in millimeters (mm) by (2) the previous measurement, and (3) multiplying by 100.

Client: Joyce Age: 54   Scale Weight: 154   Testing Date: 8/1

Fat Fold Measurement Site	Previous Fat Fold Measurement in Millimeters (mm)	New Measurement in Millimeters (mm)	New & Previous Measurement Change in Millimeters (mm); (+ or -)	Percentage of Change
Scapula	13.8	13.0	- 0.8	5.8 %
Triceps	21.2	20.0	- 1.2	5.7 %
Chest	n/a	n/a	n/a	n/a
Axilla	17.0	15.2	- 1.8	10.6 %
Iliac Crest	18.2	13.1	- 5.1	28.0 %
Abdomen	23.2	15.8	- 7.4	31.9 %
Thigh	29.0	26.5	- 2.5	8.6 %
Sum of Fat Fold Measures	115.4	100.6	- 14.8	12.8 %

Flexibility and Postural Assessment

Trainers must go beyond the simple sit-and-reach test to assess flexibility. Some experts, including Plowman (1992) and Kendall (1993), are beginning to question whether the sit-and-reach test can be administered safely to a variety of populations and if it actually gives you any specific and/or valuable information about flexibility in the low back, hamstrings and gastrocnemius muscle groups. Functional hamstring flexibility is easily assessed by having your client lie supine. One leg is lifted while the other is kept flat on the ground. Neither knee should be bent. Sufficient hamstring flexibility is exhibited when the raised leg can reach a vertical position (90 degrees of hip flexion) with no outside assistance.

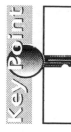

Flexibility is joint specific. This implies that a number of *specific* flexibility and/or postural assessment tests are needed to adequately evaluate your client's range of motion needs.

An effective approach must address *all* of the body's postural misalignments and areas of insufficient flexibility. For example, is your client's chin forward and shoulders rounded? If so, the muscles of the chest and anterior shoulder must be stretched and the muscles of the upper back strengthened. This determination results when you look at flexibility from the context of posture.

Postural assessment is essential to inform and motivate your client, and for gathering critical information for the program. Is their skeletal alignment normal? Are there postural imbalances that need to be addressed through proper selection of strengthening and stretching exercises? Excellent sources for developing this type of flexibility and postural assessment approach include Francis and Francis, 1988; Kendall, 1993; and Plowman, 1992.

Poor posture can place an excessive burden on bones, joints, muscles, tendons and ligaments. Therefore, it is important to identify any significant postural imperfections that might predispose your client to injuries. Improvements in posture will probably involve several different areas of the body. Correcting only a single misalignment will be unsuccessful. In addition, an evaluative process must be in place that effectively measures and reevaluates exercise-related postural and range-of-motion changes over specific time periods.

The Bridge

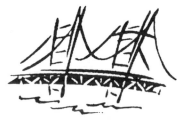

The key to success is to *individualize* and to know your client's needs and goals. Fitness assessment may or may not be a tool that will motivate your clients. But the health history information and your interview will enable you to detect health risks that require referral to medical professionals. Consult with your advisory board if your client's needs go beyond your area of knowledge and expertise. Stay within your knowledge base and listen to the client, and you'll have safe and successful programs.

Parts of this chapter originally appeared in, The Business of Personal Training, Chapter 12, "The Art and Science of Program Design," by Douglas Brooks, published by Human Kinetics Publishers, 1995. Reprinted with permission.

SPECIAL SECTION
SAMPLE HEALTH AND FITNESS ASSESSMENT FORMS
A. Sample Short Form Medical Questionnaire

Name _____

Address _____

Contact Phone Numbers _____

Age _____ Birthdate _____

Primary Health Care Provider _____

Provider's Phone _____

Health History

1. Do you smoke? _____ How much? _____

2. Has your doctor ever said your blood pressure was too high or low? _____

3. Have you (or a family member) ever been told that you have diabetes? _____

4. Do you have any known cardiovascular problems (abnormal ECG, previous heart attack, atherosclerosis, etc.)? _____

If so, what? _____

5. Has your doctor ever told you your cholesterol level was high?_____

6. Are you overweight? _____ How much? _____

7. Do you have any injuries or orthopedic problems (bursitis, bad back, bad knees, etc.)? _____

8. Are you taking any prescribed medications or dietary supplements? _____

9. Are you pregnant or post-partum less than six weeks? _____

10. Date of last physical examination _____

11. Do you have any other medical conditions or problems not previously mentioned? _____

12. Are you currently involved in a regular exercise program? _____

13. What are your goals within this program? _____

_____

Consent Form

I acknowledge, to the best of my ability, that I am in good health and have no known medical problems that would restrict my ability to participate in this exercise program.

Signed _____ Date _____

Author's Note: This form would be appropriate to use with low-risk clients or short-term clients (consulting/program design only). If you are not comfortable using an involved medical history questionnaire, a short form like this makes more sense.

B. Sample Long Form Medical Questionnaire

MEDICAL HISTORY QUESTIONNAIRE
(History, health, smoking, diet, exercise, risk factor and stress analysis)
Douglas S. Brooks, M.S.
Exercise Physiologist

This is your medical history form, to be completed prior to your first training session with Brooks - The Training Edge. All information will be kept confidential. This information will be used for the evaluation of your health and readiness to begin our exercise program. Your answers will help us design a comprehensive program that meets your individual needs. You will want to make it as accurate and complete as possible, yet free from meaningless details. Please fill out the form carefully and thoroughly, then review it to be certain you have not left anything out.

Name: _____

Date: _____

B. Long Medical History Questionnaire (continued)

MEDICAL HISTORY AND SCREENING FORM

General Information

Participant:

Name _____

Address _____

Contact phone numbers _____

Birthdate _____

Family Physician and/or Primary Health Care Provider:

Doctor/Other _____ Phone _____

Address _____ City _____

May I send a copy of your consultation to your physician or
primary health care provider?   ❑ Yes   ❑ No

Marital Status:

❑ Single   ❑ Married   ❑ Divorced   ❑ Widowed

Sex:

❑ Male   ❑ Female

Education:

❑ Grade School   ❑ Jr. High School   ❑ High School

❑ College (2-4 years)   ❑ Graduate School   ❑ Degree _____

Occupation:

Position _____ Employer _____

Address _____

Phone _____

**What is (are) your purpose(s)
for participation in this Fitness Program?**

❑ To determine my current level of physical fitness and to receive recommendations
for an exercise program.

❑ Other (please explain) _____

_____

_____

_____

_____

_____

B. Long Medical History Questionnaire (continued)

Present Medical History

Check those questions to which your answer is yes (leave the others blank).
❑ Has a doctor ever said your blood pressure was too high?
❑ Do you ever have pain in your chest or heart?
❑ Are you often bothered by a thumping of the heart?
❑ Does your heart often race like mad?
❑ Do you ever notice extra heartbeats or skipped beats?
❑ Are your ankles often badly swollen?
❑ Do cold hands or feet trouble you even in hot weather?
❑ Has a doctor ever said that you have or had heart trouble, an abnormal electrocardiogram (ECG or EKG), heart attack or coronary?
❑ Do you suffer from frequent cramps in your legs?
❑ Do you often have difficulty breathing?
❑ Do you get out of breath long before anyone else?
❑ Do you sometimes get out of breath when sitting still or sleeping?
❑ Has a doctor ever told you your cholesterol level was high?
Comments: _____

_____

Do you now have or have you recently experienced:
❑ Chronic, recurrent or morning cough?
❑ Episode of coughing up blood?
❑ Increased anxiety or depression?
❑ Problems with recurrent fatigue, trouble sleeping or increased irritability?
❑ Migraine or recurrent headaches?
❑ Swollen or painful knees or ankles?
❑ Swollen, stiff or painful joints?
❑ Pain in your legs after walking short distances?
❑ Foot problems?
❑ Back problems?
❑ Stomach or intestinal problems, such as recurrent heartburn, ulcers, constipation or diarrhea?
❑ Significant vision or hearing problems?
❑ Recent change in a wart or a mole?
❑ Glaucoma or increased pressure in the eyes?
❑ Exposure to loud noises for long periods?
Comments: _____

_____

B. Long Medical History Questionnaire (continued)

Women only answer the following. Do you have:

❏ Menstrual period problems?

❏ Significant childbirth-related problems?

❏ Urine loss when you cough, sneeze or laugh?

Date of last pelvic exam and/or Pap smear _____

Comments: _____

_____

Are you on any type of hormone replacement therapy? _____

_____

Men and women answer the following:

List any prescription medications you are now taking: _____

_____

List any self-prescribed medications or dietary supplements you are now taking: ____

_____

Date of last complete physical examination: _____

❏ Normal   ❏ Abnormal   ❏ Never   ❏ Can't remember

Date of last chest X-ray: _____

❏ Normal   ❏ Abnormal   ❏ Never   ❏ Can't remember

Date of last electrocardiogram (EKG or ECG): _____

❏ Normal   ❏ Abnormal   ❏ Never   ❏ Can't remember

Date of last dental checkup: _____

❏ Normal   ❏ Abnormal   ❏ Never   ❏ Can't remember

List any other medical or diagnostic test you have had in the past two years: _____

_____

List hospitalizations, including dates of and reasons for hospitalization: _____

_____

_____

List any drug allergies: _____

_____

_____

B. Long Medical History Questionnaire (continued)

Past Medical History

Check those questions to which your answer is yes (leave others blank).

❑ Heart attack If so, how many years ago?_____

❑ Rheumatic fever

❑ Heart murmur

❑ Diseases of the arteries

❑ Varicose veins

❑ Arthritis of legs or arms

❑ Diabetes or abnormal blood-sugar tests

❑ Phlebitis (inflammation of a vein)

❑ Dizziness or fainting spells

❑ Epilepsy or seizures

❑ Stroke

❑ Diphtheria

❑ Scarlet fever

❑ Infectious mononucleosis

❑ Nervous or emotional problems

❑ Anemia

❑ Thyroid problems

❑ Pneumonia

❑ Bronchitis

❑ Asthma

❑ Abnormal chest X-ray

❑ Other lung disease

❑ Injuries to back, arms, legs or joints

❑ Broken bones

❑ Jaundice or gall bladder problems

Comments:_____

_____

_____

_____

B. Long Medical History Questionnaire (continued)

Family Medical History

Father:
❏ Alive   Current age _____
My father's general health is:
❏ Excellent   ❏ Good   ❏ Fair   ❏ Poor
Reason for poor health:
❏ Deceased   ❏ Age at death _____
Cause of death: _____

Mother:
❏ Alive   Current age _____
My mother's general health is:
❏ Excellent   ❏ Good   ❏ Fair   ❏ Poor
Reason for poor health: _____
❏ Deceased   ❏ Age at death _____
Cause of death: _____

Siblings:
Number of brothers _____Number of sisters _____Age range _____
Health problems _____

Familial Diseases

Have you or your blood relatives had any of the following (include grandparents, aunts and uncles, but exclude cousins, relatives by marriage and half-relatives)?

Check those to which the answer is yes (leave others blank).

❏ Heart attacks under age 50
❏ Strokes under age 50
❏ High blood pressure
❏ Elevated cholesterol
❏ Diabetes
❏ Asthma or hay fever
❏ Congenital heart disease (existing at birth but not hereditary)
❏ Heart operations
❏ Glaucoma
❏ Obesity (20 or more pounds overweight)
❏ Leukemia or cancer under age 60
Comments: _____
_____
_____
_____

B. Long Medical History Questionnaire (continued)

Other Heart Disease Risk Factors

Smoking

Have you ever smoked cigarettes, cigars or a pipe?

❏ Yes   ❏ No

(If no, skip to Diet section)

If you did or now smoke cigarettes, how many per day? _____ Age started ____

If you did or now smoke cigars, how many per day? _____ Age started ____

If you did or now smoke a pipe, how many pipefuls a day? _____ Age started ____

If you have stopped smoking, when was it? _____

If you now smoke, how long ago did you start? _____

Diet

What do you consider a good weight for yourself? _____

What is the most you ever weighed (including when pregnant)? _____

How old were you? _____

My current weight is: _____

One year ago my weight was: ____

At age 21 my weight was: _____

Number of meals you usually eat per day: _____

Average number of eggs you eat per week: _____

Number of times per week you usually eat the following:

Beef _____ Fish _____ Desserts _____

Pork _____ Fowl _____ Fried foods _____

Number of servings (cups, glasses or containers) per week you usually consume of:

Homogenized (whole) milk _____Buttermilk _____Skim (nonfat) milk _____

2% (low-fat) milk _____ 1% (low-fat) milk _____Coffee _____

Tea (iced or hot) _____Regular or diet sodas _____ Glasses of water _____

B. Long Medical History Questionnaire (continued)

Do you ever drink alcoholic beverages?   ❑ Yes   ❑ No

If yes, what is your approximate intake of these beverages?

Beer:

❑ None   ❑ Occasional   ❑ Often   If often, _____ per week

Wine:

❑ None   ❑ Occasional   ❑ Often   If often, _____ per week

Hard Liquor:

❑ None   ❑ Occasional   ❑ Often   If often, _____ per week

At any time in the past, were you a heavy drinker (consumption of six ounces of hard liquor per day or more)?

   ❑ Yes   ❑ No

Comments: _____

_____

_____

Do you usually use oil or margarine in place of high cholesterol shortening or butter?

   ❑ Yes   ❑ No

Do you usually abstain from extra sugar usage?

   ❑ Yes   ❑ No

Do you usually eat salt at the table?

   ❑ Yes   ❑ No

Do you eat differently on weekends as compared to weekdays?

   ❑ Yes   ❑ No

Comments: _____

_____

_____

_____

_____

_____

C. Sample Nutritional Profile

This form can be used with either the Short Screening Form or the Long Medical History Questionnaire

Write down everything you typically eat or drink in a 24-hour period. Indicate approximate amounts, being as specific as possible. Indicate where eaten as well.

Typical Workday

Breakfast:
Where eaten: _____

Mid-Morning:
Where eaten: _____

Lunch:
Where eaten: _____

Cocktails:
Where: _____

Dinner:
Where eaten: _____

Bedtime Snack:
Where eaten: _____

Typical Weekend or Holiday

Breakfast:
Where eaten: _____

Mid-Morning:
Where eaten: _____

Lunch:
Where eaten: _____

Mid-Afternoon:
Where eaten: _____

Cocktails:
Where: _____

Dinner:
Where eaten: _____

Dessert:
Where eaten: _____

Bedtime Snack:
Where eaten: _____

D. Sample Exercise Profile

This form can be used with either the Short Screening Form or the Long Medical History Questionnaire

Are you currently involved in a regular exercise program?

❑ Yes ❑ No

Do you regularly walk or run one or more miles continuously?

❑ Yes ❑ No

If yes, average number of miles covered per workout day: _____

Average time per mile? (minutes and seconds)_____ ❑ Unsure

Do you practice weight lifting or home calisthenics?

❑ Yes ❑ No

Are you involved in an aerobic program?

❑ Yes ❑ No

Do you frequently participate in competitive sports?

❑ Yes ❑ No

If yes, check those sports you participate in:

❑ Golf	❑ Basketball	❑ Bowling	❑ Volleyball
❑ Tennis	❑ Football	❑ Handball	❑ Baseball
❑ Racquetball	❑ Soccer	❑ Track	❑ Road racing

Other(s): _____

Average time per month: _____

In which of the following high school or college athletics did you participate?

❑ Track	❑ Football	❑ Swimming	❑ Basketball
❑ Tennis	❑ Baseball	❑ Wrestling	❑ Soccer
❑ Cross Country		❑ Gymnastics	

Other(s): _____

What activities would you prefer in a regular exercise program for yourself?

❑ Walking and/or running	❑ Tennis	❑ Bicycling (outside)
❑ Stationary running (treadmill)	❑ Swimming	❑ Jumping rope
❑ Handball, squash, racquetball	❑ Basketball	❑ Stationary cycling
❑ Other(s)? _____		

Comments: _____

_____

E. Sample Activities Questionnaire

This form can be used with either the Short Screening Form or the Long Medical History Questionnaire

Do you consider yourself:

❑ Sedentary (little, if any, vigorous physical activity)

❑ Lightly active (sporadic workouts, lawn work, other kinds of activity; little aerobic)

❑ Moderately active (work out 1-2 days per week for at least 15-30 minutes/day; aerobic work)

❑ Highly active (work out 3 or more days/week, at least 30-45 minutes/day; aerobic work)

How many minutes per week do you spend in exercise?

❑ 0	❑ 1-15	❑ 15-30	❑ 30-60
❑ 61-90	❑ 91-120	❑121-180	❑181 and above

How physically fit are you?

❑ Not	❑ Less than average	❑ Average
❑ Above average	❑ Outstanding	❑ Don't know

At the job, do you sit more than you are on the move?

❑ Yes   ❑ No

Indicate the main reason why you exercise (select only one).

❑ I do not exercise.	❑ It is good for my health.
❑ It makes me feel good.	❑ I am required to exercise.
❑ I'm trying to lose weight.	❑ My doctor told me to exercise.

Other: _____

_____

Do you know what cardiovascular or aerobic fitness means?

❑ Yes   ❑ No

If yes, please explain your interpretation: _____

_____

_____

Using your understanding, discuss what aerobic activity involves: List examples of aerobic activities: _____

_____

_____

What is the importance of strength or resistance training? _____

_____

_____

F. Sample Physical Activity Index

This form can be used with either the Short Screening Form or the Long Medical History Questionnaire

Evaluate your current exercise program by selecting your score for each category.

	Score	Activity
Intensity	5	Sustained heavy breathing and perspiration
	4	Intermittent heavy breathing and perspiration, as in tennis
	3	Moderately heavy, as in cycling and other recreational sports
	2	Moderate, as in volleyball, softball
	1	Light, as in fishing
Duration	4	Over 30 minutes
	3	20 to 30 minutes
	2	10 to 20 minutes
	1	less than 10 minutes
Frequency	5	6 to 7 times per week
	4	3 to 5 times per week
	3	1 to 2 times per week
	2	A few times per month
	1	Less than once a month

Intensity X Duration X Frequency = Score Total

Your Score: _____ X _____ X _____ = _____

Evaluation of Activity Score

Score	Evaluation	Activity Category
81 to 100	Very active lifestyle	High
60 to 80	Active and healthy	Very good
40 to 59	Acceptable but could be better	Fair
20 to 39	Not good enough	Poor
Under 20	Sedentary	

G. Sample Overview and Consent/Release Form

This program consists of various phases designed to determine your readiness to engage in physical activity, measure your functional fitness capacity in several areas, record objective data in relation to your current fitness levels, and on an ongoing basis, regularly update and evaluate your current health and fitness status.

During the first phase you will undergo a **screening evaluation** process designed to identify risk factors that are associated with increased risk for incurring cardiovascular disease. This will include having you fill out a written medical history/questionnaire form and an informal interview. This written form of assessment and verbal interaction will assist with evaluation of your overall health. Several major risk factors related to coronary heart disease will be evaluated. These include: smoking; blood cholesterol and lipids; blood pressure; obesity or extreme over-fatness; and inactivity.

To complement these factors, blood pressure, percent body fat, height and weight, and resting heart rate will be determined.

Additionally, self-evaluation of stress levels, activity levels, diet and a summary of overall risk to injury and ill health will be determined by questionnaire.

To determine blood lipid (i.e., cholesterol, HDL and LDL) levels it is necessary to have blood samples taken. If you have already been tested, these results, with your consent, will be requested from the appropriate medical facility and attending health care provider. Blood lipid profiles are extremely useful in helping motivate you to improve dietary habits and decrease your risk of coronary heart disease.

Upon successful completion of the screening phase, you may elect to go through the second or **fitness-evaluation phase**. After consultation with your trainer and/or qualified health care specialist, fitness evaluation may, or may not, initially be encouraged. The fitness-evaluation phase is certainly not necessary for you to begin an effective, safe and exciting program. A thorough and honest approach to phase-one screening sets the stage for a safe starting point.

Fitness evaluations are administered to measure fitness levels and NOT to be confused with medical diagnostic tests. Their purpose is to evaluate your starting point with regard to current level of fitness, develop an individual exercise plan, provide incentive and note progress in the following months. Fitness evaluations should be an optional complement to phase-one screening. Fitness evaluations can include:

A. A series of evaluations to measure and assess flexibility, posture, muscular strength and muscular endurance.

B. A series of evaluations to measure and assess flexibility, posture, strength and tone of key postural muscles that are important in helping prevent orthopedic pain and discomfort associated with chronic misalignment. The lowback and neck are examples of areas of the body that will be evaluated.

C. Skinfolds to measure body fat, and various tape measurements to record girth or circumference of specific body sites. Both measurements serve as a base for future reference

G. Sample Overview and Consent/Release Form (continued)

and reflect changes in body composition, such as increases in muscle mass and losses of body fat. This may be performed in phase one.

D. Blood pressure assessment to determine resting systolic and diastolic pressures. Blood pressure is the force of your blood pushing against the walls of arteries. It is important to monitor on a regular basis to screen for hypertension or high blood pressure. It is easy to perform, painless and takes only seconds to administer.

E. Using a bike ergometer, treadmill, adjustable step platform or walking/running course, a heart-rate response to increased work (speed or resistance) will be determined. This submaximal cardiorespiratory test may be used to predict a maximal oxygen uptake and can help in determining an appropriate heart-rate training range.

The cardiorespiratory test is often described by my clients as the most physically demanding. The exercise intensity begins at a level of effort that is easily sustained. It may or may not progress in intensity. This is dependent on fitness level, personal response and the cardiorespiratory test chosen.

The test involves measuring heart rate and observing breathing (respiratory) responses to steady or increased submaximal work load. In other words, you will have the option to work increasingly harder.

Not only does this establish your present level of cardiorespiratory fitness, but it also provides a baseline for measuring future improvements. The final workload will have you working at approximately 85% or less of predicted (or actual maximal heart rate if available) maximal heart rate. The test may be stopped at any time due to signs of fatigue, strain, physiological response or other contraindications to exercise. You may also choose to stop due to personal feelings of fatigue, discomfort or any reason you deem appropriate.

During any of these fitness evaluations (A through E) there exists the possibility of heart disorders, fainting, abnormal blood pressure response and in rare instances heart attack, stroke or death. Every effort has been made to minimize these risks by gathering preliminary information relating to your current health and fitness, and by observations during testing.

At best, all of these fitness-testing evaluation procedures are a general measure of your degree of fitness, but they do NOT state whether or not you have heart disease. Furthermore, you agree to look to your physician or qualified primary health care provider for any medical care. It is generally recommended, though not always necessary, to have both a physical exam and a diagnostic fitness evaluation conducted by qualified personnel on an annual basis. Discuss this with your health care provider(s).

A short period of time must pass before the appropriate data can be compiled. At this point, a meeting between you and your trainer will occur. All pertinent information will be explained with an accompanying personal exercise prescription or exercise plan. You may then elect to enter (or continue) our personal training program, which is valuable in motivating and helping you adhere to your exercise plan. Reevaluation and assessment of your

G. Sample Overview and Consent/Release Form (continued)

progress and program plan is encouraged, and performed on a regular basis.

Any questions you have about the procedures, risks or benefits to be expected are welcome. If you have any reservations or doubts, please voice these concerns and ask for an explanation or clarification.

Participation in any tests and this program is voluntary. You are free to deny consent or withdraw consent at any time after consenting. However, it is important that you promptly report any unusual feelings and/or other information that can assist the testing staff with any difficulties you perceive or are experiencing. It is your responsibility to fully disclose such information as relegated by your feelings and as requested by questionnaire or staff.

I, the undersigned, being aware of my own health and physical condition, and having knowledge that my participation in this program and fitness testing procedures may be injurious to my health, am voluntarily participating in the *Training Edge Program*, which has been explained to me verbally, as well as presented in written form.

Having such knowledge, I hereby release *Brooks...The Training Edge*, its representatives, agents, employees and successors from liability for accidental injury or illness which I may incur as a result of participating in said fitness program or in the testing and/or screening procedures. I hereby assume all risks connected therewith and consent to participate in said program.

Signature_____Date_____

References and Recommended Reading

Personality and Needs Assessment:

The Personal Fitness System: Interactive Wellness© (PFS), The Fitness Company, 7127 E. Becker Lane, Suite 168, Scottsdale, AZ, 85254 or contact Deby Harper at (602) 951-8149.

Fitness Testing and Assessment:

American College of Sports Medicine—ACSM (1991). Guidelines for Exercise Testing and Prescription. 4th edition, Lea and Febiger, Philadelphia, PA.

American Council on Exercise (ACE) (1991). Personal Trainer Manual. Published by ACE, San Diego, CA.

Anderson, Owen (1993). "Running Research News" (general reference). Published Lansing, MI. (517) 371-4897

Baechle, Tom, and Groves, Barney (1992). Weight Training - Steps To Success. Human Kinetics Publishers, Champaign, IL. (800) 747-4457

Basmajian, John, and DeLuca, Carlo (1979). Muscles Alive - Their Functions Revealed By Electromyography. 4th edition, Williams and Wilkins, Baltimore, MD. (800) 638-0672

Brittingham, Mark (1996). The Fitness Analyst. Information on this excellent software is available through Brittingham Software Design Inc., 15 Pheasant Court, Flanders, NJ 07836 (908) 879-4991

Brooks, Douglas (1990). Going Solo—The Art of Personal Training. 2nd edition, Moves International Publishing, Mammoth Lakes, CA (619) 934-0312

Cailliet, R. (1988). Low Back Pain Syndrome. 4th edition, F.A. Davis Company, Philadelphia, PA.

Carter Center (1988). "Healthier People: Health Risk Appraisal Program," The Carter Center of Emory University, Atlanta, GA, July.

Evans, William, and Rosenberg, Irwin (1991). Biomarkers. Simon & Schuster, New York, NY.

Fair, Erik (1992). "Fitness Software." IDEA Today, San Diego, CA. June, pg. 27.

Francis, Peter, and Francis, Lorna (1988). If It Hurts, Don't Do It. Prima Publishing, Rocklin, CA. (916) 624-5718

Giese, M. (1988). "Organization of an exercise session." In American College of Sports Medicine Resource Manual, for guidelines for exercise testing and prescription. pp. 244-247, Philadelphia: Lea and Febiger.

Golding, Lawrence et al. (1989). The Y's Way to Physical Fitness. Human Kinetics Publishers, Champaign, IL. 1-800-747-4457

Heyward, Vivian (1991). Advanced Fitness Assessment and Exercise Prescription. 2nd edition, Human Kinetics Books, Champaign, IL.

Jackson, Andrew S., Pollock, Michael L., (1985) "Practical Assessment of Body Composition," The Physician and Sports Medicine, Vol. 13, No. 5, May 1985, pp. 76-90

Kendall, Florence, et al. (1993). *Muscles - Testing and Function*. 4th edition, Williams and Wilkins, Baltimore, MD. (800) 638-0672

Komi, P.V., editor (1992). *Strength and Power in Sport*. Distributed by Human Kinetics Publishers, Champaign, IL. (800) 747-4457

Lohman, Timothy, et al. (1988). *Anthropometric Standardization Reference Manual*. Human Kinetics Books, Champaign, IL.

MacDougal, J. Duncan et al. (1991). *Physiological Testing of the High-Performance Athlete*. Champaign, IL: Human Kinetics Publishers.

McArdle, William et al. (1991). *Exercise Physiology - Energy, Nutrition, and Human Performance*. 3rd edition, Lea and Febiger, Philadelphia, PA.

Meyers, Jill (1994). "The Art of Needs Assessment." *IDEA Personal Trainer* magazine, September.

Plowman, Sharon (1992). "Physical Activity, Physical Fitness, and Low Back Pain." *Exercise and Sport Sciences Reviews*, Volume 20, pp. 221-242.

Pollock, Michael, and Wilmore, Jack (1990). *Exercise in Health and Disease*. 2nd edition, W.B. Saunders, Philadelphia, PA.

Roberts, Scott, editor (1996). *The Business of Personal Training*. Champaign, IL: Human Kinetics Publishers.

Sharkey, Brian (1991). *New Dimensions in Aerobic Fitness*. Human Kinetics Publishers, Champaign, IL.

Sharkey, Brian (1990). *Physiology of Fitness*. 3rd edition, Human Kinetics Publishers, Champaign, IL.

Thompson, Clem (1989). *Manual of Structural Kinesiology*. 11th edition, Times Mirror/Mosby, St. Louis, MO. (314) 872-8370

Wilmore, Jack, and Costill, David (1994). *Physiology of Sport and Exercise*. Human Kinetics Publishers, Champaign, IL. (800) 747-4457

Wilmore, Jack, and Costill, David (1988). *Training for Sport and Activity: The Physisological Basis of Conditioning*, 3rd edition, William Brown Publishers, Dubuque, IA.

CHAPTER 3

PLANNING FOR OVERALL HEALTH

Have you met a client like Mrs. Delpino? She is 51 years of age, claims to love exercise and has a personality that is irresistible. You learn that her mom is obese, diabetic and has high blood pressure. Her father died from a heart attack. Upon meeting her, it is obvious that she is overfat and deconditioned. Yet, she doesn't see her current health as a risk. With her glowing and infectious personality, she says, "So basically, even though my family is unhealthy and hates to exercise, I love it. I'm in perfect health except for a knee that always bothers me and my back that goes out occasionally."

Through further dialogue and a written health history, you confirm that she is 34% fat, has a blood pressure of 140/90 and a low level of cardiovascular conditioning. As you wrap up your introductory meeting, Mrs. Delpino enthusiastically exclaims, "And I love aerobic dance. Not that low-impact stuff. You know, more like what you see on television. When can we start?"

Even though you may be chuckling through this scenario, Mrs. Delpino represents a composite of many clients whom I have worked with over the years. She is positive and her enthusiasm is unbridled. And her self-assessment of her current health/fitness status is inaccurate because she feels she has no particular health weakness or "red flags."

Personal trainers have the opportunity to look beyond "activity only" to broader health issues. Physical activity is not your only approach to encouraging a healthy and balanced lifestyle for your clientele. Do you help your client implement lifestyle behavior changes related to stress, a family history of coronary heart disease, obesity, lack of regular exercise, smoking, high blood pressure or high cholesterol?

Personally, I think the significance of health risks is lost on the general public because of an attitude of denial, or "I don't really want to know." This leads to reasoning that begins with "Hopefully it won't...," or "It can't happen to me." Yet statistics pull all of us into the law of averages. It is the rare individual who is the exception to the rule. Thus, it is increasingly important that the personal trainer take on the role and responsibility of driving home, to the client, the *personal* importance of risk factor information.

The Carter Center (1988) estimates that 2 of 3 deaths in the United States are linked to only 6 health hazards: cigarette smoking/tobacco, alcohol, high blood pressure, obesity, high cholesterol and gaps in medical care for pregnant women and newborn babies. These are largely controllable hazards. By being aware of the health risks that confront them, at least your clients can make an informed decision about their lifestyles.

Once you understand health risk factors, you can explain to a client what blood cholesterol numbers mean. You can explain how physical activity fits into a preventative program for coronary heart disease (CHD). You can become the bridge between your client and the medical and preventive health community, where practitioners may not have the time, or may not use simple language, to make risk factors easily understood and controlled.

By using this type of approach, you are working with clients for their optimal benefit. And you are positioning your business for success by helping clients see results, and establishing a link with physicians and health promotion specialists. This raises your perceived value to both client and health practitioner.

What Is Atherosclerotic Disease?

When cholesterol and/or plaque are deposited in the arteries of the body, it can result in various vascular diseases, called atherosclerotic disease. Vascular or blood vessel disease can be one of, or a combination of, coronary heart disease, stroke or peripheral vascular disease (PVD). Vascular disease is most often caused by atherosclerotic plaque accumulations in the arteries of the brain, legs and heart.

Coronary artery disease (CAD) is caused by plaque accumulation in the heart's coronary arteries. Examples of CAD-influenced CHD disease include myocardial infarctions (heart attacks), angina (chest pains) and sudden cardiac death. **Strokes** represent blood vessel disease in the small arteries of the brain. Strokes can result in severe brain damage and disability, or death. And, **peripheral vascular disease** is manifested by cramp-like (claudication) leg pain. PVD can lead to gangrene and amputation of the affected extremity. CHD, stroke and PVD are usually manifestations of **atherosclerotic disease**, which can be defined as cholesterol deposits in the arteries of the heart, brain or legs. All artery disease can be housed under the atherosclerotic-disease umbrella.

Essentially, CHD is an imbalance between oxygen available to the heart tissue and the heart's demand for oxygen. Coronary artery circulation is often compromised by a combination of **atherosclerosis** and **arteriosclerosis**. **Atherosclerosis** affects the diameter of the artery because of changes in the intima (inner most lining) and media (inner layer) of the artery. Accumulation of fats (lipids), blood products, fibrous tissue and calcium deposits is associated with these changes, which cause a narrowing of the arteries. It is obvious a decrease in diameter would compromise blood delivery by the coronary arteries to the heart. **Arteriosclerosis** can result in thickening of the artery walls, calcium deposits and loss of elasticity. This "hardening" of arteries or loss of flexibility may contribute significantly to decreased blood flow to the heart muscle.

An enlightening though often-unknown fact is that blood returning to the heart is totally dependent on the arteries that "feed" the heart (coronary circulation), if oxygen and nutrients are to be used by the heart muscle. Many lay people assume that once blood is returned to the heart, after being oxygenated and delivered to the left ventricle (one of 4 heart chambers), the heart's oxygen and energy needs are assured. You would think that the blood rushing through the chambers of the heart would nourish the heart. This is not the case.

Blood is carried to the heart through 2 coronary arteries that branch off the aorta, just after it leaves the heart. The blood must be ejected from the left ventricle into the aorta, and it is not until this point that oxygenated blood has an opportunity to enter the coronary circulation or arteries. These arteries divide into smaller and smaller branches, like all blood vessels, eventually culminating in capillaries. After the blood has passed through the capillaries and the heart tissue has extracted the needed oxygen, it returns by way of venules and veins, which become larger and larger until they, like all other veins in the body, empty in the right atrium of the heart.

In most organs or tissues of the body there is a "reserve" or collateral blood supply. In other words, there are often 2 arteries that "feed" blood to a similar area. These arteries are connected by many cross-channels or collateral vessels. If one artery is blocked, the collateral circulation can compensate and deliver the needed blood to sustain tissue function. Unfortunately, this situation does not exist in the wall of the heart. The coronary arteries are referred to as "end arteries." Each branch follows its own course with very few cross connections with other nearby branches. The amount of cross-connections depends on the individual, and activity patterns may influence this to some degree.

If the arteries are inelastic, narrowed, partially blocked or totally blocked, blood flow will be compromised. If the nature of the activity, whether rest or vigorous activity, places a demand for oxygen to the heart muscle, and it is not met because of compromised coronary circulation, angina (pain associated with ischemia or lack of oxygen to the heart muscle) or a heart attack may occur.

The heart is only as strong as its weakest link, which is usually the 2 coronary arteries that branch off from the aorta and can compromise coronary circulation.

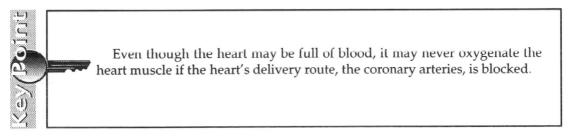

Even though the heart may be full of blood, it may never oxygenate the heart muscle if the heart's delivery route, the coronary arteries, is blocked.

Another little known fact about CHD sheds light on the insidious and extremely dangerous nature of it. The heart's coronary circulation branches off the aorta and splits into 3 main delivery routes. These delivery routes further divide to cover the surface area of the heart and bring necessary nutrition and oxygen to the heart muscle. Significant (up to 80-85%) occlusion or blockage of the main coronary arteries may bring no symptoms or warning signs. In fact, total occlusion may be present in one or more of the branching, smaller arteries with no symptoms. Unfortunately, the first outward sign of heart disease for many individuals is death.

Understanding CHD Risk

Even though a person has marked and progressive coronary heart disease, it may go undiagnosed and remain asymptomatic. Then finally, a situation such as stress or physical activity occurs where the oxygen demands of the heart are not met. Does your client get a warning sign such as chest pains or rapid breathing? Here is the reality. Often, the first symptom of heart disease is *death*. There is no second chance.

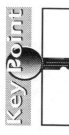

Only 18% of adults are free of commonly identified, major risk factors, reports the Centers for Disease Control. Heart attacks still account for 500,000 deaths per year, and 20% of those deaths occur in people under the age of 65 (*Berkeley Wellness Letter*, May 1994).

This is why I believe a keen awareness of risk factors and taking preventive steps toward correcting modifiable risk factors related to CHD is so important. You can lead this charge and make it important to your clients.

Risk-factor analysis begins with identifying the 6 factors that increase an individual's risk for coronary artery disease (CAD) and coronary heart disease (CHD). CAD is caused by plaque accumulation in the heart's coronary arteries. CHD refers to heart attack, angina and sudden cardiac death. CHD is caused by CAD. Does your health/medical history ask about these risks (in no particular order of importance)?

- smoking
- high blood pressure
- high blood cholesterol
- obesity
- diabetes
- inactivity

A risk factor(s) does not guarantee a certain outcome. However, when risk factors accumulate for a person, the statistical probability of developing some form of CAD increases exponentially. The combined impact of several risk factors is greater than adding them together. For example, 2 risk factors result in 3.3 times the risk and 3 risk factors result in 10 times the risk.

CAD claims the lives of more than 500,000 women each year, which is more than twice the number killed by all types of cancer combined (American Heart Association). Risk factors for CAD vary in women and are especially dependent on whether women have gone through menopause.

Premenopausal (before the cessation of menstruation) women are less likely to suffer from a heart attack. However, if they have diabetes, a predisposition to high cholesterol, hypertension, family history of CHD or smoke cigarettes, there is an increased risk of heart disease for perimenopausal (the phase of declining menstrual function before menopause) women. Furthermore, once estrogen production begins to slow, women begin to catch up to and exhibit the same risk for heart disease as men. A 60-year-old postmenopausal (menstrual function has stopped) woman has the same risk for heart attack as a 50-year-old man.

CHD Risk Factors That *Cannot* Be Changed

When speaking with clients, cite the unchangeable factors, but emphasize the risks that *can* be controlled and changed. Coupled with the information on the exponential effect of coronary risk factors, you can motivate their behavior changes. The following are out of our control:

Heredity. A parent or sibling who has had a heart attack before the age of 55 if a man, or 65 if a woman.

Increasing age. 80% of fatal heart attacks, and 55% of all heart attacks, occur after the age of 65.

Gender. Before age 55, men have a much higher incidence of CAD than women. At about age 60, women begin to develop a similar level of risk.

Race. Because they have a higher risk for hypertension and diabetes, African-Americans have an increased risk for CAD.

CHD Risk Factors That *Can* Be Changed

These are key points that you can relay to your clients when educating them about risk factors. They were reported in the May 1994 issue of the *Berkeley Wellness Letter* and constitute one of the best synopses I've read. In 1992, Dr. JoAnn Manson and her colleagues from Harvard analyzed about 200 studies on CAD to evaluate the role of known preventive measures on the incidence of CAD. Their results were published in the *New England Journal of Medicine* and reported in the *Berkeley Wellness Letter*.

Smoking. The best advice to smokers: quit! This is the single most-effective step that can be taken to reduce the risk of CAD-related deaths. Most medical professionals would rather deal with an increase in weight than with the effects of smoking. Between 20-40% of all deaths attributed to CAD are directly related to smoking.

The exciting news about smoking is that the risk for CAD starts to decrease almost immediately after quitting. It is estimated that within 5-10 years, the risk for heart attack declines in the person who has stopped smoking to a level that is similar to someone's who has never smoked.

Cholesterol. There is a 2-3% decline in the risk of heart attack for every 1% reduction in blood cholesterol. A "desirable" level of cholesterol is below 200 mg/dl. The best approach to improving blood lipid and cholesterol levels is to lower cholesterol through diet and raise the protective, or "good guy," high-density lipoprotein (HDL) through regular exercise.

High blood pressure (hypertension). High blood pressure is a risk factor for heart attack and stroke. A borderline high blood pressure reading is 130 systolic over 90 diastolic. For each one point drop in diastolic blood pressure, a 2-3% drop in the risk of heart attack occurs. The easiest way to lower blood pressure is through lifestyle changes. By limiting sodium (salt), losing weight and decreasing alcohol consumption, significant reductions in blood pressure may be gained. After conservative measures have failed, medication may be required in conjunction with lifestyle modifications.

Inactivity. Numerous epidemiological studies demonstrate that exercise protects against CAD. A sedentary lifestyle carries with it the same risks as, for example, smoking or high cholesterol. A regular exercise program can reduce the risk of heart attack by 35-55%. Furthermore, research supports the fact that even low-intensity activities, such as gardening or strolling on a regular and consistent basis, can decrease the risk for heart disease and increase HDL levels. (This contradicts previous research which indicated only *vigorous* activity would decrease risk and increase HDL levels.)

This is powerful information that can be used to effectively motivate your clients. Activity, at any level, can:

- increase the efficiency of the heart
- make the heart stronger
- reduce blood pressure
- help control stress levels
- reduce the likelihood of blood clot formation
- help maintain or lose weight
- increase the HDL, or "good guy," cholesterol carrier

Obesity/extreme overweight. About one in 3 Americans is seriously overweight or obese. This doubles the risk of CAD at any age. Being obese also increases the risk for diabetes, hypertension and high blood pressure.

Diabetes. Diabetes increases the risk for CAD, high blood pressure and other health-related risks. Non-insulin-dependent diabetes mellitus (NIDDM) or Type II diabetes (commonly referred to as adult-onset diabetes) afflicts about 12 million Americans and is often preventable. Weight control, regular aerobic exercise, good nutrition, stress reduction and other forms of exercise can improve insulin sensitivity, sugar utilization and help control diabetes.

Quick Index:

Understanding Cholesterol Levels

Many clients think that fat (triglyceride) or cholesterol equals heart attack. Though a focus on cholesterol is important, it need not be obsessive. "Total" cholesterol (TC) is an important gauge, however. This measurement includes both high-density lipoprotein (HDL) and low-density lipoprotein (LDL) cholesterol in the blood, as well as very-low-density lipoproteins (VLDL). VLDLs are commonly called triglycerides or fat.

It is generally desirable to have a TC reading of below 200 mg/dl. Borderline is between 200-239 and high is 240 or greater (*Nutrition Action Health Letter*, October 1995). The National Cholesterol Education Program (NCEP) now recommends testing for HDL, along with TC. A high HDL reading may balance any potential negative effects of a high TC reading.

When TC is divided by HDL, a number called the **TC/HDL ratio** is derived. An ideal value is less than 3.5, though a range of 3.5-4.5 is commonly cited as acceptable. The importance of the TC/HDL ratio lies in its ability to reflect how the body is managing individual cholesterol amounts. For example, a low cholesterol level does not make you immune to heart disease. A 180 TC reading, coupled with an HDL of 30, results in a ratio of 5. This level indicates an increased risk for heart disease even though the cholesterol reading, if interpreted by itself, would indicate otherwise.

A client with a TC or cholesterol reading of 240 and HDL value of 70 would have a TC/HDL ratio of less than 3.5. This indicates a low risk for heart disease, as related to this one risk factor. Look at the whole picture within each risk factor, as well as across the board for every contributing risk factor.

Table 4. Terminology and Total Cholesterol (TC) Equation

Total Cholesterol (TC) =	•reflection of 3 lipoprotein transport vehicles
High-Density Lipoprotein (HDL)	•"Good guy" •Available to scavenge •Can reverse transport of cholesterol •Transports mostly cholesterol
Low-Density Lipoprotein (LDL)	•"Bad guy" •Deposits cholesterol in arterial wall •Transports 3/4 of total blood cholesterol
Very-Low-Density Lipoprotein (VLDL)	•Is the same as triglycerides •Carries mostly fat •Carries both saturated and unsaturated fat

Therefore, the TC equation is: TC = HDL + LDL + VLDL

Structure and Function of Lipoproteins

Cholesterol, fats and fat-like substances are not soluble in water. They must be packaged as lipoproteins to be transported in the watery medium of blood. Lipoproteins have 2 important functions:

1. They transport cholesterol and blood lipids. Cholesterol is a derivative of fat and is not considered a lipid.

2. They regulate cholesterol and blood lipid levels.

Nearly all of the cholesterol in the blood is carried by HDL and LDL. About three-fourths of all blood cholesterol is carried by LDL. It is apparent why a low LDL is preferred in the body. LDL is the prime carrier of cholesterol and has a tendency to deposit it in arteries, contributing to CAD. VLDLs and chylomicrons carry primarily triglycerides or fat (Byrne, 1991).

Low-Density Lipoprotein (LDL). High levels of LDL are associated with increased risk for CAD, CHD, stroke and peripheral vascular disease (PVD), thus its characterization as the villain or "bad guy." Byrne (1991) reports that if LDL concentration increases above 100 mg/dl, some of its cholesterol is deposited in the arterial walls as plaque.

Diet greatly affects the rate of both LDL production and removal. An intake of dietary saturated fat and cholesterol increases the liver's production of VLDLs to transport the lipids in the fat, and ultimately, some of the VLDLs (triglycerides) are converted into LDLs (Byrne, 1991). To compound the problem, saturated fat and cholesterol decrease the ability of the liver to pull LDL out of the blood stream by literally absorbing the cholesterol-loaded lipoprotein and "digesting" it. This situation further elevates LDL levels (Byrne, 1991).

High-density lipoproteins (HDL). HDLs are appropriately called the "good guys," or good cholesterol. Their importance as a protective factor in decreasing the risk for CAD is highly documented. HDL protects the arterial walls from atherosclerosis by removing some cholesterol from the arterial wall and possibly by inhibiting the entry of cholesterol, to some degree, into arterial-wall tissues (Byrne, 1991). Byrne also reports that HDL promotes the production of prostacycline, a substance that inhibits clotting along the inner walls of arteries. The reduced tendency toward clotting because of elevated HDL levels has important implications for occurrence of stroke, heart attack and PVD, which are often caused by blood particles or debris breaking away from diseased arteries where blood coagulation (clotting) has taken place.

High levels of HDL are associated with a lower rate of CHD. As little as a 10 mg/dl increase in HDL can decrease the risk of heart disease by almost half (Byrne, 1991). Most HDL is generated by the liver and small intestine.

> While diet has little effect on increased HDL production, exercise and weight reduction seem to be the most effective approach for increasing HDLs. It should be noted that an increase in HDL may take several months and could be preceded by an initial drop. As for most health gains, patience, consistency and moderation rule.

Intake of alcohol has been touted, quite popularly, as a means for increasing the "good cholesterol." Byrne reports that moderate intake of alcohol can raise HDL by about 5 mg/dl. An increase of HDL from 30 to 35, equals a 16.7% increase. An increase from 60 to 65 equals an increase of 8.3%. As noted above, an increase in HDL by as little as 10 mg/dl may halve one's risk for heart disease. Statistically, the importance of these numbers deserves consideration, but be sure to look at the total health picture before recommending this approach to your clients.

First, "moderate" is described as 3 beers, or 2 glasses of wine or 2 ounces of 100-proof whiskey. The increase occurs in a type called HDL-3. Its role in prevention of CHD is not clearly proven. Since the protective benefit is not 100% proven, many professionals find it difficult to recommend alcohol intake as a general preventive measure to the public. On the other hand, the negative health consequences of excessive alcohol intake are well documented.

HDL is the key in making the body's reverse cholesterol transport system operate. The outcome of this process is a healing and reversal of the atherosclerotic process. Once HDL picks up cholesterol (free cholesterol or non-esterified) from the other tissues, blood and arterial walls, it is converted to a cholesterol ester which prevents it from reentering the arterial wall (Byrne, 1991). The cholesterol eventually ends up at the liver, where it is removed or absorbed.

Even though a high HDL level of 60 mg/dl or greater seems to be protective, the deposit of cholesterol is caused by LDL. Many professionals contend that the primary focus of a cholesterol management program is to maintain ideal or lower levels of LDLs. High HDL levels do not exclude the possibility of simultaneous cholesterol deposition by LDLs. All factors of the blood cholesterol and lipid profile must be managed.

Very-low-density lipoproteins (and chylomicrons). Fat or triglycerides are carried by 2 lipoproteins. Chylomicrons transport absorbed dietary fat from the intestines to the liver, whereas VLDLs carry triglycerides manufactured in the liver to the rest of the body (Byrne, 1991).

Chylomicrons have no impact on CHD and atherosclerosis. Their biggest presence is up to several hours after a meal. Because blood is drawn after at least an overnight or 12-hour fast for an individual blood panel, nearly all of the triglycerides present in the blood will be contained in VLDL. Generally, triglycerides refer only to VLDL triglycerides (Byrne, 1991).

VLDL contains little cholesterol but large amounts of tri's or fat. A large intake of simple sugars, a high-fat diet, excessive consumption of alcohol and being overweight can contribute to high VLDL levels.

Triglycerides are regulated by hormonal influence and eventually release their fat to the cells of the body. In doing so, these large lipoproteins shrink into smaller LDLs. This physiological link between a high VLDL level and the resultant transformation to LDLs is good reason to keep triglyceride levels down. Triglycerides do not accumulate in the blood stream like cholesterol because they can be used for energy with resultant end products of carbon dioxide and water. But if the VLDL is degraded to the "bad guy" LDL, there are more receptor sites for cholesterol to attach. In combination with the fact that high VLDL levels are associated with depressed HDLs, it seems prudent to keep triglyceride levels below 200, and preferably below 150 mg/dl.

Table 5. Cholesterol and Blood-Borne Fats
Ideal Levels and Commonly Cited Ranges

	(IDEAL)	(RANGE)
Total Cholesterol (TC)	less than 160 mg/dl	140-240
HDL	greater than 60 mg/dl	35-75
LDL	less than 100 mg/dl	100-130
Triglycerides	less than 150 mg/dl	150-250
VLDL (triglycerides/5)	less than 30 mg/dl	30-50
TC/HDL Ratio	less than 3.5	3.5-4.5

Lowering Cholesterol

After receiving this type of information, your clients are going to want to know how to lower their cholesterol. That is natural, and you are in the perfect position to facilitate this interest. Here is what your clients have to do.

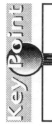

> To lower cholesterol—lose weight, exercise regularly, eat less saturated fat, cut back on cholesterol in foods, eat less trans fat (partially hydrogenated oil) and eat more fruits, vegetables and other foods high in fiber.

Losing as little as 5-10 pounds can make a difference. Losing weight can raise HDL levels and lower LDLs, triglycerides, blood pressure and help prevent diabetes. Exercise that raises your heart rate, done as little as 3 times per week for a total of 30-90 minutes per week, can raise HDLs, lower LDLs and triglycerides and blood pressure, help maintain weight and help prevent diabetes.

A diet low in saturated fat and cholesterol will lower LDL, triglycerides and cholesterol. Diets rich in **soluble fiber** may lower LDL (blood cholesterol) and help control blood sugar levels of people who have diabetes. Soluble fiber is found in oat bran, barley, kidney beans, fruits and vegetables. Diets rich in **insoluble fiber**, mainly the indigestible cellulose commonly found in the skins of fruits and vegetables, and in the coverings of whole grains, such as wheat bran and some cereals, encourages good intestinal function and elimination. A diet low in saturated fat and cholesterol, and high in fiber and vegetables may also reduce the risk of cancer, and the high amounts of folic acid (good sources are cereals, lentils, beans, spinach, romaine lettuce, wheat germ, peas, orange juice and broccoli) present in this type of diet may further lessen your risk for heart disease. Eating less hydrogenated or trans fats will decrease LDL levels (*Nutrition Action Heath Letter*, October 1995).

You can help your clients identify these foods, or refer them to a registered dietitian.

Quick Index:

Chapter 19, dietary impact on cholesterol

Increasing HDL ("good guy") Cholesterol

HDL levels of 60 or more are considered desirable. A reading of 35-39 is intermediate and below 35 is low. HDLs are described as the cholesterol carrier that scours the blood for debris that could lead to CHD, attaches to it and transports it out of your arteries. An HDL below 35 is a heart attack risk even if your cholesterol is below 200. This is evident from a TC/HDL ratio that equals 5.7, when using a value of 200 for cholesterol that is divided by an HDL of 35. A low HDL reading indicates that even small amounts of cholesterol in the blood stream are not being handled effectively by the body. To raise HDL:

- lose weight
- exercise on a regular basis
- quit smoking

The impact of moderate to regular activity on CHD, and a healthy lifestyle, cannot be overstated.

Lowering Triglycerides (VLDLs), the Fat in Your Blood

Your clients can lower their triglycerides by losing weight, exercising—even at a moderate intensity—decreasing saturated fat intake, and cutting back on cholesterol-laden foods. An exception to these rules follows.

Your clients may already be eating a low-fat, high-carbohydrate diet. If they still have high triglycerides and low HDLs, consider adding a tablespoon of oil to their diet. A tablespoon of oil has 120 calories and may be used in food preparation, or for example, add a quarter cup of nuts to the diet. This strategy may raise HDL and lower triglycerides. However, weight gain still needs to be avoided, and a dietary increase in fat is what most Americans do not need.

Blood Pressure

The National Cholesterol Education Program (NCEP) does not recognize blood pressure as a risk until it is greater than 140 systolic and 90 diastolic. However, the fact remains that if your blood pressure is not below 120 systolic and 80 diastolic, an increased risk for CHD and heart attack is present.

The following preventive steps may keep blood pressure from rising, or lower it. Losing weight and exercising are 2 important first steps. Eating more fruits and vegetables increases potassium intake, which is good. And sodium intake should be reduced to at least 2,400 mg per day, or preferably less.

Alcohol consumption should be limited to moderate or occasional use. Research indicates that people who limit themselves to one (women) or 2 (men) drinks per day have a lower risk of CHD than people who do not drink. However, even a drink per day may increase the risk for breast cancer in women, and more than 2 drinks per day may increase the risk of high blood pressure in women and men. Alcohol abuse should also be considered when weighing the option to drink or not to drink.

Meditation on CHD Therapies

Since in most cases the controllable risk factors can be improved—sometimes dramatically—with a healthy diet and exercise, why don't people "just do it?" Perhaps the answer lies both in human nature and the capabilities of modern medicine.

When faced with the uncertainty of how to minimize their risk for CAD, many clients make their first choice drugs. Often this decision is made because of fear and lack of information and professional direction on how to control these risks.

The NCEP suggests drug prescription for high LDL levels only after an exhaustive attempt to use exercise and diet has failed. However, many people fail to follow this more conservative recommendation, and opt for the "quick fix." In my opinion, drugs should be reserved for special circumstances where honest attempts at diet and exercise have failed. Even if drugs are required, they should not be used to the exclusion of healthy lifestyle choices related to diet, proper food selection and moderate and regular exercise.

In a study that was once thought to be highly provocative, physician Dean Ornish showed people with CHD were motivated to make profound changes in their lifestyle and were able to *reverse* arterial blockage (Ornish, 1990).

The control group was asked to quit smoking, exercise more and cut dietary fat intake to 30% of calories. The experimental group ate a vegetarian diet with almost no cholesterol and 7% fat. They also participated in stress reduction by practicing meditation, stretches and deep relaxation. Smoking was prohibited and they exercised at least 3 hours per week.

The results were dramatic. In one year, the participants in the stricter regimen improved their hearts and arteries, whereas CHD worsened in 50% of the control subjects. On an average, coronary blockage dropped 10% in the experimental or stricter group, but increased slightly in the control group. Also, the experimental group lost an average of 24 pounds, whereas the control group gained 2 pounds. What contributed most? Was it diet, exercise, weight loss, stress reduction, group support or a synergistic total? Diet and exercise surely played a big role, in addition to the experimental groups' commitment and dedication to significant changes in their lifestyles.

Will this work for your clients? Skepticism remains toward this approach because compliance is the key. Can this type of lifestyle intervention be effective for a population that resists cutting fat to a recommended 30% level? Ornish argues that it is easier to motivate people to make big lifestyle changes as opposed to small ones. Individuals who make small changes still feel deprived, and they usually get no reductions in cholesterol or angina symptoms. On the other hand, many experts feel that less extreme changes will lead to a decreased risk in CHD. Any change is better than no change. Sometimes your clients can be set up for failure if a strict, all-or-none approach is communicated as the only remedy.

Many physicians and nurse cardiac specialists prefer primary intervention programming similar to Ornish's, but prefer less drastic measures. **Primary intervention** is characterized by a conservative, less invasive, lifestyle/behavior change approach. This is in contrast to more radical treatments like drugs and surgery. Effective primary intervention can involve less drastic lifestyle and behavior changes than those used in Ornish's program, which he felt were necessary to reverse CAD. However, if your client wants significant results or is facing life-threatening CHD, the Ornish approach may be a perfect fit. With your support, motivation and knowledge, your clients will succeed. By and large, the most important factors for most apparently non-diseased participants in the prevention of CAD are consistency, adherence and moderation in their approach to diet and exercise.

The Bridge

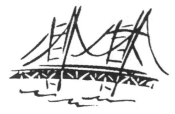

By understanding the risk factors for cardiovascular disease, you have the potential to improve each client's health status far beyond fitness. Plus, you can spend sufficient time during a session to explain the terminology and issues surrounding fats, cholesterol and blood pressure, whereas the physician probably does not. Exercise and diet significantly impact risk factors. While helping to improve your client's overall health, you are strengthening links to the medical profession.

SPECIAL SECTION
INTERPRETING BLOOD PANEL REPORTS

Recently, my 65-year-old mother added a P.S. about her blood panel in a letter she had written to me.

P.S. I had my checkup. My cholesterol is down from 257 to 247 (I know this is still too high). HDL was 76, now 78; LDL was 139, is now 135; triglycerides were 211 and now 172. What do you think? Bye for now, Mom

How would you advise and encourage my Mom? Regardless of gender, there is a set of specific questions that need to be answered:

- Is Mom on the right track?
- Is her cholesterol too high in relation to HDL?
- Should she increase her HDL?
- How can she decrease her triglycerides?

You'll be able to figure out the answers by reading the following information and reviewing previous sections in this chapter. At the end of this section, you'll have a chance to compare your analysis with mine.

How the Report Looks

A typical blood profile, blood "work-up" or lipid panel, consists of a total cholesterol (TC) reading that reflects how cholesterol and fat are carried in the blood. Lipoproteins include HDL, LDL, VLDL and chylomicrons. They allow cholesterol and other blood lipids, which are fat soluble, to exist in the watery medium of blood. Lipoproteins transport and regulate blood lipids (Byrne, 1991).

In Table 6, Sample Lab Analysis, VLDL, LDL and TC/HDL ratio are calculated by using the given values for TC, HDL and triglycerides (VLDL), as determined by a blood analysis.

Table 6: Sample Lab Analysis

CLIENT: JoAnn   Date: 6/15
Lab Analysis Report: TC=210;   HDL=42;   TRIGLYCERIDE=110
VLDL = 110 (triglycerides)/5 = 22
LDL = 210 (TC) -{42 (HDL) + 22 (VLDL)}; LDL = 146 (IDEAL < 130)
TC/HDL = 210/42 = 5 (Ideal ratio is < 3.5)

CLIENT: JoAnn   Date 9/15
Lab Analysis Report: TC=210;   HDL=65;   TRIGLYCERIDE=110
VLDL = 110/5 = 22
LDL = 210 -(65 + 22); LDL = 123 (IDEAL < 130)
TC/HDL = 210/65 = 3.23 (Ideal ratio is < 3.5)

Note the difference in risk for CHD between the 2 measurement dates because of the increase in HDL. HDLs have increased to a protective level and LDLs have decreased to 123 mg/dl, which is below the ideal level of 130 mg/dl. Though the 5 ratio for TC/HDL exhibited in the first test date is considered "normal" or an average risk for CHD in the United States, your clients can hardly afford being lumped into "normal." Statistically, "normal" is neither safe nor protective in this instance. The second test date reveals a TC/HDL ratio which has changed to 3.23, which reflects an ideal level.

How the Lab Reports Triglycerides

Triglycerides are simply fat. Very-low-density lipoproteins (VLDLs) are the same as triglycerides but are an expression of triglycerides divided by 5. Many labs give triglyceride information in the form of VLDLs. To convert this to a standard that is more understandable or familiar to most consumers, VLDLs are multiplied by 5. For example, a 30 mg/dl VLDL reading is converted to triglycerides by multiplying by 5. The resultant 150 mg/dl triglyceride reading is the same, in terms of blood fat levels, as a 30 mg/dl VLDL reading.

Converting Blood Values to International Units

The following conversion factors are used to convert blood cholesterol and lipid values reported in milligrams per deciliter (mg/dl) to international lipid units, which are expressed in millimoles per liter (mmol/L). Converting blood measurements into units of measurement that are familiar will help you accurately interpret research and individual lab reports.

Cholesterol (representation includes values for TC, or HDL, or LDL levels times the conversion factor)

- when reported in mg/dl x .02586 = cholesterol in mmol/L

Triglycerides or VLDL (representation includes reported triglycerides or VLDL level times the conversion factor)

- when reported in mg/dl x .01129 = triglycerides in mmol/L

Conversely, if you need to convert measurements in mmol/L to mg/dl, multiply the cholesterol level in mmol/L by 38.67. Multiply the triglyceride level in mmol/L by 88.57 (Byrne, 1991).

Explaining the Letters and Numbers

To help your clients interpret cholesterol and blood fat information, provide the information in Table 4, Terminology and Total Cholesterol Equation and Table 5, Cholesterol and Blood-Borne Fats. Most blood reports from labs show a value for TC, and this represents cholesterol and fat contained in LDL, HDL and VLDL. However, only HDL and VLDL (remember, triglycerides equal VLDL value times 5) are measured directly. LDL is usually calculated using the following formula (Byrne, 1991), as opposed to actually being measured.

To calculate LDL, use this formula and the blood values derived from the laboratory for TC, HDL and triglycerides (VLDLs). See Table 6.

LDL Formula:

LDL = TC (total cholesterol) - {HDL + VLDL (triglycerides /5)}.

LDL = TC - (HDL + VLDL)

Evaluating Mom's Report

How did you do? Here's my analysis:

Mom is certainly on the right track. Though some of her improvements are small, even maintenance should be applauded because it's better than regression of any sort. She has decreased her total cholesterol, raised her HDL 2 points, decreased her LDL and significantly lowered her triglycerides. Her HDL increase from 76 to 78 remains in the ideal range. This is a very important protective factor.

In fact, even though her cholesterol reading of 247 is well above 200 and the ideal of 160 mg/dl or less, Mom's TC/HDL ratio is only 3.17 (247 divided by 78). Her total cholesterol (TC) to HDL ratio falls in the ideal range. This information reveals that her body, because of her excellent HDL levels, is handling the higher amounts of cholesterol in her blood effectively. Even though her total cholesterol reading is high, she is at no apparent increased risk for heart disease. She needs to continue working on dropping her cholesterol, LDL and triglycerides.

Mom can decrease her tri's by continuing to decrease her saturated and trans fat (hydrogenated oils) intake, as well as any excessive simple sugar (refined) or alcohol consumption. Since some triglycerides (VLDLs) are converted to LDLs (the "bad guy" cholesterol), controlling triglycerides will help decrease LDL.

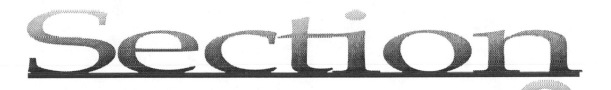

Section 2

The Science Behind Exercise Programs

"You will ask, I have often been asked, what happens to the body in training? I am sorry, I do not know. Perhaps the blood supply to the active muscles becomes better, the capillaries responding more rapidly to the needs of the muscles; perhaps more alkali is deposited in the fibres to neutralize the acid formed by exertion. More glycogen seems to be deposited in them as a store of energy, and certainly, ... the nervous system which governs them learns in training to work more economically. Perhaps by training the recovery process is quickened. Maybe the actual mechanical strength of the muscle fibre and its surrounding membrane (sarcolemma) is increased by training so that it can stand, without injury, the strains and stresses of violent effort. All these factors may be at work, but at present we can only point to the importance and interest of the problem, and suggest that someone should investigate it properly."

A. V. Hill (1927), quoted in the Lore of Running, Noakes (1991)

CHAPTER 4

THE BODY'S ENERGY SYSTEMS

Depending on the intensity and duration of an activity, as well as the fitness level of your client, the body utilizes energy from 3 metabolic, or energy-producing, pathways. That's why understanding how the body makes energy is useful regardless of the component of fitness you are training—cardiorespiratory, muscular strength and endurance or flexibility.

The diversity of the 3 energy systems allows you to accommodate a variety of energy needs based on the type and intensity of the activity.

1. Immediate energy. The ATP-CP System (phosphagen system). This immediate energy system allows your client to snatch a toppling child, spike a volleyball and react immediately to a given situation that requires movement.

2. Short-term energy. The Lactic Acid System (anaerobic glycolysis). This is the system that is largely responsible for creating the energy needed for a client to walk up a 100-yard hill as fast as possible, or pass another participant in a 5K race with a burst of speed.

3. Long-term energy. The Aerobic System. This system supplies the energy needed to walk or cycle continuously. In fact, any activity where you "just keep going" or sustain the activity beyond 3-5 minutes relies primarily on the long-term energy system.

At any given time, all 3 energy systems are functioning simultaneously. The percentage of contribution from each system, termed the **energy spectrum,** is determined primarily by the intensity and duration of the activity, and the participant's fitness level. The energy needs of the body's musculature are not satisfied by an "all or nothing" approach. Instead, there is a smooth merging of one system into the other, with all systems functioning simultaneously, regardless of intensity, with considerable overlap.

You can compare the energy systems' use in the body to a light dimmer's effect on the brightness of bulbs. Depending on the energy demands placed on the muscles of the body, one of the 3 energy systems will glow more brightly than another. As exercise intensity and energy demands change, another system may shine more or less brightly, as the "dimmer switch of intensity" is turned either up or down. Regardless, there will *always* be at least a low-level glow, or energy contribution, from all 3 energy systems.

Energy for physical activity and for sustaining all cellular function is derived from food—carbohydrate, fat and protein. Energy that is synthesized from food is chemically released by breaking the food molecule bonds and then stored in a high-energy compound called ATP (adenosine triphosphate). ATP is called "the energy currency" of the cell because it is required for *all* processes related to cellular function. Without ATP, energy from food could not be harnessed to perform work. ATP is essential to form and conserve potential energy. All 3 energy systems have ATP as their foundation and work on the premise that potential energy is released by splitting molecular bonds and conserved by the formation of new bonds. This process is repeated over and over in the 3 energy systems.

Immediate Energy: ATP-CP System

Adenosine triphosphate (ATP) is the immediately available form of energy needed for muscular contraction and motor movement. The energy in food *can not* be directly transferred to cells for work. Instead, the energy stored in food is converted and delivered through ATP. ATP is used for *all* energy-requiring processes in the cells of the body. This includes energy for muscle contraction, nerve transmission, circulation, tissue synthesis, digestion and glandular secretion (McArdle et al., 1991).

Only small amounts of ATP are stored in the body at any one time—about 85 grams, or 3 ounces. This allows for just a few seconds of muscular work performed at maximum effort. Beyond this point, ATP must be resynthesized continuously to sustain muscular contraction and movement.

To release energy, ATP is broken down to form a new compound called adenosine diphosphate (ADP). Since ADP *can not* be further split to release energy, and ATP *can not* be supplied by the blood or from other tissues, it must be recycled continuously within each cell. Over and over again, ATP is re-created by reforming ADP to ATP. This is the body's way to capture, store and release energy.

It is because of ATP's critical role that it is characterized as the "energy currency" of the cell. Without ATP, there would be no energy production and muscle contraction. But, since only small quantities are stored in the body's cells, it must be resynthesized from ADP to ATP at the rate it is being utilized, or work effort will be limited rather quickly. The body's 3 energy systems contribute to solving this challenge of maintaining ATP availability in the body, regardless of the level of intensity.

Creatin phosphate (CP) is a molecule similar to ATP in that a large amount of energy is released when the bond between the creatin and phosphate molecules splits. Potential energy in the cells of the body is released by splitting bonds. For example, ATP is broken down to ADP + P and CP is broken down to C + P. Energy is liberated in both of these situations. Some of the energy for **ATP resynthesis** can be provided by the breakdown of CP. This energy is provided rapidly and without oxygen, which makes it useful in high-intensity situations where adequate oxygen is not available to produce ATP.

Energy is reconstructed, or conserved, by creating new bonds. For example, ADP is converted back to ATP and C + P is converted back to CP. Once the bonds are reformed, energy is now available for release once again. You can imagine the complexity and sheer volume of energy transfer that must occur every second in exercising muscles to maintain high energy outputs.

Table 7. Important Energy System Characteristics

	Immediate Energy/ ATP-CP System	Short-term Energy/ Lactic Acid or Glycolytic System	Long-term Energy or Oxidative System
	Anaerobic System	Anaerobic System	Aerobic System
Fuel or Substrate	• Creatin Phosphate • Stored ATP	• Blood Glucose • Glycogen	• Fatty Acids • Blood Glucose • Glycogen
Intensity	• Very, very hard • 9-10 Borg scale	• Very hard • 7 Borg scale	• Moderate to somewhat hard • 3-4 Borg scale*
% VO2 =	• > 95% max	• 85-95% max	• < 85% max
Time to Fatigue	• Very short duration • 1-10 seconds	• Short duration • 60-180 seconds	• Longer duration • > 3 minutes
Limits to ATP Production	• Limited muscle stores of CP and ATP	• Lactic acid accumulation • Rapid fatigue	• Depletion of muscle glycogen and glucose • Insufficient oxygen delivery/utilization

* Modified Borg Scale

The energy for movement is ultimately generated by the **oxidation** of the fats, carbohydrates and proteins that are consumed in our diet. Through aerobic processes, ATP and CP are ultimately replenished during recovery or lesser intensities. This occurs when ADP and C + P create new bonds to reform ATP and CP. This restoration occurs even though stored ATP and CP may have been depleted through anaerobic (without adequate oxygen) energy production.

The splitting of the ATP molecule can take place whether or not oxygen is available. The anaerobic systems of the body allow you to perform all types of exercises and necessary movements on a temporary basis without consuming, delivering and utilizing oxygen (aerobic metabolism). Remember, ATP supplies are limited and sustain activity for short duration.

The immediate energy ATP-CP system is utilized for activities of short duration and high intensity, such as lifting a heavy weight once. At the onset of an activity, or when an activity requires a sudden burst of instantaneous energy, the phosphagen system provides that energy from very limited ATP and CP stores in the muscles.

Key Point

Enough energy is provided by the ATP-CP system for about 10 seconds of maximal effort.

In situations where intramuscular ATP-CP energy stores may limit performance, a common goal is to improve these quantities with activity-specific training. Activities such as Olympic weight lifting, power lifting and short sprints require an immediate and rapid energy supply to ensure competitive levels of performance and personal safety during the performance of these sports. The energy provided for this type of effort comes from the ATP-CP stored in the specific muscles utilized for the activity.

It is easy to see why training the ATP-CP system may not be a necessary goal for many of your clients. It takes a highly motivated, highly skilled individual, with specific, short-term, all-out performance efforts in mind to desire this type of energy system improvement. Needless to say, this type of effort would never be labeled "easy" or "enjoyable" by most of your clients.

Short-term Energy: Lactic Acid or Glycolytic System

Since there is only a small amount of ATP available in your body, the body must continually resynthesize ATP or physical effort would be limited quickly. The short-term lactic acid system allows ATP and CP to be resynthesized at a rapid rate.

During a period of vigorous activity, energy to reconstruct ATP and CP comes mainly from glucose and glycogen. ATP, in turn, is directly available to reconstruct C and P back to CP. Utilization of glucose in this metabolic pathway comes from an anaerobic process called glycolysis.

Anaerobic glycolysis is used when energy from ATP is needed for activities requiring high-intensity effort for periods longer than the phosphagen system (ATP-CP) can provide. For example, the energy needed to walk up a 100-yard hill as fast as possible, slide (lateral training) performed in an athletic position at 60 slides per minute for 90 seconds, or passing a participant in a 5K race with a 60-second burst of speed.

Anaerobic glycolysis ultimately leads to the formation and significant accumulation of lactic acid. This creates a "burning" sensation in the exercising muscles and eventually requires a decrease in intensity or cessation of activity. But, even though anaerobic glycolysis ultimately has limitations in terms of exercise duration, it allows for the rapid resynthesis of ADP to ATP and continuation of vigorous activity when neither the ATP-CP or long-term aerobic energy systems could contribute significantly.

The short-term energy system is important because it supplies energy beyond that which the ATP-CP system is capable of supplying.

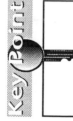

> The most rapidly accumulated and highest lactic acid levels are reached during maximal exercise that can be sustained for 60-180 seconds (McArdle et al., 1991).

It is obvious that all-out effort from several seconds to 3 minutes relies almost exclusively on the ATP-CP and lactic acid systems. If all-out effort is moderated to a less-intense effort, the period of activity that can be sustained will be extended, with both anaerobic and aerobic energy pathways contributing to sustenance of the particular exercise intensity.

Lactic Acid, Aerobic and Anaerobic Energy Production

Lactic acid does not accumulate *significantly* at all levels of activity. During light to moderate levels of activity, ATP energy production is met by processes that predominantly utilize oxygen (aerobic). The small amount of lactic acid that is produced under these conditions is easily oxidized (used for energy) in the muscle or liver.

It should be reemphasized that at *all* times, even at rest or during mild exercise, both aerobic and anaerobic processes are active in the body. For example, the red blood cells (RBCs) of the body contain no mitochondria, the "aerobic powerhouses" of cells. Because RBCs cannot produce energy aerobically, lactic acid is continually formed to supply the energy they require. Conversely, even at the highest of maximal efforts, though anaerobic metabolism predominates, some aerobic metabolism is sustaining some type of cellular function. However, in the case of the RBCs or low-level activity, lactic acid does not build up because its production rate equals its removal rate. As exercise intensity increases, the role of lactic acid becomes more significant.

> **Key Point**
>
> Lactic acid begins to accumulate and rise quickly at about 50-55% of a healthy, untrained client's maximal aerobic capacity, max VO2, or heart rate reserve (HRR). This is comparable to 60-65% of maximum heart rate. In a conditioned participant, significant lactate accumulation may not occur until 80-85% of max VO2. The increase in lactic acid becomes *exponentially* pronounced as the activity becomes more intense relative to current fitness level, and indicates that the aerobic energy system can no longer meet the additional energy requirements of the exercising muscles.

At some point, whether at 50%, 85% or some other percentage of maximal aerobic capacity, the participant will reach a threshold or a limiting factor in continued performance. This is commonly associated with **anaerobic threshold (AT)**, but more precisely labeled **blood lactate threshold (BLT)** or **onset of blood lactate accumulation (OBLA)**. As BLT is reached, the demands of exercise can no longer be met by available aerobic sources and the anaerobic lactic acid system begins to play a predominant role. This is reflected by a blood lactate concentration well above resting values and eventually results in an inability to sustain that level of intensity.

Through training that is sufficiently intense but still appropriate to a client's current fitness level, specific local muscular adaptations account for a lower production rate, increased tolerance and a quicker removal rate of lactic acid at *any* exercise intensity. Changes related to these adaptations allow an individual to work at increasingly more intense paces, and for longer duration.

Quick Index:

Long-term Energy: The Aerobic or Oxidative System

The aerobic system is the last of the 3 important stages of energy transfer in the body. It is the most complex of the 3 energy systems, but it is not necessary to go into lengthy detail with regard to its complexity.

The long-term energy system is an **oxidative system.** With the aid of oxygen this system breaks down fuels to generate energy. This disassembling of mainly carbohydrates and fats is referred to as **cellular respiration.** (Protein does not contribute significantly to total energy expenditure. Though protein, or specifically its amino acids, can enter into oxidative metabolism and be converted to glucose through gluconeogenesis, proteins are not a "preferred fuel" by the body. Protein metabolism accounts for less than 5-10% of energy needs in a healthy body. Protein is generally ignored when estimating total energy expenditure during rest and exercise.) This aerobic process (cellular respiration) of ATP production occurs within special cell organelles—the mitochondria. The lactic acid and ATP-CP systems are not very efficient at producing a large amount of ATP. A large percentage of the total *potential* ATP produced via the lactic acid and ATP-CP systems is never realized from the breakdown of their primary energy substrate, carbohydrate. It is wasted or fails to be preserved. This inefficiency is a result of an inability of these systems to completely oxidize fuel or metabolic fragments.

On the other hand, a large amount of ATP is created efficiently by the aerobic system because of its capacity to completely oxidize carbohydrate, fat and other fuel fragments created by incomplete oxidation of these substrates during anaerobic metabolism. Of course, complete oxidation of the nutrients will never occur in the ATP-CP and the lactic acid systems since these are anaerobic systems.

If the body is oxidizing or disassembling carbohydrate, the processes of aerobic glycolysis, Krebs cycle and electron transport chain are involved. The end product of **anaerobic** and **aerobic glycolysis** is the same—pyruvic acid. However, in the case of *anaerobic* glycolysis, and without the involvement of adequate oxygen, the pyruvic acid is converted to lactic acid. In the presence of sufficient oxygen, pyruvic acid is converted to acetyl coenzyme A (acetyl CoA). This conversion in the presence of oxygen allows acetyl CoA to enter the **Krebs** or **citric acid cycle**. The Krebs cycle is a very complex series of chemical reactions that permits complete oxidation of acetyl CoA. The remaining carbon of the original carbohydrate combines with oxygen and forms carbon dioxide (CO_2). CO_2 is carried to the lungs by the blood and easily expelled.

During glycolysis, hydrogen is released as the carbohydrate (glucose) is metabolized to pyruvic acid and enters into the Krebs cycle. This accumulation of hydrogen in the cell must be eliminated or the cell will become too acidic. The Krebs cycle is closely associated with a series of chemical reactions know as the **electron transport chain.** Hydrogen released during aerobic glycolysis and during the Krebs cycle combines with 2 coenzymes (NAD and FAD) that carry the hydrogen to the electron transport chain. At the end of this chain of reactions the hydrogen combines with oxygen to form water. This prevents an acidic cell environment and water is easily eliminated from the body. The energy yield from complete oxidation of a single molecule of glycogen is 38 or 39 ATP versus only 3 ATP from anaerobic glycolysis.

Oxidation of fat is important because muscle and liver glycogen stores may be able to provide only 1,200-2,000 kcal of energy. Energy from fat is virtually unlimited in the presence of sufficient oxygen. Triglycerides are the major energy source and are stored in fat cells and skeletal muscle fibers. If a triglyceride is to be used for energy, it must be broken down to one molecule of glycerol and 3 molecules of free fatty acids (FFAs) in a process called **lypolysis**. Once the FFAs are free of the glycerol molecule, they can easily enter the blood and be used by skeletal muscle. FFAs enter muscle cells and are broken down within the mitochondria. This breakdown of the fat within the mitochondria is called **beta oxidation**. It results in the formation of acetic acid and ultimately acetyl CoA.

At this point, as with carbohydrate oxidation, acetyl CoA that is formed by beta oxidation enters the Krebs cycle. Hydrogen that is generated in the Krebs cycle is transported to the electron transport chain and, as in carbohydrate metabolism, the end-products of FFA oxidation are a high yield of ATP, water and carbon dioxide.

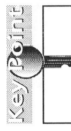

> Fat metabolism can generate even more energy than oxidative carbohydrate metabolism, but it requires more oxygen. That is why carbohydrate is generally the preferred fuel of the body during high-intensity exercise. However, with specific training adaptations the body can become a more efficient fat user, even at higher intensities, thus sparing precious glycogen stores and blood glucose.

Oxidative processes, as related to endurance activities and recovery from anaerobic activity, rely on the body's ability to effectively deliver and utilize oxygen in the working muscles. Vigorous activity could not extend beyond several minutes, and recovery from anaerobic efforts would not be possible, if not for the long-term oxidative system.

Quick Index:

Training Energy Systems

Many participants will not have a need, or the desire, to train all 3 energy systems. For example, most people will not focus on the ATP-CP system because to train, it requires intense, short, maximal bursts of activity. Most of your clients do not have a functional use for this type of training, though the ATP system is regularly called upon in day-to-day tasks.

When training energy systems it is important to ask this question: "Are the characteristics required to train this specific energy system compatible with my client's training and health-related goals?" The answer should dictate the specific type of energy system training.

Quick Index:

The Bridge

The intensity of an activity determines which of the body's 3 energy systems will predominate. Each system has a purpose that can translate to a client's goals. Understanding the aerobic and anaerobic energy systems allows you to choose which one to emphasize, and will be the foundation of interval and strength training programs. Training the systems will impact your client's ability to get specific results.

CHAPTER 5

CARDIORESPIRATORY PHYSIOLOGY AND CONDITIONING

Although exercise to challenge the cardiorespiratory system may seem like the simple part of an exercise program, that's not necessarily the case. Changing the training regimen allows you to break up the boredom many people feel toward aerobic exercise while improving their results. A more sophisticated approach enhances your value to clients who need you to help with program variations. And it's a good mental challenge for you, too.

Most types of cells—including the heart, nerves and brain—can produce energy only aerobically. That is why a constant supply of oxygen to these cells is necessary. For example, if the delivery of oxygen to a portion of the heart is stopped, that area of the heart suffers a heart attack or myocardial infarction. If the brain stops getting oxygen, a stroke occurs in the deprived area. Nearly all cells in the body require a constant supply of oxygen. Because of this, the aerobic energy system is the predominant energy system in the body. (Refer to Table 7 in Chapter 4.)

A healthy cardiorespiratory system that is challenged by appropriate physical activity and not compromised by a poor diet ensures an adequate supply and use of oxygen for most of the body's functions and oxygen-demanding tissues. Cardiorespiratory training or aerobic conditioning moves the body toward being a more "efficient machine" in relation to its ability to carry out everyday tasks and recreation.

The **cardiorespiratory (C-R) system** (often referred to as the cardiovascular system) is really a transport network in the body. **Cardio** refers to the heart and its pumping force that circulates the blood through an amazing network of blood vessels. **Respiratory** refers to the lungs and the exchange of gases. Oxygen and carbon dioxide are exchanged in the lungs, as well as in the cells of the body.

The C-R system consists of the heart, lungs, arteries (carrying oxygen-loaded blood away from the heart throughout the body), capillaries (exchanging gases, nutrients and byproducts between the bloodstream and cells) and veins (carrying oxygen-depleted blood back to the heart). An important purpose of the cardiorespiratory system is to deliver oxygen to the various tissues of the body, both at rest and during a broad spectrum of exercise intensities, from low level to high level.

Blood is the vehicle that delivers oxygen and nutrients (like fat and carbohydrate) to the cells in the body where they are needed to produce ATP. Blood also picks up **metabolic byproducts** of energy metabolism, including lactic acid, water and carbon dioxide. In contrast to a **waste product** that has no usefulness and is difficult to dispose of, byproducts such as carbon dioxide can easily be carried to the lungs and breathed out of the body, and water can be sweated out of the body or breathed out (expelled air is saturated with humidity or water). And, lactic acid is carried to the liver where it is metabolized or oxidized.

Lactic acid is *not* a waste product. Its production at higher intensity levels allows you to work out at harder levels than can be sustained with aerobic metabolism. During recovery, or when the activity is slowed, sufficient oxygen becomes available again and lactic acid is oxidized and converted to **pyruvic acid**, which is eventually used as an energy source. In the presence of oxygen, lactate enters the glycolytic pathway, is converted to pyruvic acid, enters the Krebs cycle and is oxidized for energy. Furthermore, the potential energy in the lactate and pyruvate molecules formed during strenuous activity can be used for the resynthesis of glucose (gluconeogenesis) in the liver through a process called the Cori cycle (McArdle et al., 1991). The Cori cycle provides an additional means for lactic acid removal, as well as a source for meeting blood glucose and muscle glycogen needs.

Quick Index:

Chapter 4, discussion of lactic acid utilization

Energy for Cardiorespiratory Conditioning

Think of your body as a factory. It processes different raw materials to make its final product, which is energy. Energy is used by every cell in the body, including skeletal muscle cells, which produce movement. Oxygen, carbohydrates (sugar and starches), fat and protein are the raw materials available in virtually an unlimited supply.

Adenosine triphosphate (ATP) is a high-energy compound formed from the oxidation of fat and carbohydrate. It is used as the energy supply for muscles and body functions. When a muscle contracts and exerts force, the energy used to drive the contraction comes from ATP. However, since the amount of ATP stored in the muscle is small, your body begins to immediately produce more ATP by breaking down carbohydrate and fat. Otherwise, the duration of activity would be severely limited. ATP is ultimately the body's only energy source, and is supplied both aerobically and anaerobically.

To understand how a muscle cell produces energy for cardiorespiratory effort, let's tie together the 2 primary energy systems of the body. **Aerobic** means "with oxygen." Energy is produced aerobically as long as *enough* oxygen is supplied to the exercising muscles by the cardiorespiratory (C-R) system. Even when the C-R system is unable to supply enough oxygen, your skeletal muscles can still produce energy via a process called **anaerobic metabolism**. The muscles produce energy "without oxygen," or more accurately, without sufficient oxygen. The immediate energy (ATP-CP) and short-term energy (lactic acid) systems contribute to anaerobic metabolism.

In intense exercise of short duration (100-yard dash, traditional resistance training, shot-put), the energy is predominantly derived from the already-present stores of intramuscular ATP and CP using the immediate and short-term anaerobic energy systems. After several minutes, oxygen consumption becomes an important factor if the activity is to be sustained and the predominant energy pathway is the long-term, aerobic energy system.

To totally develop the C-R system, *both* aerobic and anaerobic energy systems must be trained. And, if reducing body fat is a goal of the exercise program, include both. Why? The anaerobic systems use stored ATP-CP and burn glucose, a simple sugar derived from carbohydrates. The aerobic system also uses glucose but in the process, it burns fat as well. Stored body fat is released into the bloodstream and sent to the muscles, where, in the presence of oxygen and glucose, it is burned aerobically to produce energy. Fat can only be burned aerobically (in the presence of oxygen) and the byproducts of the aerobic system—carbon dioxide and water—do not lead to premature muscle fatigue.

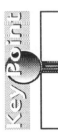

Aerobic or anaerobic exercise is neither "good" or "bad." Which type of exercise is appropriate to your client's needs and exercise goals?

Even though we say that we're "aerobic" or "anaerobic," these terms actually refer to the *muscles being used for the activity* since the energy for muscle contraction and movement is produced inside the muscle cells. Aerobic exercise means that the muscles you are using to perform the activity are getting enough oxygen to meet the energy needs via aerobic processes. Anaerobic exercise occurs when the exercising muscles no longer get enough oxygen to produce the necessary energy aerobically and must rely on the anaerobic system.

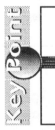

The more fit you are, the more capable your C-R system is of delivering adequate oxygen to sustain aerobic energy production at increasingly higher levels of intensity.

Moving Along the Energy Spectrum

At rest your muscles are *aerobic*. Remember, your body is always aerobic, as the cells of the heart, brain and nerves need a constant supply of oxygen to meet their energy demands and sustain cellular life. Rest is an exercise intensity and requires a volume of oxygen (VO2) to sustain resting-energy demands of the body.

As exercise intensity increases from rest to walking to running 6-minute miles, the demand for oxygen continues to increase. It becomes more of a challenge for the C-R system to get enough oxygen to the working muscles. And, unless the muscle cells are trained to do so, they may not be able to extract available oxygen from the blood as exercise intensity increases. Somewhere between about 50-85% of maximum aerobic capacity (depending on fitness level and specific genetic factors), the delivery and utilization of oxygen to the exercising muscles becomes inadequate.

It is at this point muscles shift largely to the anaerobic energy system to support continued contractions. For example, anaerobic metabolism is used when strength training to fatigue in 8-12 repetitions and other strenuous efforts that last from 30-seconds to about 2 or 3 minutes.

The intensity at which the muscles no longer get enough oxygen (they are getting some) to produce energy predominantly by aerobic metabolism is commonly referred to as **anaerobic threshold**. Crossing over anaerobic threshold is usually accompanied by a significant increase in breathing or respiration, burning muscles (accumulation of lactate from anaerobic energy-system contribution), a feeling by the participant that she would like to slow down or that she could not continue this activity at the current pace indefinitely. She probably will not be able to string together 3 or 4 words without gasping.

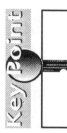

Even the recovery from traditional anaerobic strength efforts (muscle fatigue in about 90 seconds) could not be accomplished without the long-term aerobic system.

I sometimes use this information to motivate clients who "only want to strength train." I explain that their anaerobic strength training may be enhanced by more effective and quicker recovery as a result of aerobic conditioning. For many clients it is difficult to understand how aerobic effort enhances anaerobic effort, recovery and total well-being. This explanation helps answer your clients' questions related to the importance of a balanced approach to fitness.

While one energy system will predominate over the other, both aerobic and anaerobic energy systems are *always* working, regardless of intensity or type of activity. The aerobic system produces a great deal of energy compared to the anaerobic system. It is the predominant energy system at rest, during mild to moderate, or even high-intensity activity if you are highly conditioned, and during recovery from anaerobic efforts. Also, carbon dioxide and water, the primary byproducts of the aerobic system, are easily eliminated by breathing and sweating.

The anaerobic system can produce energy quickly for powerful and immediate muscle contractions—without the need for "sufficient" amounts of oxygen. However, the trade-off for immediate muscular response is susceptibility to quicker fatigue.

Of course, your body does not switch over to the anaerobic system all at once—or in fact totally—but *gradually shifts gears* to produce energy at a faster rate than can aerobically be supplied, as demanded by relative intensity of exercise. Any activity that can be performed at an "aerobic" pace can also be pushed to an "anaerobic" level of intensity. As one becomes more fit, surges of increased intensity above what is comfortable might be appropriate for a variety of fitness levels.

Physiological Adjustments to Energy Demand

There are several physiological adjustments made by your body to meet the increased energy requirements of exercising skeletal muscles during cardiorespiratory effort and during recovery from anaerobic effort. The primary objective of these adjustments is to provide an exercising muscle with oxygenated blood that can be used for the production of energy (ATP). Your endurance capabilities will be greatly influenced by the magnitude and direction of these changes.

Cardiac output. Cardiac output (Q) is the product of stroke volume (SV) and heart rate (HR), where Q = HR x SV. This measure is indicative of the rate of oxygen delivery to your exercising muscles. The more work performed (large-muscle, rhythmic, sustained activity), the more blood that will be pumped per minute by your heart. With training, you are able to deliver the same amount of blood and oxygen needed to accomplish the given workload with fewer heart beats per minute because of the increased amount of blood the heart can pump each beat (SV).

Heart rate (HR) is the number of times the heart beats per minute. As you become more fit for a *given* amount of work, HR decreases and an increased stroke volume accomplishes the necessary delivery of oxygen and blood. As exercise intensity (work load) increases heart-rate will increase up to a point. At or near your max VO2 heart rate begins to level off and is referred to as **maximal heart rate** (MHR).

As the equation "220 minus your age" implies, your MHR declines with age. Training can not affect this aging consequence. But, staying fit as you age allows you to work at a higher percentage of your attainable maximum, thus attenuating the greatest of aging effects—inactivity!

Stroke volume. Stroke volume (SV) is the other primary determinant of Q and represents the amount of blood ejected from the heart during each beat. Unlike HR and Q, SV does not increase linearly with work rate. SV increases progressively until a work rate equivalent to approximately 50 75% of max VO2 is reached. Thereafter, continued increases in work rate cause little or no increase in SV.

Exercise-induced increases in SV are believed to be the result of factors that are both intrinsic and extrinsic to the heart. According to the Frank-Starling law, a greater stretch is placed on the muscle fibers of the heart due to a greater venous return of blood to the heart, resulting in a more forceful contraction of those fibers and consequently a greater SV. Extrinsic factors such as increased nervous (sympathetic) or endocrine (release of adrenal hormones epinephrine and norepinephrine) stimulation to the heart can also contribute to the increased SV that occurs during exercise.

Blood Pressure (BP)

Blood pressure (BP) is the amount of force exerted on the arterial wall. **Systolic blood pressure (SBP)** represents the force developed by your heart during left ventricular contraction (ejection of blood from the heart's left ventricle). SBP increases linearly with work rate increases. **Diastolic blood pressure (DBP)** is indicative of the pressure in the arterial system during ventricular relaxation and reflects *lowest* resistance to blood flow. It changes little from rest to maximal levels of exercise in healthy people.

Pulse pressure is the difference between SBP and DBP. It increases in direct proportion to the intensity of exercise. Pulse pressure is significant since it reflects the driving force for blood flow in the arteries.

Total peripheral resistance (TPR). The sum of all the forces that oppose blood flow in the systemic circulation is called **total peripheral resistance (TPR)**. Numerous factors affect TPR, including blood viscosity (thickness), vessel length, hydrostatic pressure (pressure created in a fluid system or environment such as is present in the body) and vessel diameter.

Vessel diameter is by far the most important of these factors, since TPR is inversely proportional to the fourth power of the radius of the vessel. To emphasize what impact this has, if one vessel has one-half the radius of another and if all other factors are equal, the larger vessel would have 16 times (i.e., 2 or whatever radius to the 4th power) less resistance than the smaller vessel. As a result, 16 times more blood would flow through the larger vessel at the same pressure.

Implications for exercise. Certain organs require more blood flow than others during physical activity. The same is true for skeletal muscle. During activity the active muscles demand a greater flow and generally, during rest, do not require a large volume of blood. During exercise, resistance in the vessels supplying the muscle and skin is *decreased*. This implies that blood flow to these parts of the body is *enhanced*.

Resistance in vessels supplying visceral organs (the liver, gastrointestinal tract, kidneys) is *increased*. Increased resistance indicates that blood flow to the visceral organs is reduced, thus "freeing" up oxygen for more immediate and demanding needs of the exercising body.

These changes are due almost entirely to intrinsic factors such as the increased demand of the muscle and the requirement of skin blood flow to facilitate heat dissipation. Nerves and local metabolic conditions act on the smooth muscular band of arteriole walls and cause them to alter their internal diameter almost instantaneously. When the diameter is increased, this is termed **vasodilation**. Total peripheral resistance (TPR) tends to *decrease* during progressive, dynamic exercise, because vasodilation is occurring in the muscles and skin. This seems to override the **vasoconstriction** (narrowing of the internal diameter of the lumen or blood vessel) which is occurring in the visceral organs and the net result is *less* total resistance to blood flow.

In addition, stimulation of nerves to the venous vessels causes them to "stiffen." Such **venoconstriction** permits large quantities of blood to move from peripheral (toward the extremities) veins into the central circulation.

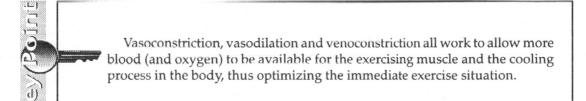

Vasoconstriction, vasodilation and venoconstriction all work to allow more blood (and oxygen) to be available for the exercising muscle and the cooling process in the body, thus optimizing the immediate exercise situation.

All of these factors contribute to **blood shunting**, which helps the body prioritize the flow of blood based on the demands of the activity and the needs of the body. The capability of large portions of the body's vasculature (especially the arterioles, capillaries, veins and venules) to either constrict or dilate provides a rapid redistribution of blood to meet the tissue's (muscles, organs) metabolic requirements while maintaining an appropriate blood pressure throughout the entire system (McArdle et al., 1991).

Owing to neural and hormonal vascular regulation and the local (specific muscle sites) metabolic conditions of the muscles themselves, blood is redistributed and directed through working muscles *from* areas that can temporarily tolerate a reduction in normal blood flow. This shunting of blood from specific tissues occurs most dramatically during high-intensity exercise.

Any increase in the maximum cardiac output directly affects your client's capacity to circulate oxygen. An increase in maximum cardiac output clearly results in a proportionate increase in the potential for aerobic metabolism. Proper C-R training conditions the entire cardiorespiratory system and maximizes the availability of oxygen to the body's systems.

Quick Index:

Chapter 3, explains how the heart works

Energy Production and Physiological Adaptations to Exercise

Let's take a look at how the body makes energy and the body's physiological adjustments to exercise (overload). This understanding will go a long way in bridging theory and practical application when faced with program design choices.

In a healthy person, resting energy needs are predominantly and easily met by the aerobic energy system. When the activity demands placed on the body increase, your body immediately needs greater amounts of energy to sustain this new level of work. Unfortunately, the rate of aerobic energy production is sluggish when moving from low levels of activity to higher levels that demand more oxygen. Oxygen must be breathed in, transferred from your lungs to the blood, carried to your heart and then pumped to your muscles where it is needed.

Because of the mechanics in getting oxygen to your muscles, a delay exists in the delivery of oxygen from the heart and vascular system. This is termed **oxygen deficit** and is associated with the beginning phases of exercise—even with low-intensity levels to some extent. (See Figure 1, Oxygen Deficit/Oxygen Debt)

Oxygen deficit occurs because oxygen consumption requires several minutes to reach the "required oxygen intake" for a given, submaximal exercise intensity. Even though the oxygen requirement for the given activity is constant from the very start of the exercise, this initial period of exercise has an oxygen consumption that is below the needed level.

This lag in oxygen uptake isn't surprising when you consider that the *immediate* energy for muscular work is *always* provided directly by the immediate and non-oxygen consuming (anaerobic) breakdown of ATP in the muscle. Oxygen deficit is the difference between the total oxygen consumed during exercise and the total that would have been consumed had a steady-rate of aerobic metabolism been reached immediately at the start (McArdle et al., 1991).

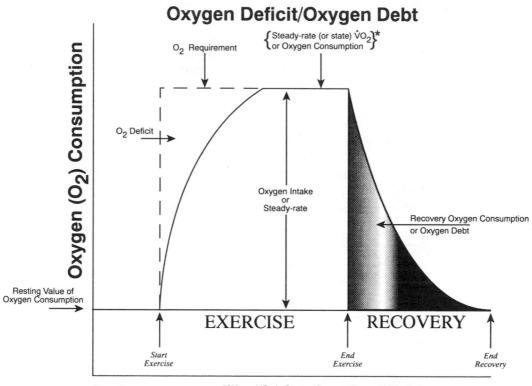

Figure 1   *(Where VO_2 is Oxygen Consumption and Utilization)

Oxygen deficit may be minimized by a slower, progressive warm-up as opposed to a quick acceleration to training pace. It takes the body time to shunt blood flow away from the visceral organs to meet the new demands that are being placed on exercising muscle. However, oxygen deficit can not be eliminated totally because of the necessity of using nonoxygen-consuming processes that break down ATP for initiating immediate muscular work.

Though oxygen deficit will occur, effects such as breathlessness can be diminished with a proper warm-up.

Oxygen consumption rises rapidly during the first minutes of exercise. Generally, during any kind of steady exercise, a plateau in oxygen consumption is reached between the third and fourth minute. After this plateau is reached and intensity remains constant, oxygen consumption is relatively stable for the rest of the exercise period. The flat portion (plateau) of the oxygen consumption curve is considered the steady-state or, more precisely, the steady-rate. (Refer to Figure 1.)

Steady-rate reflects a balance between the energy required by the working muscles and the rate of ATP production by the aerobic energy system. If exercise is started at a "slow" pace, a steady-rate is reached in about the third or fourth minute. Steady-rate activity can be described as a level of cardiorespiratory effort that is relatively easy to maintain. Your clients may describe this level of intensity as "cruising," or characterize it by saying, "I could keep this up all day long!" Another good indicator of steady-rate is a pace of activity that is easily maintained for a sustained duration of 5 minutes or longer.

Under steady-rate metabolic conditions, lactate accumulation is minimal because there is an abundance of available oxygen. The energy demands of steady-rate activity are met predominantly by aerobic metabolism of carbohydrates and fat. Steady-rate occurs during *aerobic* glycolysis and submaximal levels of exercise.

It is important for your clients to understand steady-rate and how they feel during a steady-rate effort. There will be instances, such as during interval training, that you will encourage your clients to work beyond this comfort zone, and at times during recovery from vigorous effort, they may be asked to work at or below this level of perceived effort.

Maximum steady-rate or state (MSR or MSS) levels, which equate with anaerobic threshold and blood lactate threshold, vary from one individual to the next. Differences depend primarily on a person's ability to deliver and utilize oxygen according to her current cardiorespiratory fitness level. For a sedentary client, going from rest to slow walking at about a 20-minute-per-mile pace may push the need for energy (ATP) by the muscle into anaerobic metabolism. Her MSR exists at very low-intensity levels of activity. Contrast this to a highly conditioned client, where the energy balance can be maintained aerobically at very intense levels of exercise. For example, in a highly conditioned and genetically blessed marathon runner, steady-rate aerobic metabolism can be maintained at a pace well under 6-minute miles, for 26 miles!

> Steady-rate exercise is the highest exercise intensity your client can maintain for prolonged periods of time.

Recovery Oxygen Consumption

In **recovery** from either light, moderate or strenuous exercise, the oxygen consumed in excess of the resting value of oxygen consumption has been termed the oxygen debt or recovery oxygen consumption. (Refer to Figure 1.) **Recovery oxygen debt** is calculated as the total oxygen consumed in recovery minus the total oxygen theoretically consumed at rest during the recovery period. To understand this concept in manageable terms, I'll utilize a discussion by scientist A.V. Hill, as reported in McArdle et al., 1991.

In 1922, Hill and others discussed energy metabolism during exercise and recovery in financial-accounting terms. Within his characterization, the body's carbohydrate stores were likened to energy "credits." If these stored credits were expended during exercise, then a "debt" was incurred. The greater the energy deficit, or use of available stored energy credits, the larger the energy debt incurred. The accumulation of lactic acid during the anaerobic component of exercise represented the utilization of the stored energy credit, glycogen. Though scientists now know that recovery oxygen uptake is a more complex issue, this was thought to represent the metabolic cost of repaying this debt—thus the term oxygen debt.

There is no doubt that the elevated aerobic metabolism in recovery is necessary. When you are breathing harder after activity, more oxygen is being taken in to restore the body's level of energy prior to activity. In recovery from strenuous exercise, recovery oxygen consumption (oxygen debt) serves to replenish the high-energy phosphates (ATP-CP/anaerobic energy) depleted by exercise. In recovery from strenuous to moderate exercise, recovery oxygen is also used to resynthesize a portion of lactic acid to glycogen. The main source for reestablished pre-exercise glycogen levels, however, is carbohydrate in the diet, *not* resynthesized lactic acid.

Oxygen debt includes oxygen deficit (Figure 1). Furthermore, it reflects the energy costs of both (1) anaerobic metabolism during exercise and (2) the respiratory, circulatory, hormonal, tissue repair, ionic (redistribution of calcium, potassium, and sodium within the muscle and other body parts) and thermal adjustments that occur in recovery. During recovery, all of these processes require oxygen in amounts well above resting rates to return the body to normal.

After any kind of exercise the body does not return immediately to a resting level of oxygen consumption. One function of a cool-down is to safely and/or with the least amount of physiological stress return the body to resting VO2 level. During submaximal (easy to moderate) efforts the return to resting level, after exercise, is hardly noticeable. During strenuous activity, the return to pre-activity metabolic rate (resting oxygen consumption) is perceptible in terms of, for example breathing rate, possibly sweat rate, and increased time necessary to return to pre-exercise levels.

Implications of Oxygen Debt for Exercise and Recovery
Procedures for speeding recovery from exercise can generally be labeled as either active or passive. In **active recovery**, which is often called "cooling-down" or "tapering-off," submaximal exercise is performed in the belief that this continued movement in some way prevents muscle cramps and stiffness and facilitates the recovery process. With **passive recovery**, the person usually lies down or is totally inactive, with the hope that complete inactivity may reduce the resting energy requirements and thus "free" oxygen for the recovery process.

From *steady-rate exercise*, the recovery is more rapid with *passive* procedures. No appreciable lactic acid accumulates with either steady-rate aerobic exercise or brief 5- to 10-second bouts of all-out exercise. Therefore, recovery is rapid and additional exercise can begin again without the hindering effects of fatigue.

It may be argued that both lying down or low-level activity will facilitate recovery fairly quickly. Even though research indicates that the passive method is optimal, it may be more appropriate if a cardiac event (heart attack or symptoms indicating a potential for one) has occurred or if you are trying to optimize a training response. Realize that low-level activity will not hinder your client's recovery in most instances.

When exercise intensity for the *average* individual exceeds about 55-60% of max VO2 (about 70-75% of max heart rate), regardless of fitness level, a steady-rate of aerobic metabolism is usually no longer maintained. Lactic acid formation exceeds its rate of removal and accumulates. Soon the exerciser becomes exhausted. (It should be noted that some highly trained endurance athletes can maintain 85% or greater of their max VO2 at steady-rate.)

Lactic acid removal is accelerated by *active recovery*. Large-muscle, rhythmic activity that is at about steady-rate or lower is clearly more effective in facilitating lactate removal when compared to passive recovery (McArdle et al., 1991). Though the reasons are not clear for the benefits of active recovery, the facilitated removal of lactate may be the result of an increased circulation of blood through "lactate using" organs like the liver and heart. Also, increased blood flow through the muscles in active recovery would certainly enhance lactic acid removal because muscle tissue can use this substrate (lactate) and oxidize it via Krebs (aerobic energy pathway) cycle metabolism. However, if the exercise in recovery is too intense and above the lactate or steady-rate threshold, it may prolong recovery by increasing lactic acid formation.

This has a potential impact on sports such as basketball, soccer and tennis. If you are pushed to a high level of anaerobic metabolism, you may not fully recover during the brief rest periods inherent to a particular activity. This may affect performance or increase the risk for injury. Regardless, specific training can improve the situation.

If left to their own choice, most of your clients will naturally select their own optimal recovery exercise intensity. This is at a level just below their lactate-accumulation threshold—in other words, at a level of exercise intensity they can easily maintain without breathlessness, can speak 3 or 4 words at a time without gasping and do not report that their muscles ache or burn (from lactic acid accumulation).

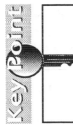

Cool-down helps return the body's systems to "normal" or resting levels. Less demand is placed on the heart muscle during recovery if an appropriate cool-down is used following exercise.

Quick Index:

Energy Spectrum Chronology for Submaximal C-R Conditioning

1. Exercise begins. First 10 seconds. Only a limited supply of energy is present in the muscle for *immediate* use. Energy can be produced anaerobically from stored creatine phosphate (CP) and ATP in the immediate energy system. Because muscles store very little CP and ATP, energy production is limited when this energy pathway is called upon. This immediate, anaerobic system supports high-intensity activity for about 10 seconds, but also may be drawn on in less-intense efforts to a lesser degree. Regardless of start-up exercise intensity, the ATP-CP and lactic acid systems will be used to some degree in at least the first few minutes of activity.

Note that no lactic acid is produced with the ATP-CP system. However, if the ATP-CP system is operating in conjunction with the lactic acid system, lactic acid could be produced and accumulated. Because they are required to help with start-up activity until a steady-rate has been achieved and the aerobic system can predominate, an oxygen deficit is created.

2. Next 1 to 3 minutes. Either glycogen stored in the muscle or glucose transported by the blood from the liver *can* be used without oxygen to provide a limited supply of energy via a process termed anaerobic glycolysis. Intensity of effort will dictate whether this anaerobic energy source is heavily relied upon. This second, short-term anaerobic pathway involves the breakdown of glucose or glycogen under certain conditions. Lactic acid is the byproduct of this anaerobic chemical reaction. Because of lactic acid's rapid buildup, which causes fatigue, it is generally the limiting factor in high-intensity activities. Most of the lactic acid formed during an anaerobic reaction is released into the blood and transported to the liver, where it is converted back to glycogen and stored.

3. About 3 minutes into activity. As additional oxygen becomes available (e.g., during steady-rate, recovery or a slowed pace), the aerobic system is used more. After a few minutes, the aerobic system is able to supply most of the energy needed for mild exercise and reaches steady-rate.

At this time, liver glycogen is converted to glucose and released into the blood to provide fuel for both the aerobic and anaerobic systems. The nature or intensity of activity will dictate whether the glucose is used in an aerobic or anaerobic energy pathway. If steady-rate has been achieved, aerobic glycolysis will predominate.

4. Steady-rate activity of 3 minutes to hours. Finally, adipocytes (fat cells) release more fat, the preferred fuel for the aerobic system. The aerobic pathway primarily utilizes fatty acids, glucose and glycogen as its key substrates to produce ATP. Limitations to aerobic energy production include depletion of muscle glycogen and sugar (glucose), and insufficient oxygen delivery and utilization. Generally, aerobic pathways will sustain long-duration, sub-anaerobic threshold activities lasting longer than 3 minutes.

5. Recovery. Lactic acid must be metabolized in the presence of adequate oxygen, and stored ATP and CP that were used and broken down to liberate energy for muscular effort must be reconstructed by oxidative or aerobic processes. The importance of the aerobic system during recovery from anaerobic work, such as anaerobic cardiorespiratory intervals or strength training, is often overlooked.

Energy Chronology for High-Intensity Activity

Beginning of exercise bout. If the exercise bout is intense (relative to fitness level), there is an attempt by the body to deliver the energy demands of the exercising muscles through the aerobic pathway. The speed of the aerobic reactions and respiration (through increases in breathing rate) increase to provide more energy. However, because the body does not have the proper "chemistry" in place as a result of training adaptations, the body no longer has the capacity to deliver and/or extract additional oxygen to meet the demands of the exercise intensity aerobically.

Anaerobic threshold. As the cardiorespiratory exercise becomes more intense, the anaerobic systems dominate, especially the lactic acid system, and supply an increasing amount of energy. The intensity of the muscle contractions may cause compression of small arteries, thus allowing very limited blood flow to the exercising muscle. Because of this vascular bed compression, restricted amounts of oxygen, glucose or fat, if any, can enter the muscle cell. Thus, the majority of the carbohydrate needed comes from glycogen already stored in the muscle. Lactic acid begins to accumulate as your client approaches and/or surpasses her steady-rate or anaerobic threshold.

Eventually, more lactic acid is formed and increased amounts of lactic acid are released into the bloodstream. As lactic acid levels within the muscle increase, the efficiency of aerobic chemical reactions is inhibited, and in general, efficiency of muscular contraction starts to decrease.

If you slow down or stop exercise, and oxygen becomes available to the formed lactic acid, it can be converted to a usable glucose energy source or transformed into glycogen (stored energy) by a process called gluconeogenesis. In fact, almost all of the lactic acid produced by an intense exercise bout is cleared from the blood in about 30-45 minutes.

The amount of energy produced anaerobically is relatively high per unit of time, but peaks after only about 40-50 seconds of all-out work. It does not last long because of the body's limited tolerance to significant accumulation of lactic acid and limited stores of ATP-CP. In contrast, after 5-6 minutes of continuous exercise at steady-rate or lower, the majority of energy required by the body is produced aerobically. The longer the duration of exercise, the greater the contribution from the aerobic system.

Anaerobic Threshold and Interval Training

All of this seemingly complex information becomes of real value when planning cardiorespiratory exercise programs. Several approaches can be taken to enable a client to perform significant amounts of normally exhaustive exercise, while at the same time reducing the contribution from anaerobic energy transfer through glycolysis and subsequent lactic acid buildup. These science-based approaches enable your clients to perform more total work, reach their desired fitness levels and burn more calories. Yet, the work doses are in tolerable amounts, so client compliance remains high.

Anaerobic threshold training. (Anaerobic threshold is the point beyond which significant amounts of lactic acid start to accumulate and lead to fairly rapid onset of fatigue.) By keeping intensity at or just below anaerobic or steady-rate threshold, you can train the body to have a high rate of aerobic energy transfer. A dramatic example of this is a marathon runner who can sustain sub 5-minute miles, for 26.2 miles, at or just below anaerobic threshold.

Interval training. A second approach involves training intermittently (interval training) above the lactate or steady-rate threshold and recovering just below it. Improving anaerobic threshold is directly dependent on high-intensity cardiorespiratory training. During interval training, various work-to-rest intervals are used. This type of training enables you to push back the threshold at which lactate accumulates significantly. This translates into a higher intensity of work accomplished aerobically, greater fitness gains and more calories burned.

If you train only at low-intensity exercise levels, your max VO2 may or may not be relatively high, but it will not increase. Also, your ability to work at a higher percentage of your max VO2 will not change. (Working at a higher percentage of max VO2 is often referred to as "functional percentage of max VO2," and is a good indicator of cardiorespiratory fitness.)

This especially has implications for optimizing fitness gains and performance, although it may not be as important from a health standpoint. Interval training, in a milder form, can optimize fitness gains and weight loss in even the most deconditioned person. The key is to make the training relative to your client's current fitness level.

Quick Index:

Chapter 12, how to make interval training applicable to all fitness levels

Applying Overload to Cardiorespiratory Fitness

When designing exercise programs, your concern is applying the appropriate amount of overload to improve the cardiorespiratory system. **Overload** is defined as a rhythmic, continuous, large-muscle activity that promotes a *simultaneous* increase in heart-rate and return of blood (venous return) to the heart. If continued improvements are to be realized, the overload must be progressive in nature.

Many factors may increase heart rate without increasing blood return to the heart, such as the influence of drugs, excitement, heat or traditional resistance training. Yet sustaining a large volume of venous return is essential for a significant training effect to occur in cardiorespiratory fitness.

To further define the cardiorespiratory overload definition, **frequency**, **intensity** and **duration** must be considered. Once you have identified the "right kind of activity" that satisfies the overload definition, it is generally recommended that your client exercise and challenge this component of fitness 3-5 times per week.

ACSM (1991) intensity guidelines for healthy adults are set at 50-85% of their max VO2 or heart-rate reserve (HRR). This compares to 60-90% of maximum heart-rate (MHR). The recommended duration is 20-60 minutes.

The *minimum* threshold for increasing max VO2 is 50% of max VO2 or heart-rate reserve (HRR). This compares to about 60% of max HR. However, an increase in max VO2 is not essential for substantial and beneficial effects on your health or cardiorespiratory endurance.

The ability to work at a higher percentage of max VO2 (not necessarily increasing maximum VO2), and your client's health, is enhanced by *moderate and consistent* C-R training. This includes both continuous training (aerobic) and interval training (largely anaerobic) to optimize cardiorespiratory fitness. The correct exercise overload may have the following effects in creating a more efficient cardiorespiratory system that is able to better deliver and extract oxygen.

It is well documented that:

1. **Capillary density** increases with endurance-type training. This increased capillarization allows for better distribution of nutrients and oxygen to the working muscle, and enhanced metabolic byproduct (lactic acid, carbon dioxide, water) removal.

2. The size and number of **mitochondria**, which are characterized as the aerobic "power houses" in the cell, *increase* with endurance training. This allows a higher level of aerobic metabolism to be maintained.

3. **Aerobic enzymes** (protein substances in the cell that facilitate energy production) *increase* with endurance training and enhance the ability to use oxygen more efficiently. This adaptation facilitates the energy-production process.

4. High-intensity interval conditioning has a positive training effect on shifting the metabolic profile of fast-twitch, Type IIa muscle fibers toward a more endurant fiber.

5. **Blood delivery (cardiac output)** is improved by a stronger heart that has a greater pumping or volume capacity per heart beat.

6. **Oxygen extraction (a-v02 difference)** is improved by regular and specific training.

Such physiologic and biochemical changes in the muscle cells of the body enhance the cell's capacity to generate ATP aerobically while working at increasingly higher levels of exercise intensity.

Case Study—VO2 and Cardiorespiratory Fitness

The *correct* activity, frequency, duration and intensity have the biggest impact on your clients' accomplishment of their specific fitness goals. Let's look at the following scenario to explain the relationship of VO2 to heart rate, stroke volume and oxygen extraction.

Jill and Jan, who are the same size, are jogging at about a 9-minute mile. This is a submaximal exercise pace for both women. Since they weigh the same, let's assume they will use approximately the same amount of oxygen when exercising at this pace. Why does Jill, who is less trained aerobically, have so much trouble running with Jan, who is more highly trained aerobically?

The most important factor related to answering this question is VO2, and how oxygen is delivered and utilized. VO2 is related directly to cardiac output (Q). Since cardiac output equals heart rate times stroke volume (Q = HR x SV), the person with the larger stroke volume will need fewer beats of the heart to pump the same amount of blood. That's Jan, the more highly trained person. Furthermore, Jan will be better able to use (a-v02 difference) oxygen at the site of oxygen delivery to the exercising muscles.

Jill, the lesser trained person, will have a much higher heart rate at any given workload and will be "tired" or "panting" because she is less efficient at oxygen delivery and extraction when compared to Jan. Both Jan and Jill will deliver about the same amount of oxygen to satisfy the oxygen demands of the given submaximal activity, but Jan (more fit) will deliver the oxygen in a more efficient manner. That is why Jan's perceived effort is much less than Jill's, even though they are accomplishing the same amount of absolute work and burning about the same number of calories.

Additionally, Jan and Jill have different anaerobic or steady-rate thresholds. Here is where Jan's fitness advantage is really highlighted. If exercise intensity is increased above the 9-minute pace which is submaximal for both women, eventually Jill would not be able to tolerate and sustain as high an intensity as Jan. Because of Jan's better conditioning, her anaerobic threshold occurs later than Jill's, allowing her to work harder and longer at higher levels of effort that are very manageable. Jan probably has a higher max VO2 and can work at a higher percentage of her max VO2.

Bottom line: Jan can work harder over given time periods, and harder and longer in general when compared to Jill. And, she can sustain these higher intensity and/or longer duration efforts predominantly with the long-term aerobic pathway. In a given time period, Jan can optimize fitness gains and calorie burning by working at an optimal yet manageable level of intensity in relation to her better level of conditioning.

Choosing the Training Method

When cardiorespiratory fitness levels improve, goals change or client interests vary, you can utilize any large-muscle, rhythmic activity to challenge the client. There is no one cardiorespiratory activity that is better than another.

The appropriate approach to exercise training in general is to analyze an activity in terms of its specific energy requirements and then train specifically to improve those systems. An improved capacity for energy transfer (oxygen delivery and utilization) usually translates into improved exercise performance and/or health.

Optimizing cardiorespiratory conditioning requires training of both aerobic and anaerobic pathways. Interval conditioning can increase your client's ability to delay the need for anaerobic glycolysis by increasing an individual's anaerobic threshold or maximum steady-rate (MSR). This adaptation to intermittent cardiorespiratory work efforts (interval training) that are above what your client normally works at (steady-rate) increases your client's ability to work at increasingly intense workloads without requiring anaerobic metabolism as quickly as needed in a less-trained state. Interval conditioning also increases the body's ability to tolerate higher levels of lactate.

The final selection(s) depends on whether the activity "fits" your client and she is motivated to pursue it. Then, check to make sure it follows the overload definition for effective cardiorespiratory conditioning. In terms of intensity or level of effort, it helps to answer the question, "Right intensity for what?" Consider such issues as your client's current fitness level and personal goals. Do not forget to ask whether she is training for performance, improved fitness, maximal caloric expenditure, "fat burning" or other health-related issues.

Excellent cardiorespiratory activities include, but are not limited to: walking, swimming, water fitness, jogging, running, cross-country skiing, skate skiing, in-line skating, lateral movement training (slide), cycling, mountain biking and stair/step training.

As with all programming decisions, take a realistic look at your client's time availability and psychological profile. Work within her parameters, emphasizing individual make-up and drive, and identify activities she truly enjoys.

Quick Index:

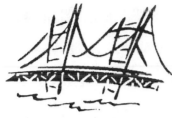

The Bridge
Cardiorespiratory training does not have to be boring or repetitive. By choosing regimens that enhance both the aerobic and anaerobic energy systems, you can keep C-R conditioning motivating. You need to know how the energy systems interact to set the appropriate intensity levels.

SPECIAL SECTION
Oxygen Delivery and Max VO_2

Volume of oxygen (VO2), is the scientific representation of how the body delivers and utilizes oxygen. It is important to comprehend VO2 when discussing the terms "cardiorespiratory conditioning," "aerobic" and "anaerobic."

The ability to "use" or extract oxygen (a-vO2 difference) depends on the amount of blood pumped per minute by your heart. The amount of blood that can be pumped per minute is termed **cardiac output** (represented by Q). It is the product of heart rate (HR) and stroke volume (SV). **Heart rate** is defined as the number of times your heart beats per minute and **stroke volume** is defined as the amount of blood that is ejected from the heart during each beat. The formula for cardiac output is $Q = HR \times SV$.

This combination of delivery (Q) of blood and extraction (a-vO2 difference) of oxygen from blood can be represented by the Fick equation.

FICK EQUATION
VO2 = Q x a-vO2 difference (arteriovenous oxygen difference) or simply,
VO2 = Delivery (Q) x Extraction (a-vO2 difference)
VO2 = Delivery x Extraction

VO2 represents a volume of oxygen consumed by the body on a continuum from death (no oxygen requirements), rest (low-level oxygen requirements), and submaximal activity (moderate to high oxygen requirements), to all-out maximal effort (very high oxygen requirements either during and/or after the activity). Fick's equation represents the body's ability to deliver blood that is loaded with oxygen, and then extract the oxygen needed for activity as well as other bodily functions such as cell repair and growth.

Cardiac output can be characterized as the blood delivery component of VO2. You can liken this to a truck leaving a loading dock (the heart), loaded with marbles (oxygen-laden red blood cells), headed for a delivery point (in the case of activity, the exercising muscles). Generally, the more fit an individual is and the more she is accustomed to the specific type of activity, the more likely the load will be accepted at the **delivery point (extraction)** or working muscle.

The ability to extract oxygen efficiently is an example of the complexities of biochemistry and training specificity. When you increase both anaerobic and aerobic enzymes, capillary density and mitochondria through training adaptations, you are affecting the body's biochemistry and its ability to effectively deliver and use oxygen. This increases the body's efficiency for producing energy.

Arterial-venous oxygen difference (a-vO2 difference) is the technical characterization for **oxygen extraction**. It is the other critical component of VO2. It is your muscle cells' ability to *utilize* oxygen. The oxygen content of blood *at rest* varies from 20 milliliters (ml) of oxygen for every 100 ml of arterial blood to 14 ml of oxygen for every 100 ml of venous blood. The difference between these 2 values, 20 ml - 14 ml = 6 ml, is referred to as the arterial-venous oxygen difference (a-vO2 difference).

The arterial-venous oxygen difference is the difference between the oxygen content of the arterial blood (oxygenated blood as it leaves the heart) and mixed venous blood (after it has passed skeletal muscle and given some of its original oxygen content). This value reflects the extent to which oxygen is extracted or removed from the blood as it passes through the body. Cardiorespiratory conditioning that utilizes proper exercise intensity and duration results in a progressive increase in the a-vO2 difference. This reflects a decreasing venous (blood that is returned to the heart) oxygen content and indicates a greater utilization of oxygen by the working muscles. Exercising muscles can reduce the oxygen content of venous blood from one-half to one-third of resting levels. This indicates that your muscles are extracting a much higher proportion of the oxygen delivered to them in the arterial blood. As much as 85% of the oxygen in arterial blood can be removed during maximal exercise in highly trained individuals. It is apparent that effective delivery and transport of the "oxygen molecule cargo" is not very helpful if it cannot be accepted (extracted/a-vO2 difference) at the delivery site (working muscles).

At this point, since we have discussed VO2 you may be asking yourself, "So, what is **maximum oxygen uptake (max VO2)?**" When you increase the intensity of exercise above what you are accustomed, heart rate, respiration and oxygen intake increase. However, a point occurs beyond which oxygen intake cannot increase, even though more work is being performed. At this point, you have reached a level that is commonly referred to as maximal oxygen uptake (maximal oxygen consumption, maximal aerobic power or simply max VO2). It is generally assumed that this represents your capacity for the *aerobic resynthesis* (production) of ATP.

This is considered by many experts as the single best indicator of cardiorespiratory fitness, since it involves the optimal ability of 3 major systems (pulmonary—lungs; cardiovascular—heart and blood vessels; and muscular—skeletal muscles) of your body to take in, transport and utilize oxygen. The higher your level of maximal oxygen uptake, the greater your potential level of physical working capacity.

Your ability to deliver and utilize a large volume of oxygen (VO2) at *sustained* levels of intensity above rest determines your work capacity or how efficient and effective your body can be during activity. In other words, though max VO2 is important, what percentage of your max you can use and sustain is also important.

Most important, at any level below max VO2, a fit person is able to deliver more efficiently that particular volume of oxygen required by the body's systems for that particular activity and intensity. This translates into a more effective and efficient person in terms of physical work capacity. In addition, the individual may have created what I call a "fitness margin." A fitness margin translates into a client who has energy left over for daily activities, including time with family, recreation and hobbies, as well as a higher tolerance for dealing with life's accumulated stress.

CHAPTER 6

MEASURING EXERCISE INTENSITY

When I discussed the value of fitness assessments in Chapter 2, I communicated the results very differently to John, a sedentary and overfat new client, than to Sally, a triathlete. You'll need the same blend of scientific measurements and subjective judgment when determining exercise intensity.

What's the value in measuring exercise intensity? Knowing the appropriate "training sensitive zone" allows you to guide clients' efforts to a level that improves their conditioning while keeping heart rate in a safe range. It also enables you to demonstrate fitness improvements in your clients, such as a decrease in resting heart rate and a decrease in heart rate response for any given submaximal work load (effort). While the term "training sensitive zone" is almost cliché, there is still considerable confusion about appropriate training intensities, especially in the areas of fat burning and exercise for health versus fitness.

There are numerous methods for monitoring exercise intensity. Most trainers will use one or more of these 5 methods:

• Percentage of Maximal Heart Rate (MHR), counting heart beats and using a formula based on age-related norms to estimate a preferred intensity level.

• Heart Rate Maximum Reserve (HRR), using the Karvonen formula to estimate a preferred intensity level.

• Rating Perceived Exertion (RPE), using the client's perception of effort measured on a scale.

• "Talk Test," identifying the level of breathlessness, often used in combination with RPE.

• Preferred Exertion (PE), a concept where the exerciser chooses a preferred exertion level, often used in combination with RPE.

These methods are used to estimate a target heart rate (THR) or training heart rate range (THRR). Which is the right method for your client? How important is an exacting intensity level for achieving results?

How Accurately Does Heart Rate Reflect Oxygen Consumption?

Training sensitive zone has its physiological basis in the laboratory. **Heart rate (HR)** is the number of heart beats within a time frame. As a general rule, **maximal aerobic capacity**—maximum capacity to generate ATP aerobically—improves if exercise intensity is sufficient to increase heart rate to about 70% of maximum heart rate (MHR). This is equivalent to about 50-55% of max VO2 (McArdle et al., 1991).

This level of effort appears to be the *minimal* stimulus required for training improvements in maximal aerobic capacity. However, this level of effort is not necessary for improvements in health-related goals. For relatively deconditioned clients, the training threshold may be closer to 60% of MHR, which corresponds to about 40-45% of max VO2. The lower limits for a training-sensitive threshold related to improved aerobic capacity (but not necessarily improved max VO2) depend on the client's *current* fitness capacity and state of training.

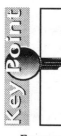

> Seemingly minimal efforts should be encouraged. Work efforts that take clients beyond what they are accustomed can contribute significantly to positive conditioning effects and health gains.

For nearly all levels of **submaximal exercise**, the percentage of MHR does *not* equal the same percentage of max VO2 or aerobic capacity. On the other hand, the Karvonen formula explained later in this chapter is used to predict **heart rate maximum reserve (HRR)** and correlates directly to max VO2. Calculating HRR may more accurately accommodate various fitness level differences based upon the individual **resting heart rate (RHR)** that is entered into the formula. The difference between resting and maximal heart rates for any given client reflects the "reserve" of the heart for increasing heart rate and stroke volume, or cardiac output (LaForge, 1991 and McArdle et al., 1991).

Let's look at the conditions that influence heart rate increases and/or decreases:

• Rhythmic, continuous, large-muscle activity that simultaneously increases heart rate and venous return (overload definition for cardiorespiratory fitness, Chapter 5).

• Metabolism requirements of large amounts of muscle mass.

• Arm movement overhead that elicits pressor response (heart rate increases without a matching increase in oxygen consumption) with or without light hand-held weights.

• Strong resistive efforts that increase resistance to blood flow. This includes traditional resistance training, and may or may not be combined with a **Valsalva maneuver** (a momentary or sustained holding of the breath upon strenuous effort).

• Dehydration, temperature, emotions and pharmacological (drugs and medication) effects.

Now let's place these many variables that can affect HR against the capabilities of a training heart rate range (THRR) to accurately reflect exercise intensity as measured by actual oxygen consumption. Training heart rate (THR) is a useful indicator—if measured accurately—of oxygen consumption, calorie burning and metabolism in continuous, dynamic activity, that involves a large amount of muscle mass, and simultaneously increases heart rate (HR) and blood flow (venous return) back to the heart. Remember, oxygen consumption stimulates cardiorespiratory system training adaptations, not just a fast or increased heart rate.

You can see why heart rate measurement can be an accurate reflection of work performed for the average person with no special concerns, *if* he is engaged in rhythmic, continuous, large-muscle activity. But, while heart rate may be a good indicator of training intensity in generally healthy adults, heart rate may not be a good indicator of intensity for others.

Training heart rate may *not* be the best choice to monitor exercise intensity for:

• People taking medication, which may, for example, slow HR. If HR is used, the exercising HR must be determined while the client is medicated and under medical supervision.

• Clients who are unable to accurately monitor HR.

• Clients, such as those in postcardiac rehabilitation, who require very accurate heart rate monitoring. Prediction equations such as 220 minus age for estimating training or target heart rate have a large amount of error, often plus or minus 10-12 beats per minute.

Additionally, standard HR response may not apply when swimming or participating in activities that may invoke a pressor response.

Swimming usually elicits a *lower* maximal heart rate response (10-13 beats per minute when compared to running or cycling (McArdle et al., 1991; *Berkeley Wellness Letter*, June 1994). The combined effects of a prone body position, which may allow the heart to distribute blood more uniformly and not have to pump against gravity, and submersion in water probably account for swimming's slightly lower exercise heart rate. Being submersed in water may facilitate blood return to the heart, and rapid heat dissipation in cool water may require less work from the heart if hydration is maintained.

On the other hand, excessively warm water temperatures will *increase* HR. Furthermore, swimming involves more arm work and uses smaller muscle mass than, for example, running and cycling. Use of less muscle mass would also elicit a *lower* maximal heart rate response when compared to running and cycling. Because of the information cited, it may be impossible for your client to reach land-based THRR or MHR.

> When figuring THR for swimming, subtract about 13 beats from either an actual land-based MHR, or from a predicted MHR. (An upper and lower limit THR must be calculated to create a THRR.)

In contrast to swimming, **aerobic dance** can elicit a *higher* maximal heart rate response for given exercise efforts, when compared to running and cycling. This probably results from the use of overhead arm movements and the upright posture associated with aerobic dance.

When arms are moved overhead, with or without light hand-held weights, a pressor response may be elicited. **Pressor response** is a physiological response of the body where heart rate may increase without a linear or matching increase in oxygen consumption. The occurrence of a pressor response results in an *inaccurate* reflection of cardiorespiratory work effort because oxygen consumption increase does not parallel the elevated HR response.

Pressor response also occurs during traditional resistance training exercise. Resistance training (8-12 reps to fatigue) has erroneously been identified on several occasions as effective cardiorespiratory activity because HR can remain elevated during this type of training. However, when oxygen consumption is measured during this type of resistance training, it is found that HR is an inaccurate measurement of exercise intensity.

Because of these limitations, there is mounting evidence that rating of perceived exertion (RPE) may be the better choice, in terms of effectiveness and safety (Ebbeling et al., 1991), once the relationship between heart rate (cardiac response) and RPE (physiologic response) has been accurately established. Ultimately, using *both* RPE and heart rate may be the best approach.

Quick Index:

Chapters 2 and 3, health-related versus fitness goals
Chapter 5, about max VO2 and heart rate

Quick List of Abbreviations

THR	Training or Target Heart Rate
THRR	Training or Target Heart Rate Range (includes an upper and lower limit THR)
EHR	Exercise/Exercising Heart Rate
MHR	Maximum/Maximal Heart Rate
HRR	Heart Rate Reserve or Heart Rate Maximum Reserve
RPE	Rating Perceived Exertion
PE	Preferred Exertion
bpm	Beats Per Minute

Has Heart Rate Monitoring Been Overemphasized?

Many experts feel that target heart rate (THR) has been overemphasized for average exercise participants, and may have led to inappropriate exercise intensities in many instances. This includes exercising too hard as well as exercising with too little effort. The resultant effects can be injury, lawsuits, lack of results for time invested and an alarmingly high number of exercise dropouts.

Monitoring exercise heart rates in a precise and accurate manner is probably of greatest importance to competitive athletes and cardiac patients. High-intensity interval training for highly conditioned athletes is very structured. Both the effort and recovery of the interval are closely monitored in the belief that this will produce optimal training result. After a thorough diagnostic evaluation, cardiac patients are assigned a precise THRR. The THRR for the cardiac patient is critical for the continued ability of the patient to exercise without occurrence of angina and heart arrhythmia, or even death.

For a generally healthy adult, many experts are recommending a combination of rating of perceived exertion (RPE) and "preferred exertion." A research team (Dishman et al., 1994) recently suggested a **preferred exertion (PE)** protocol where the *client's preference* for exercise intensity dictates effort. The authors recommend that this preferred effort fall between some minimal range of not too hard or easy. In other words, encourage your clients to exercise according to how they *feel*, rather than to a strict exercise heart rate which may not reflect a preferred level of effort.

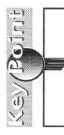

> In my opinion, what is most important is that the client perceive the effort as manageable and enjoyable, since such a wide range of exercise intensities confers health benefits. It seems this approach may be safer and promote long-term exercise compliance, as opposed to traditional approaches which focus on precise physiological criteria, such as heart rate, to dictate effort.

With exercise dropout rates as high as 45% and 8-22% of United States adults not exercising with sufficient intensity and regularity to satisfy conventional training guidelines for improvement in fitness, it is obvious another approach is needed (Dishman et al., 1994). Traditional criteria that set exercise intensity often conflict with an individual's effort preference. Dishman (1994) states, "If inactive people select, or are prescribed, an intensity that is perceived as very effortful relative to their physiological responses, they may be less attracted to continued participation." And, on the other hand, some clients may prefer to exceed the conventional or prescribed exercise plan.

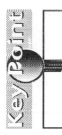

> Teach your clients how to "tune in" to their bodies. I recommend using a combination of heart rate monitoring, RPE and preferred exertion to produce the safest, most effective and time-efficient results.

Methods for Determining Target Heart Rate (THR) and THRR

To work in a training sensitive zone, a **maximal heart rate (MHR)** must be determined so that your client can work at some preferred or targeted percentage of MHR. A percentage of MHR is referred to as THR. To determine a **training heart rate range (THRR)**, a percentage that represents an upper limit THR and a lower limit THR must be chosen.

An actual MHR is more useful and accurate than one you predict. Actual MHR for a specific activity can easily be determined after 2-4 minutes of all-out effort if peak heart rate is accurately monitored. However, this involves considerable motivation and is not advisable for clients who do not have medical clearance or are at any kind of risk. A maximal aerobic capacity test or "max stress test" performed in a clinical and properly supervised setting is another excellent way to determine actual MHR. However, as with any maximal test, there is some risk of injury or even death. Additionally, many clients do not wish to incur the cost or do not have easy access to this type of testing.

Because of these reasons, most trainers and consumers alike use a simple formula to *predict* age-adjusted maximal heart rates. However, this method for determining age-adjusted maximal heart rates has limitations because individuals of a particular age do not all possess the same MHR. This is certainly not reason enough to never use predicted MHR, but you do need to recognize the limitations of prediction.

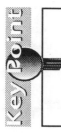

With age-predicted MHR, there is a standard deviation of plus or minus 10-12 beats per minute.

For example, about 95% of men and women aged 40 have an MHR between 160 and 200 beats per minute (McArdle et al., 1991). Because of this large variance in measured MHRs, it is important to take into account individual responses to assigned training heart rate ranges. Some will be too easy, and some too hard, based on the predicted training range. Necessary adjustments must be made with regard to individual effort so that the THRR best "fits" your client's current fitness level and health needs. This information lends additional support for the argument of using THRR and RPE simultaneously to gauge client exercise intensity.

Overall, heart rate is a relatively accurate means of monitoring and determining exercise intensity. When heart rates are accurately monitored, you can assure your clients of predictable and efficient results. Furthermore, you can motivate them with the fact that low-level intensity and low to moderate training heart rates can bring them significant and measurable health and fitness results.

Upper- and lower-limit training heart rates (THRs) for clients on medication should be determined in a clinical setting, under medical supervision. The client should be medicated when the determination is made as to what THR, or training heart rate range (THRR), should be observed.

An appropriate training heart rate range (THRR) that accommodates most levels of fitness, for asymptomatic individuals, is from about 40-85% of max VO2 or HRR. Remember, a given percentage of HRR corresponds directly with the same percentage of max VO2, whereas 40-85% of max VO2 or HRR corresponds to about 50-90% of maximum heart rate (MHR). This wide training range is certainly in the "training sensitive zone" for improvements in health and fitness for a majority of our inactive population.

Quick Index:

Chapter 2, when medically supervised stress tests are appropriate

Using Percentage of Maximal Heart Rate

The most common approach—though not necessarily the best—in estimating a target heart rate range (THRR), simply requires you to determine an MHR for your client. This can be determined by subtracting your client's age from 220. This number results in an *estimated* max heart rate (MHR).

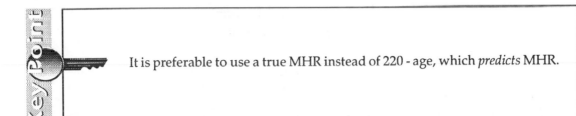

It is preferable to use a true MHR instead of 220 - age, which *predicts* MHR.

THRR results from the MHR being multiplied by an upper limit THR percentage and a lower limit THR percentage. Generally, a THRR is desired because this provides some flexibility as to the degree of effort the client will work within.

Calculating THR as a Percentage of MHR

Target Heart Rate (THR) = [(220 - age) or actual MHR] x desired % of MHR

Your 47-year-old female client, Roxanne, is a competitive, long-distance runner, so her interval training regimen benefits from a high level of accuracy in heart rate monitoring. You determine Roxanne needs a recovery THRR between intervals of 85-90% of MHR (about 80-85% of max VO2 or HRR). Therefore, to determine THRR you will calculate a THR for both 85% and 90% of Roxanne's MHR.

Her maximal heart rate, as determined on a functional capacity test, is 187. Her predicted MHR (220 minus 47) is only 173. Therefore, you use her actual MHR (187) to determine her recovery training intensity range. Note that THRR can be used for determining both proper cardiorespiratory effort *and* recovery.

THR (lower intensity limit) equals:	MHR x .85
	187 (MHR) x .85 = 159
THR (higher intensity limit) equals:	MHR x .90
	187 (MHR) x .90 = 168

Roxanne's THRR for recovery after high-intensity intervals is between 159-168 beats per minute (bpm). Her 10-second HR count is about 26-28 bpm and is determined by dividing 159 and 168 by 6. Her 15-second count is about 39-42 bpm and is determined by dividing 159 and 168 by 4.

Adapting the Range. Pollock and Wilmore (1990) believe that you should *add* 10-15% to the above calculated THRR upper and lower limits, particularly with cardiac patients who may have extremely high resting heart rates, which can result in a THRR *lower* than their resting HR. Also, you may consider adding 10-15% above calculated THRR if a *predicted* MHR is used instead of an *actual* MHR. This adjustment *may* more accurately reflect the appropriate percentage of maximal oxygen uptake as related to the THRR. Additionally, a straight percentage of MHR has been shown to less accurately reflect functional aerobic capacity or percentage of max VO2.

To add this 15%, multiply the derived percentage(s) of MHR by 1.15.

The adapted formula for percentage of MHR looks like this:

Target Heart Rate (THR) = [(220 - age) or actual MHR] x desired training
percentage intensity or THRs x 1.15

How does this adjustment work for Roxanne? Roxanne's THRR for recovery, using the conversion factor of 1.15, is now between 182-193 beats per minute (multiply THRs 159 and 168 by 1.15 to derive these higher numbers). Her previous recovery heart rate range was 159-168. However, since her actual MHR is only 187, *this formula has overestimated* her recovery THRR, which will have her exercising at close to 100% of her capacity. Obviously, she will not recover using this.

However, the use of this formula for *lesser intensities*, cardiac patients and in cases where actual MHR is not known may prove helpful for some clients and encourage them to train at more aggressive, yet appropriate exercise heart rates or intensities. Your best bet will be to use a combination of RPE and HR, whether or not you choose to use Pollock and Wilmore's method for adjusting THRR. Your client's feelings and feedback will most accurately guide adjustments in level of effort.

Using Heart Rate Maximum Reserve Method (Karvonen's Formula)

The Karvonen formula is used to predict heart rate maximum reserve (HRR). HRR accommodates various fitness level differences and more accurately predicts training heart rate range because individual resting heart rate (RHR) is entered into the formula. HRR is based on a simple concept. As your client becomes more fit, his heart becomes stronger and more efficient so that for any given submaximal workload, HR will be lower. This includes resting heart rate (RHR). Utilizing RHR helps avoid lumping people into statistical averages, which can be less effective and dangerous when calculating THRRs.

Furthermore, the use of an *actual* MHR in the HRR equation is important. According to exercise physiologist Tom LaFontaine, Ph.D., maximum HR for 100 men aged 30 may vary from 166-214. Based on the age equation, 220 - 30, all of these individuals would have THRs predicted from an estimated MHR of 190. The use of *actual MHR* and RHR in predicting THRR in the Karvonen equation has profound implications in terms of personalizing training to the client's current fitness level.

Karvonen's formula is probably the most widely used method to calculate target heart rate (THR) for cardiorespiratory conditioning. Using this formula, the percentage of heart rate reserve (HRR) that a participant should be working at, or within, corresponds directly with max VO2. For example, an individual working at 80-85% of his HRR would be exercising at an intensity of about 80-85% of his maximum VO2.

In order to use Karvonen's formula and calculate HRR, a trainer must know the client's resting heart rate (RHR) and actual maximal heart rate or predicted maximal heart rate. The Karvonen formula is more effective if actual MHR is known, as opposed to using predicted MHR.

Table 8. Relation Between Percent Maximum Heart Rate, HRR and Percent Maximum VO2

For any given percentage of MHR, the corresponding percentage of max VO2 is at least 5-10% less. Note that the corresponding HRR, as predicted by the Karvonen formula, matches perfectly with max VO2 or aerobic capacity. Thus, Karvonen predictions more closely reflect actual percentage of max VO2.

Percent Maximum HR	Percent HR Maximum Reserve (HRR)	Percent Maximum VO2 or Aerobic Capacity
50	28	28
60	42	42
70	56	56
80	70	70
90	83	83
100	100	100

Adapted from McArdle et al., 1991, pg. 435

Calculating THR Using the Karvonen Formula

Training Heart Rate (THR) = [(Max HR; predicted or actual) - Resting Heart Rate] x % of Desired Training Intensity (DTI) + Resting Heart Rate
Or simply: THR = [MHR (predicted or actual) - RHR] x DTI + RHR

RHR must also accurately be monitored and recorded by your client so that it can be used in the Karvonen formula.

Maury is a 48-year-old man with a resting heart rate of 79 who you wish to train at 80% of heart rate reserve (HRR). First, his age must be subtracted from 220 to predict maximal heart rate (MHR) since his actual MHR is not available. Next, his resting heart rate (RHR) is subtracted from the estimated MHR. This number is multiplied by a percentage (THR of 80%) or, if a training *range* is desired, by upper and lower percentages.

The following example illustrates a prediction training heart rate (THR) for 80%, as estimated by the Karvonen formula.

> 220 - 48 (age) = 172 (predicted MHR)
> 172 (predicted MHR) - 79 (RHR) = 93 (heart rate reserve or HRR)
> 93 (HRR) x .8 (desired intensity or THR) = 74.4
> 74.4 + 79 (RHR) = 153.4 beats per minute (bpm)
> **THR ='s 153 bpm at 80% of HRR**

For a **10-second heart rate count**, (which reflects the number of heart beats that would occur over a one minute time period) divide 153.4 by 6, which equals 25.6 beats per 10 seconds.

As with any formula, the results are only as accurate as the information that is entered into it. The relationship of HRR as a direct reflection of max VO2 percentage is compromised when *predicted* MHR is used instead of *actual* MHR that is determined from a maximal stress test or field test.

Counting Heart Beats With Manual Palpation

One of the easiest and most practical ways to measure HR is by palpation technique, immediately after exercise is stopped. (Manual palpation during certain types of exercise, for example running or walking, is more difficult to accurately monitor though it is not impossible.) Palpation involves a manual touch to feel the pulse. The pulse of the heart is most often palpated at the carotid artery (located anteriorly on the neck, and adjacent to either side of the throat) and the radial artery at the wrist (located thumb side). The pulse may also be monitored by placing the heel of your hand (or your client's) on the left side of the chest at the apex of the heart, and counting pulsations. It should be noted that you may not be able to count the pulse of some of your clients using palpation, regardless of site chosen. This may necessitate the use of a heart rate monitor or stethoscope (Pollock and Wilmore, 1990).

The preferred location for manual monitoring of HR may be the **radial artery**. It is an easy palpation site for you and your client to access. And, sudden drops in HR are not observed when pressure is placed at this measurement site as they are at the carotid artery. To assess the radial pulse, place the index and middle finger lightly on the under side (wrist flexors) and thumb side of the wrist.

When palpating pulse at either **carotid artery** it is important to *gently* place the index and middle fingers over the artery, which is located just to either side, and slightly vertical, of the "Adam's apple" on the front of the neck.

> **Key Point**
>
> Too much finger pressure on the carotid artery may cause the carotid sensors in these arteries to respond, causing a sudden drop in heart rate by the resultant reflex action.

Be sure to exert slight pressure on only one side of the throat. If palpating to the right of your Adam's apple, use your right hand. Using the right hand to palpate the left carotid may result in pressure on both carotid arteries from your finger and thumb. This could result in an inaccurate pulse count and could even cause your client to faint if blood flow is inhibited by pressure on both arteries.

Do not use your thumb to monitor pulse, as it has an arterial pulse of its own and may confuse you or your client's heart rate count, resulting in an inaccurate assessment of beats per minute (bpm) of the heart.

Accurate pulse count assessment is essential when monitoring exercise intensity. Inaccuracies may arise from starting the counts incorrectly, not starting and ending on the correct time frame, improper hand placement and mis-counting the pulse during the timed pulse monitoring period.

Time intervals. It is well known that the longer the time interval used to measure pulse, the more accurate the reading. When monitoring bpm during a 60-second count, missing the starting beat, a middle beat and the ending beat is not critical. This results in an error of 3. However, during a 10-second count, every beat missed results in a counting error of 6. The above example of 3 missed beats in a 60-second count would result in a pulse count error of 18 beats if you were counting bpm for 10 seconds.

Whether you use 10 seconds and multiply the count by 6, 15 seconds and multiply the count by 4, 30 seconds and multiply the count by 2, or a full 60-second count, standardize and be consistent with your approach for determining bpm that reflects a one-minute count.

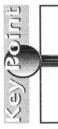

Resting heart rate is probably best recorded when using a 60-second count, although using a 30-second count is acceptable. *During activity*, a 10-second HR count may be ideal.

In a healthy client, exercise heart rate begins to slow quickly, usually after only 15 seconds, once exercise is stopped. Wilmore and Pollock (1990) recommend a 10-second count based on the following rationale. It takes about 2-4 seconds to properly position finger placement for detection of the heartbeat as represented by the pulse that is felt. By counting beats per 10 seconds, it is possible to complete the count within the crucial window of 15 seconds. This will avoid error as a result of heartbeat deceleration if longer counts are used.

Counting Technique. Locate the pulse and repeatedly count "one, one, one..." to establish **heart rate rhythm**. Begin when you (or your client) have established a sense for the heart beat pattern or rhythm. This will ensure a more accurate post exercise and actual exercise HR count. However, the pulse should be located and the HR rhythm established within seconds after exercise is completed, or slowed for a count during exercise.

What are you counting? Imagine 6 vertical lines representing heart beats. If you count each beat (starting with "one") at the top of each line, your count will be 6. If you count cardiac cycles in between beats, your count will be 5. This representation of heart beats as lines can help you understand whether your count should be started on "zero" or "one."

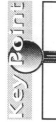

Generally, (according to Pollock and Wilmore, 1990) if a stopwatch is *not* being used, the more accurate count would begin with "one."

For the 10-second count, start on a full beat (remember the vertical line example) as you pronounce "one." After counting heart beats (pulses) during the 10 seconds, multiply by 6 to determine the heart rate in beats per minute.

Remember, this attention to counting detail is important when using a 10-second counting time because *each* one-beat error in counting results in an error of 6 beats per minute. For example, if the beginning and ending count are missed, there is an error of 12 beats per minute. Furthermore, it is easy to miss a beat or 2 in between the start and end of the count because the heart is beating rapidly upon the cessation of vigorous activity.

During a 60-second manual count, beginning the count with either "zero" or "one" is acceptable since the resultant error is only about one bpm.

Counting Heart Beats Using Heart Rate Monitors

Wireless heart rate monitors are computerized, electronic digital readout devices that are designed to be worn on the wrist like a watch or mounted on exercise equipment. The heart rate monitor constantly displays your client's heart rate, giving you and your client updated exercise intensity information every few seconds. This is an attractive alternative when the potential inaccuracies of monitoring HR by palpation are compared to the simplicity and accuracy provided by wireless telemetry.

The most important feature of a heart rate monitor is its method of pulse detection. Inexpensive—and often the least accurate—models operate by a principle called "photo-reflectance." Sensors placed on the earlobe or fingertip use a photocell and light source to detect pulse. These types of devices are sensitive to body movement and often give inaccurate readings if heart rate moves above 110 bpm.

More accurate heart rate monitors (e.g., Polar™) transmit the electrical activity of the heart through an electrode harness that is positioned on the chest to a watch-like receiver mounted on exercise equipment or the wrist. Since there are no wires connecting the transmitter to the receiver, wireless telemetry models do not interfere with upper body or arm movement.

Heart rate monitors make it easier to monitor HR during exercise and recovery. They reduce the need to stop or slow activity to get an accurate HR and replace the inaccuracy often associated with manual heart rate monitoring. There is excellent research (Leger et al., 1988) that indicates that companies such as Polar™ have a reliable heart rate measurement device. Even so, it is a good idea, in consideration of occasional erroneous readings that may result from batteries that are depleted or product malfunctions, to use RPE in conjunction with this and any type of heart rate monitoring.

Methods That Use Perception of Exertion

An easy and practical way to monitor the intensity of cardiorespiratory effort is with rating perceived exertion (RPE), a means for clients to "check in" with how they are feeling at any given moment. Since using a manual heart rate count is often difficult to perform accurately and can be distracting, RPE may be more effective and safer for many personal training situations (Ebbeling et al., 1991). Furthermore, when RPE is used in conjunction with HR monitoring, it provides a double check on the accuracy and effectiveness of training heart rate range. This is especially important if THRR is predicted using an estimated maximal heart rate.

RPE is taught by associating HR response with a particular numerical rating and its assigned descriptive term(s) on the Borg scale. For example, a moderate level of effort will probably rate 2-3 numerically and "somewhat easy" to "moderate" descriptively (See Table 9). When your clients get very skilled at this rating game—and it is a fun game to challenge your clients with— they will be able to estimate their exercising heart rates within about 5 beats. And, they will do it consistently. A wireless heart rate monitor is an excellent tool to teach this association.

RPE is especially appropriate for your clients who do not have typical heart rate responses to progressive aerobic exercise. This includes clients who are on beta blockers (and other medications), some cardiac and diabetic clients, pregnant clients and any others who may not have a predictable heart rate response to cardiorespiratory activity. In fact, using RPE with these types of clients should probably be the preferred way to monitor exercise intensity. Make this decision after consultation with your client's qualified health care provider.

Following these points will help you improve the accuracy of this method.

1. Teach accurate manual heart rate measurement. It is important to establish a relationship between physiological response (heart rate) and subjective feelings, or perceived exertion. Heart rate is a *direct* measure of physiologic response to aerobic or anaerobic cardiorespiratory effort. This is in contrast to a *predicted* measure. Poor heart rate measurement technique results in error. A wireless heart rate monitor is a good tool to help establish your client's HR relationship with the Borg scale numerical rating and associated "feeling" of effort.

2. To help establish the relationship between HR response and the Borg numerical scale (Table 9), relate a particular activity, such as walking leisurely, stair stepping vigorously, interval conditioning or steady-rate swimming, to Borg's numerical rating and descriptive term(s). For example, steady-rate swimming and leisure walking would be assigned numerical values at the lower end of intensity for most clients, whereas high-intensity interval conditioning, regardless of the activity chosen, would be at the higher end.

3. Periodically monitor HR and update the association of your client's HR response to the RPE scale. I have found that it is easy to become overly confident in your client's ability to consistently and accurately estimate RPE. It is important to "check in" because of training adaptations that take place, such as a decreased HR for a given submaximal load. To reestablish an accurate association of exercise intensity (HR) with RPE, return to heart rate. Of course, HR is an objective measure of exercise intensity and oxygen consumption only if it is recorded accurately.

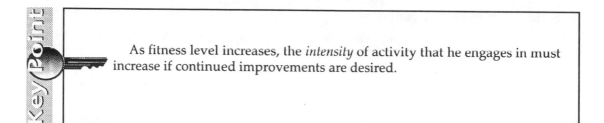

> As fitness level increases, the *intensity* of activity that he engages in must increase if continued improvements are desired.

As your client becomes better conditioned, his perception of exertion at a given RPE will remain about the same even as you increase overload. If intensity is simply maintained, he will enter a phase of cardiorespiratory maintenance, which may or may not be appropriate to his current fitness level and goals. You will have to determine its appropriateness to each client's individual training situation.

Ultimately, once empowered by you, all of your clients can take responsibility for working at the right level of cardiorespiratory aerobic or anaerobic exercise intensity that is appropriate to what *they* perceive as reasonable effort, fun and something they will likely continue with!

Quick Index:

Chapter 2, determining your client's goals over time

Case Study: Playing the Game: Associating HR With RPE

Kendall loves to walk. A main emphasis of her cardiorespiratory workout is combining recreational strolls (warm-up), fitness walking (steady-rate) and race walking (high-intensity steady-rate and interval conditioning). By using wireless telemetry to monitor heart rate (you can also use accurate manual palpation monitoring techniques), we established Kendall's heart rate and perception of effort.

Stroll. HR response to a 2-3 mile per hour (mph) stroll was 105-115 beats per minute (bpm). Using Table 9, Modified Borg Scale, she described this level of effort as "very, very easy" to "very easy" or about 0.5 to 1 on the Borg numerical scale.

Fitness walking is about 3-5 mph. Though sustainable for indefinite time periods, 5 mph (12-minute mile pace) represents about 145 bpm and represents a level of effort that is "somewhat hard," according to Kendall. The Borg numerical rating for this level of effort is 4.

Race walking. Kendall's technique allows her to complete a 10K race averaging a "race pace" that is between 10- to 11-minute miles (6 mph to about 5.5 mph) at a heart rate between 150-165 bpm. Kendall rates this effort as "somewhat hard" to "hard." The Borg numerical rating is 4-5.

A brief burst of "speed play" to pass another competitor in a race is rated at 7 or 8 and is associated with a "very hard" effort. Her HR pushes 165-170 bpm. Some of our interval conditioning drills push her to 10 on the Borg scale, or "very, very hard," and her HR may reach 180 bpm.

Initially, to learn the association between HR and RPE, we played the "game." I continually asked Kendall to guess her resting, exercising and recovery heart rates. For example, before either one of us looked at her wireless heart rate monitor during exercise, she first estimated her exercising heart rate and gave me a numerical number (Borg scale, 1-10) and descriptive term (from the Borg scale) to describe her level of effort. When we first started this fun exercise, Kendall thought her stroll elicited about a 130 heart rate. She associated it with a numerical effort of 1 and as "really easy." She was surprised to find her actual HR was only around 100 bpm, even though her description of the effort was accurate.

Eventually, by playing the game, Kendall could accurately guess her level of effort, at any intensity, within plus or minus 5 bpm. And, Kendall's choice of descriptive terms and numerical ratings (RPE) always provided the most accurate estimate of how she was feeling and of her immediate exercise intensity. It is important to use this association drill, regardless of the client or his goals, if you are to accurately and effectively use RPE.

Borg Perceived Exertion Scale

Table 9 is a useful perceived exertion scale that I have modified to assist you in teaching your clients RPE. The *numerical values* of this revised Borg scale range from 0-10, with 10 representing maximal or "very, very hard" exertion. The *C-R Conditioning* column represents recommended exertion levels for recovery (2-3), aerobic training (4-6) and anaerobic intervals (7-10). Their association with the numerical rating of the Borg scale is found by looking horizontally across the scale. The *Instructor Exertion Cues* (Brooks et al., Reebok Interval Program Manual) represent language that may be more practical to use by the trainer, as opposed to the original language suggested by Borg in the middle column.

The training-sensitive zone based on a heart rate reserve (HRR) of 40-85% (equivalent to about 50-90% of MHR) corresponds to an RPE of 3-7 on the revised Borg scale. A rating of 3-7 classifies the exercise intensity as "moderate" to "very hard." Note that a rating of 1 or 2 ("very easy" to "somewhat easy") may be sufficient to increase fitness levels in some populations, and may be well below 40% of max VO2 or HRR.

Generally, a perceived exertion of 3-7 for most personal training clients is safe and effective. Anaerobic intervals may use ratings as high as 7-10 ("very hard," to "very, very hard").

Table 9. Modified Borg Scale

C-R Conditioning	Borg Scale Numerical Rating: 0 - 10	Instructor Exertion Cues
	0 Nothing	
	0.5 Very, very weak	Very, very easy
	1 Very weak	Very easy
Recovery Effort	2 Weak	Somewhat easy
Recovery Effort	3 Moderate	Moderate
Aerobic Effort	4 Somewhat strong	Somewhat hard
Aerobic Effort	5 Strong	Hard
	6	
Anaerobic Effort	7 Very Strong	Very hard
Anaerobic Effort	8	
Anaerobic Effort	9	
Anaerobic Effort	10 Very, very strong	Very, very hard

Source: Borg, G. (1982). *Psychological Bases of Perceived Exertion, Medicine and Science in Sports and Exercise*, 14:377-387.

Talk Test

The talk test is an excellent approach for monitoring exercise intensity with clients who have a low level of conditioning or are just starting a conditioning program. (It is also effective for use with highly trained athletes, as is RPE.) For general health gains, a person should be "comfortably uncomfortable" in terms of intensity. They should be able to breathe comfortably throughout the duration of the activity. Use the talk test to ascertain if a reasonable level of effort is being maintained.

Unless anaerobic interval conditioning is being participated in, it is appropriate for most clients to *slow down* when:

1. There is a noticeable increase in respiration. Breathing occurs in gasps and it is difficult to string together 2 or 3 words of conversation. Extreme breathlessness is a sign of exceeding anaerobic threshold, and may or may not be desirable.

2. Muscles start to "burn" and participants find the activity "very uncomfortable." The client fatigues prematurely ("I can't go any longer") and wants to stop the workout.

Breathlessness and burning muscles indicate that your client is feeling the onset of blood lactate accumulation. He has reached his **anaerobic threshold** (more accurately called the respiratory threshold or blood lactate threshold). The respiratory threshold occurs as the exercise becomes more intense and the muscle cells can no longer meet the additional energy demands aerobically. Working at intensities the client is unaccustomed to is neither "good" nor "bad," but simply a matter of appropriateness.

The Bridge

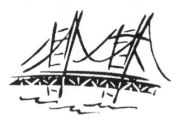

There are numerous ways to determine if your client is working at the right level of effort, and a good trainer will use most of them. These include various methods of heart rate monitoring and rating of perceived exertion. Intensity is important for clients to gain the level of conditioning they desire while still staying safe and comfortable. Your ability to accurately measure intensity will enhance your effectiveness, and increase your value in your client's eyes.

CHAPTER 7

THE PHYSIOLOGICAL BASIS OF MUSCULAR FITNESS

Adequate muscular strength and endurance is extremely beneficial for all of your clients. Everyone needs to maintain—at the very least—minimal levels of muscular fitness and muscle mass.

The process of overloading the muscular system is commonly referred to as resistance training (Fleck and Kraemer, 1987). The term **resistance training** is used to cover *all* types of "strength" or "weight" training, including: free weight (dynamic constant resistance); variable resistance (dynamic variable resistance); elastic resistance (another form of dynamic variable resistance); concentric, eccentric and isometric muscle contractions; and isokinetic training.

Resistance training not only develops muscular strength and muscular endurance, it can also improve the ability of muscles to recover from daily physical stresses of life. Physical fitness declines with age. However, many of the detrimental changes in physiological function are due to decreased physical activity that often accompanies aging. Negative, age-related changes in physiological function can be minimized with proper exercise training, especially resistance training (Evans, 1991).

Clients can see significant results from proper strength training because many people have followed ineffective or negligible strength programs. But as a personal trainer, you are in the position to design *effective* strength training programs once you have an understanding of skeletal muscle structure and function. Then you can bridge this theory into day-to-day applications to help clients achieve their goals.

Table 10. Health Benefits Associated With Resistance Training

• Fat Loss, Weight Control, Weight Maintenance	• Positive Changes in Blood Lipid Profiles
• Increased Metabolism	• Decreased Risk for Osteoporosis
• Increased Calorie Burning During Resistance Training	• Increased Bone Mineral Content
• Increased Calorie Burning After Exercise	• Improved Structural and Functional Integrity of Tendons and Ligaments
• Reductions in Resting Blood Pressure for Clients With High Blood Pressure or Borderline High Blood Pressure	• Personal Physical Independence
	• Protected from Joint and Muscle Injury
	• Enhanced Physical Activity Experiences
• Decreased Risk for Adult-Onset Diabetes or Non-Insulin Dependent Diabetes Mellitus	• Improved Posture
	• Improved Physical Image
	• Improved Self-Esteem

"Macro" or Gross Structure of Skeletal Muscle

Skeletal muscle is composed of about 75% water, 20% protein. The remaining constituents are organic salts and other substances necessary for sustaining cellular life and muscle contraction. The most abundant proteins in the muscle are actin, myosin and tropomyosin (McArdle et al., 1991).

Muscles are comprised of millions of **muscle fibers**, which are also called **muscle cells**. Individual muscle cells are wrapped and separated from adjacent fibers by a connective tissue, or fascia, called **endomysium**. A second layer of connective tissue, the **perimysium**, surrounds bundles, or groups, of fibers. Typically, each bundle includes about 150 fibers and is called a **fasciculus**. These groups of fibers which comprise the entire muscle are surrounded by a fibrous, fascial sheath of connective tissue called the **epimysium**. This protective covering of fascia tapers to form the dense and strong connective tissue of **tendons** (see Figure 2-A, Skeletal Muscle Structure and Anatomy).

Gross muscular contraction and movement. Because this fascial arrangement culminates in a tendinous attachment to bone, tension (force) developed in only one muscle cell can contribute to movement. The attachment points of muscles via the tendons are classified as an origin or insertion. Generally, the **origin** is where the tendon attaches to a more *stable* part of the skeleton. The **insertion** is characterized by attaching to a relatively more *movable* part of the skeleton. Origins are usually closer to the body's midline or proximal to the body, whereas insertions are usually distal (for example, wrist or elbow). The tendinous attachment of the muscle that is least stable (insertion) will be drawn toward the origin.

For example, the biceps muscle crosses the shoulder joint and the elbow joint. Of the 2 attachment areas, the shoulder (origin) is generally accepted to be more stable in conventional elbow flexion movements. The insertion (below the elbow) of the biceps moves toward the origin when the muscle contracts, since the muscle contracts toward its middle.

The force of muscular contraction is transmitted directly from muscle's connective tissue harness (endomysium, perimysium and epimysium culminating in tendons), via tendons, to skeletal attachment points.

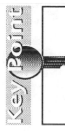

> Though the effect of origin and insertion can sometimes be reversed by stabilizing various body parts, movement relies on this relationship between origin and insertion.

Inside the fascia. Located beneath the endomysium that wraps individual muscle fibers is the **sarcolemma**. The sarcolemma is a thin, stretchable membrane (like plastic wrap) that houses the muscle fiber's contractile proteins (actin and myosin), enzymes, fat, glycogen, nuclei and specialized cellular organelles. **Sarcoplasm**, contained within the sarcolemma, bathes these cellular contents. Located within sarcoplasm is the **sarcoplasmic reticulum**. This serves as a delivery network, via interconnecting tubular channels, to help facilitate muscular contraction. The sarcoplasmic reticulum also provides the muscle fiber with additional structural integrity.

Supplying Blood to the Muscle

To accommodate the body's need—especially the needs of exercising skeletal muscles—for oxygen during exercise, local vascular beds (blood delivery vessels) control and distribute large volumes of blood.

During a *rhythmic and continuous activity* such as walking or biking, blood flow will actually fluctuate to working muscles. When muscles are contracting, blood flow decreases. During a relaxation or recovery phase (i.e., some part of the walking gait or cycling stroke), blood flow increases to the muscles. This "milking action" creates a pulse that facilitates blood delivery to exercising muscles and enhances a return of blood back to the heart. **Vasoconstriction** (narrowing) and **vasodilation** (opening or widening) of blood vessels occurs rapidly, based on the oxygen needs of the body, and also contributes to proper blood distribution in the exercising body.

In contrast, *strenuous activities*, such as traditional resistance training, may entirely stop blood flow to the muscle. Physiology texts report that when a muscle contracts to about 60% of its force-generating capacity, blood flow is actually occluded (blocked) to the working muscle(s). In my opinion, this occurs anywhere from one to about 15 reps to fatigue. I base this on the fact that a 10-repetition max (10-RM) equals about 75% of one-RM. (A one-RM equals the greatest amount of weight that can be lifted once with good technique.) This literal blockage of blood flow is a result of increases in intramuscular pressure. If a sustained or isometric contraction is maintained at this 60% intensity, or greater, blood flow to the muscle can be totally stopped for the duration that the muscle is required to, or can, produce this level of force.

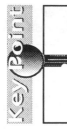

Under conditions where 60% of force-generating capacity, or greater, is being exerted, the energy source for muscular force production is mainly anaerobic. It is obvious that significant gains in *both* cardiorespiratory fitness and muscular strength and endurance cannot be simultaneously developed, based on energy system predominance and specificity.

An additional factor that affects blood flow is the **Valsalva maneuver**, which occurs when your client holds her breath momentarily during the initiation of a strenuous effort. It results in an increased heart rate and blood pressure response caused by forced expiration, or momentary breath holding, against a closed glottis. The **glottis** is the narrowest part of the larynx through which air passes into and out of the trachea. (The trachea or "windpipe" branches into the bronchi, which enter into the lungs.) The dramatic rise in blood pressure is due to increased intrathoracic pressure that forces blood from the heart into the arterial system. If the breath holding is sustained, this decreases blood flow to the active muscles and back to the heart. This reduction in blood flow increases the work load of the heart and increases its oxygen requirements at a time when coronary blood flow is potentially compromised since venous return to the heart is reduced.

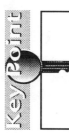

Breath holding may present a health-risk to a client with, for example, undiagnosed heart disease or high blood pressure. Increased intramuscular pressure, combined with a partial Valsalva maneuver, increases resistance to blood flow. This puts more of a load on the heart by causing an increased heart rate and additional demand for oxygen.

Though a momentary breath holding is generally a normal occurrence during the beginning of each strength exercise repetition, the key is to make sure your client does not sustain it through the entire repetition. This scenario lends additional importance to properly screening your clients and receiving medical clearance or guidance if questions arise concerning the potential for undiagnosed disease.

Quick Index:

The Microstructure of Skeletal Muscle

The electron microscope has given scientists an understanding of the microscopic anatomy of skeletal muscle. There are several levels of sub-cellular organization within single skeletal muscle fibers. To envision this sub-cellular order, let's first identify the microstructures of importance, and then view them as a series of 3 telescoping sleeves that fit into one another (Figure 2, Skeletal Muscle Structure and Anatomy).

The entire muscle is made up of many muscle fibers (Fig. 2-B). Each single muscle fiber is made of smaller functional units that lie parallel to the long axis of the muscle fiber. To visualize this relationship, envision a single muscle fiber as a straw (Fig. 2-B and C). Within this straw are smaller straws called **myofibrils** or **fibrils** (myo means muscle).

While myofibrils are only about 1/1000 of a millimeter, they are composed of even smaller subunits, called **myofilaments** or **filaments**. Myofilaments are also arranged so that they lie parallel to the long axis of myofibrils (Fig. 2-C).

Myofilaments are composed of repeating units called **sarcomeres**. The sarcomere is the smallest functional contractile unit of the muscle fiber, and is composed primarily of the proteins actin and myosin. It is the *thin* actin filaments and *thick* myosin filaments that are key players in the mechanical process of muscular contraction (Fig. 2-C, D, E and F).

Figure 2. Skeletal Muscle Structure and Anatomy

To envision the telescoping nature of the muscle, start by "seeing" a single muscle fiber as a straw (Fig. 2-B and C). Within this straw, and lying parallel, are numerous smaller straws, or myofibrils (Fig. 2-C). Looking at the end of the straw, or at a cross-sectional view, the ends of the myofibrils are peppered with small black dots. (This looks like an arrangement of *small* black dots made by a pencil point.) Within the smaller myofibril straws, as compared to a single muscle fiber, are thinner straws (small black dots) that represent the myofilaments (Fig. 2-C). Now you can see how these sub-cellular units are put together much like 3 telescoping sleeves (the straws). From a group of muscle fibers, one single fiber may be "telescoped" out, followed by a myofibril, and then a myofilament. They "slide" neatly into one another and are parallel (Fig. 2-A, B and C).

Skeletal Muscle Structure and Anatomy
(Figure 2)

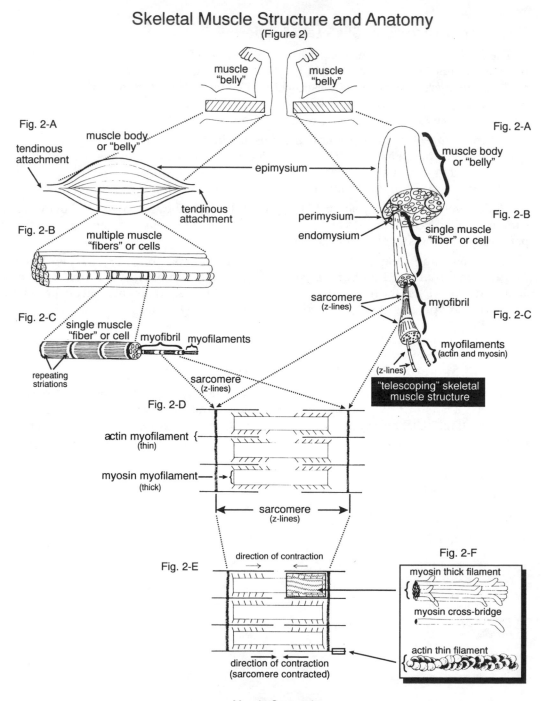

Muscle Contraction
Myosin cross-bridges contact actin and the 2 protein filaments slide past one another.
During muscle shortening, movement is toward the center of the sarcomere, see figs. D and E.

The Sliding-Filament Theory: How Muscles Contract

Each muscle contains many thousands of spaghetti-like muscle fibers (or cells), ranging from about 0.5-17 inches long. The fibers contain the contractile proteins actin and myosin, which are positioned so that they overlap. It is this overlap and contact between the hockey stick-like myosin structure and the thin actin (actin looks like a helix strand of tiny fish eggs) filaments that allow for movement and the production of muscular force (Fig. 2-D, E and F).

As long as the stimulus for contraction is strong enough, the actin and myosin filaments slide past one another by contacting and then releasing contact. This contact-release is initiated many times. The **sliding-filament theory** proposes that a muscle shortens, or lengthens, because the thick (myosin) and thin (actin) myofilaments slide past each other. The filaments themselves do not change length.

The sliding is accomplished by tiny cross-bridges that look like the curved end of a hockey stick, extending from the thicker myosin to the thinner actin filaments (Fig. 2-D, E and F). After the cross-bridges make contact, the movement of the actin over the myosin filament is similar to the action of oars (the boat is represented by myosin, the oars represent the cross-bridges extending from the myosin) pulling through water (the actin). The cross-bridges of the myosin (the oars) reach out and make contact with the actin (the water) and pull.

Each action of the cross-bridges (myosin/oars contacting the actin/water) contributes only a small amount of movement in terms of the total sliding action of the filaments (Fig. 2-D and E). This process of the oars and their hockey stick-shaped ends contacting actin and releasing has also been likened to the action of a person climbing a rope. The arms and legs of a person climbing a rope can represent the myosin cross-bridges. The rope represents the actin. Climbing (muscle contraction) is accomplished by first reaching with the arms (myosin cross-bridges), then grabbing, pulling and breaking contact with the rope (actin), reaching again, contacting the rope, pulling and sliding along the length of the rope, and then repeating this process over and over throughout the climb (muscle contraction through repeated contact and release between myosin and actin). This process equates with the muscle either shortening or lengthening through muscular-force production.

This helps you understand a very complex process and visualize why, and how, muscles contract toward the belly or middle of the muscle. When a muscle is at rest, and the position of actin and myosin in this state is compared to a fully contracted muscle (Fig 2-D and E), it is evident that the rearrangement of actin filaments sliding over the myosin filaments moves toward the middle (I-band) of the sarcomere, which is represented between two Z-lines (McArdle et al., 1991). An accumulation of many sarcomeres shortening (or changing length by the muscle lengthening during eccentric force production) a small amount contributes to bigger movements.

Key Point

It becomes apparent that the least stable end of a muscle's attachment (usually the insertion) is going to be most movable, and move toward the more stabilized attachment (usually the origin). Since a muscle contracts toward its center, as evidenced by the mechanical action of actin and myosin in the sarcomere, tension will be created on both tendinous attachments. If one is more mobile than the other, it will move toward the other attachment point. If both are fixed, such as during an isometric contraction, considerable force may be produced, but little to no movement will occur.

This is an important concept to comprehend. Its comprehension helps in understanding how movement occurs in the human body, and gives you the ability to evaluate and design strength exercises.

The Motor Unit Nerve Supply to the Muscle

The study of functional and structural characteristics of human skeletal muscle through use of the microscope and muscle biopsy has led to identification of 2 distinct types of muscle fibers. Muscle fibers are classified by their contractile and metabolic characteristics. The major muscle fiber classifications are slow-twitch (ST) and fast-twitch (FT).

Slow-twitch fibers (red, Type I) contract relatively slowly and generate energy predominantly via *aerobic* metabolism. **Fast-twitch fibers** are generally divided into 2 more categories: FT type IIa and FT type IIb (though a third FT category has been identified). **FT Type IIb** fibers (white) generate energy mainly through *anaerobic* pathways. **Type IIa**, an intermediate fast-oxidative-glycolytic fiber, has a combination of FT and ST fiber characteristics. This means its contribution to *aerobic* or *anaerobic* training can be influenced by the *type* of training. For example, traditional interval training would have very different effects on FT IIa muscle fibers when compared to the effects of traditional strength training.

Muscle fibers contract at the command of a **motor nerve**. A **motor unit** is defined as a motor nerve and all of the specific muscle fibers it commands, innervates or activates. More specifically, motor units contract, all or none, at the command of a motor nerve. This is the **functional unit** of *neuromuscular* control, whereas the smallest functional *contractile* unit of an individual muscle fiber is the sarcomere. It is these 2 mechanisms that are the key to muscular contraction.

Although each muscle fiber generally receives only one nerve fiber, a motor nerve may innervate many muscle fibers. This is because the terminal end of an axon (part of the motor nerve) forms numerous branches. One nerve and its terminal branches innervates (stimulates) one of the approximately 250 million muscle fibers in the human body. There are "only" about 420,000 motor nerves (McArdle et al., 1991). This means that a single motor nerve usually serves many individual muscle fibers through its branches.

The typical motor nerve activates 150 individual muscle fibers simultaneously. This ratio of number of muscle fibers to a single motor nerve is generally related to a muscle's particular movement function (McArdle et al., 1991). The delicate and precise work of the eye muscles, for example, requires that each motor nerve serve fewer than 10 muscle fibers. For less complex movements, a motor nerve may stimulate as many as 2,000-3,000 fibers. An example is the medial gastrocnemius (calf) muscle, which has 580 motor units and 1,030,000 muscle fibers. In this case, if 1,030,000 is divided by 580, each motor unit serves about 1,776 fibers or has a ratio of 1:1,776. However, it should be pointed out that the number of motor units and the fibers they serve cannot be calculated this simply. In actuality, each of the 580 motor units may serve *more* or *less* than 1,776 fibers. On the other hand, the first interosseous muscle of the finger which is responsible for finer motor movement contains "only" 120 motor units that control 41,000 fibers (McArdle et al., 1991; Feinstein, 1955). If 41,000 is simply divided by 120 this equals a ratio of 1 motor unit to every 342 fibers in the interosseous muscle. In this comparison, the potential for the interosseus motor units to control fewer fibers per motor unit, and thus be more suited for regulating fine motor movements, becomes apparent.

The way in which motor units activate fibers is crucial to skilled and/or powerful movement. To gain a clear understanding of how the muscle varies force, remember that each muscle has many motor nerves available to activate its many muscle fibers. The type and intensity of activity will determine which motor units are activated.

Characteristics of Motor Units

When the nervous system commands a motor unit to contract, *all the fibers of this single motor unit respond together*. There is no weak or partial contraction of a motor unit. All of the accompanying muscle fibers in the motor unit are stimulated to contract synchronously (at the same time). The *individual* motor unit fires **"all or none."**

However, innervation of a single motor unit does not mean stimulation of the entire muscle. If it did, human beings could not control movement. A single muscle may have hundreds of motor units, which innervate very few or several thousand muscle fibers. To understand how the force of contraction can be varied from slight to maximal, its important to distinguish a motor unit from the whole muscle.

Force gradation occurs in 2 ways:

- increasing the number of motor units recruited for activity, and

- increasing their frequency of discharge

By blending recruitment of motor units and the rate of their firing, optimal patterns of neural discharge permit a wide variety of graded (weak to strong) contractions (McArdle et al., 1991).

Motor units are comprised of fibers of one specific type (either FT or ST) or subdivision of a particular fiber type (FT IIa or IIb) that have the *same* metabolic profile (McArdle et al., 1991). Remember, each muscle of the body contains many motor units. If the proper and varied overload is not utilized with your clients, their training program may not be stimulating the desired motor units and optimizing the overall training result.

Motor units are classified into one of 3 categories depending on:

- their speed of contraction

- the amount of force they generate

- whether they *resist* fatigue, or conversely, fatigue relatively quickly

Table 11. Characteristics of Motor Units

Type I:	Type IIa:	Type IIb:
• slow-twitch	• fast-twitch	• fast-twitch
• slow contraction speed	• fast contraction speed	• fast contraction speed
• low force (tension) production	• fatigue resistant	• high force production
• highly resistant to fatigue	• characteristics can be influenced by the type of training	• susceptible to quick fatigue

Fast-Twitch Fibers

Fast-twitch (FT) muscle fibers, especially Type IIb, generate energy rapidly for quick, forceful contractions. Biochemical and physical characteristics suit FT IIb fibers for performance of *high-intensity, short-duration* work bouts that depend almost entirely on anaerobic metabolism for energy. These units reach greater peak tension and develop it nearly twice as fast as slow-twitch motor units. Examples of activities that would demand a large recruitment of FT IIb fibers include a 40-yard sprint and a one-RM lift. A short set of 2-10 repetitions to muscle fatigue would require significant contribution from both Type IIa and IIb fibers.

FT IIb fibers are innervated by large motor neurons that have fast conducting velocities for the nerve impulse. This motor unit may typically contain between 300 and 500 muscle fibers or more. FT fibers have a high activity of myofibrilar ATPase (myosin ATPase), the enzyme that breaks down ATP and releases energy necessary for muscle contraction. Other characteristics of FT fibers include shortening with a high contraction speed and relaxing quickly. FT fibers have high levels of ATP and CP intramuscular stores, and high glycolytic enzyme activity. All of these characteristics allow the FT fibers to develop a large amount of force quickly.

FT IIb fibers have a low aerobic capability, as evidenced by their low intramuscular stores of triglyceride, low capillary density, low mitochondrial density and low aerobic enzyme activity. However, FT IIb, and particularly IIa fibers, can be modified to either become more enduring with interval training or better able to exhibit characteristics conducive to anaerobic strength work if that type of training is emphasized. Because FT fibers generally rely predominantly on anaerobic sources of ATP and generally have low capabilities to supply ATP aerobically, they are highly susceptible to fatigue. Consequently, they are suited to perform work where a large amount of force is necessary and the activity is usually of short duration, lasting from a few seconds to several minutes.

Slow-Twitch Fibers

ST, or Type I, fibers are ideal for the performance of *low-intensity, long-duration* (endurance) activities. Activities like this include long-distance running, swimming, walking and long sets of low-intensity resistance training exercise (about 20 repetitions or more).

The ST motor units are innervated by small motor neurons with slow conduction velocities. These ST units are much more fatigue-resistant than FT units. Slow-twitch (ST) fibers generate energy for ATP resynthesis and muscle contraction by aerobic energy transfer. ST fibers are distinguished by a low activity level of myosin ATPase, a slow speed of contraction and a glycolytic capacity less well developed than in FT fibers.

However, the ST fibers contain relatively large and numerous mitochondria. The mitochondria are the muscle cells' "powerhouse" for aerobic energy production. This concentration of mitochondria, combined with high levels of **myoglobin** (myo indicates muscle and globin refers to its role as the muscle's hemoglobin or short-term oxygen storage) and mitochondrial enzymes, represents the metabolic machinery that needs to be in place to sustain aerobic metabolism.

It also appears that capacity for blood flow through muscle is determined by differences in the oxidative capacity of the fiber types, with ST fibers receiving proportionately more blood during exercise than FT fibers. Through increased capillarization as a result of training effects, ST fibers develop a greater capacity for aerobic metabolism. This ultimately influences aerobic energy metabolism during and after exercise.

ST fibers have these characteristics: high aerobic enzyme activity, high capillary density (for better oxygen delivery and byproduct removal), high intramuscular triglyceride stores and a high resistance to muscular fatigue.

Hereditary Influences and Fiber Type Distribution
The percentage of either FT or ST fibers that you have in your body is determined largely by genetics. Research indicates that what you are born with, in terms of percentage of FT versus ST, probably remains fairly constant throughout life. Since genes definitely affect performance and adaptation to training loads, you can see the significance of not being able to choose your parents!

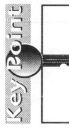

> Genetic predisposition to a predetermined ratio of ST to FT fibers will greatly affect the outer bounds of individual response to training stimuli. But, every one of your clients can realize dramatic improvements in muscular strength and endurance gains relative to their starting point.

Current scientific literature indicates that changing FT fibers to ST fibers, or vice versa, probably does not occur in humans under *normal* training conditions. However, it is interesting to note that in an extensive review of research, it was concluded that *extreme* and *prolonged* training may produce skeletal muscle fiber type conversion (Wilmore and Costill, 1994).

But, this information does not imply that, for example, FT IIa fibers physically change into ST fibers. Instead, chronic stimulation *transforms* the basic properties of the muscle fibers. High-intensity interval conditioning or strength training are examples of activities that contribute to this type of training effect on FT IIa fibers. In these cases, the fibers' training-influenced metabolic characteristics and threshold at which the motor neuron fires determines the appropriate level of intensity (and type of activity) that will engage the motor unit.

A more practical fact is that particular metabolic characteristics of *all* fiber types can be modified by specific training. High-intensity, anaerobic strength training is necessary to stimulate optimal FT fiber adaptation. This includes, for example, increases in muscle size and anaerobic enzymes. (On the other hand, the highly adaptable FT IIa fiber, with prolonged high-intensity cardiorespiratory training, can become almost as fatigue resistant as the slow-twitch units (McArdle et al., 1991).

But, high-repetition schemes (greater than about 20 reps) or endurance activities will not significantly call these FT IIa motor units into play. Because of this, your client will never realize optimal physical development unless you choose a correct and specific overload that causes these units to adapt to the load placed on the body.

Quick Index:
Chapter 12, using intervals to train different muscle fiber types

Order of Fiber-Type Recruitment or "Firing Pattern"

FT and ST motor units are selectively recruited and regulated in their firing pattern to produce desired movement and appropriate muscular-force development. Recruitment order depends upon type of activity, force required, movement pattern and position of your body. This modulatory effect is referred to as a **ramp-like recruitment effect** (Figure 3). In muscular activity requiring contractions of increasing force, ST motor units with the *lowest* functional threshold are selectively and predominantly recruited during lighter effort. This allows for activation of more powerful, higher threshold FT units when higher forces are required rather quickly.

The larger the motor neuron, the more difficult it is to stimulate that motor neuron. FT motor units have very large motor neurons in comparison to ST motor units. Because of this, FT motor units will be activated last in a muscle contraction. For example: If a light weight is being lifted slowly, predominantly ST motor units are recruited to perform this movement. If weight is increased, or if it is moved at a faster velocity, FT IIa motor units, in addition to ST units, are recruited. If weight is increased further, or moved at an even faster velocity, FT IIa and IIb motor units are recruited along with the continual contribution of ST motor units (Fig. 3).

This ramp-like order of recruitment ensures that predominantly ST motor units are recruited to perform low-intensity, long-duration endurance activities. Predominantly FT motor units are recruited for high-intensity activity. Notice that the order of recruitment holds the FT motor units, which are easily fatigued, in reserve until the ST motor units can no longer perform the particular muscular contraction.

The theoretical and simplified order of recruitment would be ST, followed by FT IIa and finally followed by FT IIb motor units. The key determining factors as to whether FT or ST motor units are recruited are the total amount of force and speed of contraction necessary to perform the movement pattern or muscular contraction.

Since an average client has a ratio of 50% FT to ST motor units, performing at workloads of low intensity will challenge half of the muscle mass in an individual's body. This has implications for both cardiorespiratory fitness and muscular strength and endurance. Steady-rate training performed exclusively will not develop a training effect in the highly adaptable FT IIa fibers, and strength training repetitions of 20 reps or higher will not significantly call into play FT motor units.

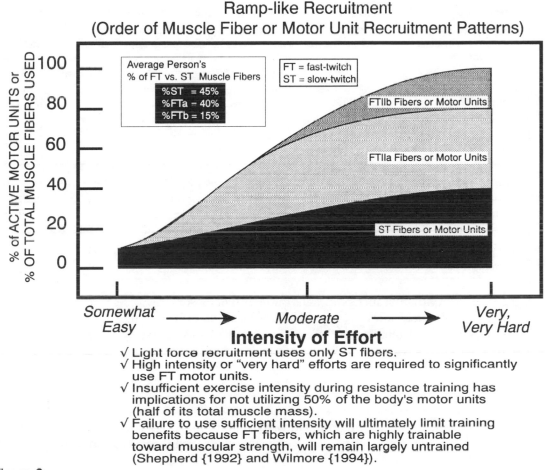

Ramp-like Recruitment
(Order of Muscle Fiber or Motor Unit Recruitment Patterns)

Average Person's
% of FT vs. ST Muscle Fibers

%ST = 45%
%FTa = 40%
%FTb = 15%

FT = fast-twitch
ST = slow-twitch

FTIIb Fibers or Motor Units

FTIIa Fibers or Motor Units

ST Fibers or Motor Units

% of ACTIVE MOTOR UNITS or % OF TOTAL MUSCLE FIBERS USED

Somewhat Easy → Moderate → Very, Very Hard

Intensity of Effort

√ Light force recruitment uses only ST fibers.
√ High intensity or "very hard" efforts are required to significantly use FT motor units.
√ Insufficient exercise intensity during resistance training has implications for not utilizing 50% of the body's motor units (half of its total muscle mass).
√ Failure to use sufficient intensity will ultimately limit training benefits because FT fibers, which are highly trainable toward muscular strength, will remain largely untrained (Shepherd {1992} and Wilmore {1994}).

Figure 3

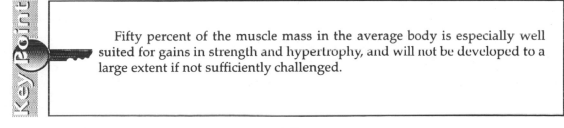

Fifty percent of the muscle mass in the average body is especially well suited for gains in strength and hypertrophy, and will not be developed to a large extent if not sufficiently challenged.

Fleck and Kraemer (1987) point out that **motor-unit recruitment order** is important from a practical standpoint for several reasons. These scientific principles should influence your program design in the area of resistance training.

1. In order to recruit FT fibers and attain a training effect, exercise must be sufficiently intense.

2. Order of recruitment is fixed for a *specific* movement (Desmedt and Godaux, 1977; as reported in Fleck and Kraemer, 1987). If the body position is changed, order of recruitment can also change (Grimby and Hannerz, 1977; as reported in Fleck and Kraemer, 1987).

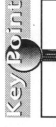

You do not necessarily have to add weight to affect motor-unit recruitment and create a new overload. Though adding weight is often a first step, simply changing the exercise movement or position of the participant will accomplish this without increasing absolute weight being lifted.

For multifunctional muscles, order of motor-unit recruitment can also change from one movement to another. For example, motor-unit recruitment order in the quadriceps is different for performance of a seated leg extension on a machine when compared to knee extension during a squat movement (Fleck and Kraemer, 1987). Variation in motor-unit recruitment order is most likely one of the factors responsible for additional strength gains even though the same muscle group(s) may be involved in a similar exercise variation or different exercises.

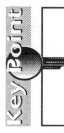

Variation in recruitment order provides some evidence that in order to completely develop a particular muscle (all the motor units), it must be exercised through several different movements. And, exercise must be of sufficient intensity to stimulate recruitment of FT IIa and IIb motor units.

If a large amount of force is necessary either to move a heavy weight slowly or to move a light weight at a fast velocity, predominantly FT motor units are recruited. More *total* force is exerted when a heavy weight is moved slowly and controlled through a range of movement. This is true even though the same amount of work is accomplished whether you move a weight slowly or quickly (for example, when performing a biceps curl, the hand is successfully brought toward the shoulder regardless of movement speed).

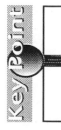

While there are some sport-specific performance issues related to speed of movement and specificity, most of your clients would probably gain the most benefit from their resistance training program by moving an appropriate overload (resistance or weight that is intense enough as related to their current fitness level to optimize training effect) through an appropriate range of movement in a controlled and steady manner.

Such information is of practical importance to help your understanding of the specific requirements along the continuum for training and competition, versus health and fitness improvements. It suggests that all training done at a slow pace *and* with light force, will emphasize the use of mostly ST fibers, inducing little training effect on FT IIa or FT IIb fibers. Long, slow training bouts using high-repetition schemes do not prepare muscle for the demands of competition or higher muscular forces, and do not optimize stimulation and training effect of your client's muscle mass. Even functional strength training, which usually emphasizes "usable" muscular endurance, balance and maintenance of correct body alignment, should incorporate some high-intensity strength training or functional strength drills. This type of training can prepare the body for high-force requirements provided by everyday challenges, such as reacting to a loss of balance on a slippery surface.

Quick Index:

Developing Muscular Strength and Muscular Endurance

Both muscular strength and muscular endurance are important to the health and well-being of your clients. **Muscular strength** refers to the muscle's ability to exert force at a given speed of movement. There is a wide continuum of muscular strength that ranges from repeated contractions to a one-RM effort, the greatest amount of weight that can be lifted once, with good form. **Muscular endurance** refers to the ability of your client to persist in physical activity or resist muscular fatigue.

Traditional muscular strength and endurance conditioning is anaerobic work that lasts about 30-90 seconds and causes the targeted muscles to fatigue or fail within this time frame. Generally, 8-20 repetitions performed in a controlled manner will fit into this time parameter.

With chronic exercise, there are a number of adaptations that occur in the neuromuscular (nerves and skeletal muscle) system. Of course, the extent of these adaptations will depend on the type of training program followed. If training is of a cardiorespiratory endurance nature, such as jogging, walking or swimming, then little or no gains in strength will occur. Likewise, a program of stretching to increase flexibility combined with light (high repetition) calisthenics, will produce substantial gains in flexibility, small to moderate gains in muscular endurance and strength, and no gain in cardiorespiratory fitness.

On the other hand, according to Wilmore and Costill (1994), properly designed strength training programs will produce substantial gains in strength, ranging from 25-100% improvement, or greater, within a period of 3-6 months. And, when cardiorespiratory fitness is the primary goal, accompanied with the appropriate training stimulus, an increase of 15-30% in max VO2 during the first 3 months of training can be accomplished. Max VO2 may rise as much as 50% over a 2-year period of intensive training (McArdle et al., 1991).

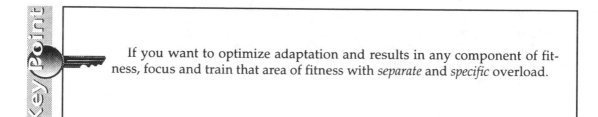

If you want to optimize adaptation and results in any component of fitness, focus and train that area of fitness with *separate* and *specific* overload.

Muscular fitness is development by placing a demand, or **overload**, on the muscles of your client in a manner in which the muscle is not accustomed. If overload is applied in a progressive and sensible manner, the neuromuscular system will adapt positively to this demand. As a result, your client becomes stronger and is better able to sustain muscular activity that may require muscle endurance and/or strength.

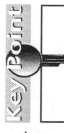

The general guideline for change (a proper and specific overload) is: exercise that uses a progressive increase in resistance over time, that causes the targeted muscle(s) to fatigue in about 30-90 seconds, and results in challenges for all major movements (joint actions) to which the muscles contribute.

A progressive increase in resistance is necessary for continued increases in muscle strength and endurance. Also, gradual increases in intensity will reduce the likelihood of injury. Appropriate intensity (attaining muscular fatigue in about 30-90 seconds) is necessary to optimize training results. All major movements of the body must be challenged to ensure balanced strength between all opposing muscle groups of the body.

Factors influencing strength. Numerous authors cite several factors that influence strength or amount of force that can be exerted during a muscle contraction. Neural inhibition, number of contracting muscle fibers (or muscle cells), contractile state of fibers and mechanical advantage or disadvantage of the lever system influence force generation.

Furthermore, a stretched muscle is capable of exerting more force, probably because of elastic recoil and because contractile proteins are aligned favorably. On the other hand, a muscle that is *overstretched* will produce less force, as the contractile proteins actin and myosin are not favorably aligned. In addition, orthopedic stress may accumulate on ligaments and other soft tissues in situations where the joint is placed in a position of excessive range of motion.

Several factors, including gender, muscle size and muscle fiber type deserve a closer look in helping to understand what effects muscular strength and endurance gains, as well as muscle hypertrophy (increased size of the muscle).

Quick Index:

Chapter 6, monitoring intensity levels and allowing for recovery periods

How Do Muscles Become Stronger?

There are many myths and misconceptions in the area of resistance training. Just how does your client become stronger? What physiological adaptations take place that allow a client to exert greater levels of strength?

For many years it was assumed that strength gains were a direct result of increases in muscle size, referred to as **hypertrophy**. This seemed a logical assumption, as many individuals who trained with free weights or other strength-training devices often developed large muscles. In addition to this, when a broken limb is placed in a cast and immobilized, in only a few days muscles begin to lose both size and strength, a process referred to as **atrophy**. Gains in strength are generally paralleled by gains in size, whereas losses in the size of a muscle correlate highly with losses in strength.

But, recent research suggests that there is more involved in understanding the basic mechanisms of strength gains than a simple relationship to the size of the muscle. Wilmore and Costill (1994) report that studies of strength training have shown that women experience gains in strength similar to men who perform the same training program, but the women do not experience the same degree of hypertrophy. Anecdotally, there are numerous stories of individuals performing superhuman feats of strength at times of great psychological and emotional stress.

There is accumulating evidence to indicate that motor-unit recruitment and neural influences are important in explaining gains in muscular strength. This is particularly true for those gains in strength that occur in the absence of hypertrophy, as well as for understanding epic, superhuman physical accomplishments ("boy lifts car off chest of trapped father").

Skeletal muscles are innervated by motor neurons. Groups of individual muscle fibers that are activated by the same motor neuron are called motor units. You will recall that the amount of force generated during muscle contraction depends on: (1) the number of motor units that are fired, and (2) the frequency of motor unit firing. **Firing frequency** refers to the number of impulses the motor unit receives per given time period. Sustained stimuli or impulses would increase the total tension/force produced in muscle for that given time period by not allowing the muscle to relax.

The preceding examples should not be taken to imply that muscle size is not an important factor in the ultimate strength potential of muscle. However, these examples indicate that mechanisms responsible for gains in strength are very complex, and at this time are not well understood by scientists.

Neural Influences on Muscular Strength

There is evidence that motor units are controlled by a number of different neurons, or **interneurons**, which have the ability to produce both excitatory and inhibitory impulses. **Inhibitory mechanisms** in the neuromuscular system are necessary to *prevent* muscles from exerting more force than can be tolerated by bones and connective tissues. During flexibility training you can take advantage of this inhibition to enhance flexibility gains. However, to increase strength gains, it is important to "push back" the reflex inhibition.

If you progressively strength train, the tendons, for example, become thicker and stronger, and more force can be exerted through the connective tissue harness before any autogenic inhibition reflex occurs. This protective reflex, causing the muscle or muscle groups to relax, is directed to a specific muscle(s) when tension on that muscle's tendons and internal connective tissue structures exceeds the threshold of **Golgi tendon organs** (GTOs).

The GTOs are sensory organs located in tendons of muscles that are sensitive to force/tension production in the tendon. If too much force is generated in relation to the GTOs' current threshold (the point at which they are activated), the associated muscle, or muscle group, will relax. This inhibition reflex keeps the tendon from tearing from its attachment or damaging other soft tissue related to the muscle complex.

At higher levels in the nervous system, the reticular formation in the brain stem and cerebral cortex both have the ability to initiate and propagate inhibitory impulses (McArdle et al., 1991). It is quite possible that these inhibitory impulses are gradually overcome or counteracted with intense resistance training. For example, the GTOs' threshold for firing is pushed back through stronger tendons and a stronger tissue "harness." This would enable muscle to reach greater levels of strength and force production, which would typically occur following a strength training program.

Whether an individual motor unit will fire and contribute to the contractile force or remain in the relaxed state also depends on the *summation of the many impulses* it receives at any one time. For instance, if excitatory impulses exceed inhibitory impulses (all or none principle specific to each individual motor unit), the unit will then be activated and contribute to the force production capabilities of that muscle (McArdle et al., 1991).

Wilmore and Costill (1994) indicate that improvement in recruitment patterns could be the result of a blocking of, or reduction in, the number of inhibitory impulses, thereby allowing more motor units to be activated simultaneously. In any case, McDonagh and Davies (1984) have concluded that there is a neurogenic component to adaptive responses to strength training, particularly during initial phases of training. Daniel Kosich, Ph.D., believes that as much as 75-80% of the increases in strength due to a resistance training program may be related to neural adaptations, whereas only about 25% of strength increases may be related to muscle hypertrophy (presented at IDEA Personal Training Conference, 1991).

Neural adaptations to resistance training predominate during the first 4 weeks of a training program. Morphological (physical changes such as hypertrophy) changes to muscle itself predominate thereafter. However, this does not mean that there are no adaptations in the neural system after this point. In fact, after years of training, *highly* trained athletes rely predominantly on neural adaptations to increase strength or power output. And finally, the contribution of both hormonal and neural influences can help us understand how significant demonstrations of extreme human strength can be exhibited without the influence of muscle hypertrophy and progressive training adaptations, that occur as a result of a strength training program.

> Gains in strength may well be the result of a gain in an ability to recruit additional motor units, sustain them in a contracted state (frequency of firing) and synchronize their firing to facilitate contraction and maximization of force production.

It is documented that nervous system adaptations and a learning curve that exists for new activities at least partially account for the ability of your client to lift more absolute weight and produce more muscular force within the early weeks of training. Because most studies typically involve training programs that last 8-20 weeks, much of the documented improvements in muscle strength are related to this combination of neural and physical adaptations.

Neural adaptations to resistance training include both an increase in number of motor units that can be fired at any give time and an increase in frequency of motor unit firing. Increasing the number of motor units that are fired may be caused by an increase in neural drive to the muscle and/or a removal of neural inhibition. Improved coordination among agonist muscles (muscles that work together to produce a specific movement) and removal of activation of antagonist muscles (muscles that produce force and movement in the opposite direction) may also contribute to an increased ability to generate greater muscular force following resistance training.

Quick Index:

Chapter 8, relationship of GTOs to flexibility training

Physical or Morphological Adaptations

An increase in muscle size, or **hypertrophy**, is probably the most readily recognized adaptation to resistance training. Such an increase is often observed following as little as 6-8 weeks of training.

Hypertrophied muscle fibers are larger because they contain more actin and myosin, the contractile proteins of muscles. Actin and myosin (myofilaments) are organized within muscle fiber in cylindrical units called myofibrils (Figure 2, Skeletal Muscle Structure and Anatomy). Myofibrils increase in both size and number (**hyperplasia**) following resistance training. Increased myofibril cross-sectional area (size) following resistance training results from an addition of actin and myosin filaments to the periphery of the myofibril. More contractile protein (actin and myosin) allows for more cross-bridges to form, and therefore, an increased potential for higher degrees of contraction force. Sarcomeres, which comprise myofibrils and are the smallest functional contractile unit of the muscle, increase in number by adding on to both the ends, and sides, of existing myofibrils.

> **Key Point**
>
> Myofibrils increase in number *within* the muscle fiber or cell; there is *no* increase in the *number* of muscle fibers under *normal* training conditions.

Even if longitudinal splitting (hyperplasia) did occur in humans—which is doubtful based upon available literature—the greatest contribution to increased muscular size with progressive resistance training occurs as a result of enlargement of existing, individual muscle fibers (McArdle et al., 1991). Trained muscles also have a thicker and tougher connective tissue harness and tendons, which also contributes to the muscle being able to exert more force.

The specific mechanism by which resistance training stimulates increased protein synthesis is unknown. There are currently 2 hypotheses which have been developed to explain the mechanism responsible for muscle hypertrophy.

One hypothesis suggests that tension developed during resistance exercise provides a signal that is read by the genetic machinery of the cell, which in turn stimulates protein synthesis. This hypothesis is supported by the fact that little or no hypertrophy will occur during resistance training when intensity is low.

McArdle et al. (1991) supports this hypothesis by stating that within the cell, myofibrils thicken and increase in number and additional sarcomeres are formed by an acceleration of **protein synthesis** and corresponding *decreases* in protein breakdown. McArdle et al. (1991) go on to state that it appears that the primary requirement for initiating muscular hypertrophy is an increase in tension, or force, that the muscle must generate.

The second hypothesis involves the theory of breakdown-and-repair. It is postulated that during each training session part of the muscle is broken down and that the repair process gradually builds up muscle to a higher level. The breakdown and repair hypothesis is supported by studies that have identified skeletal muscle damage following heavy resistance exercise through key markers in the blood.

However, muscle damage associated with a strenuous effort should not imply a "cause and effect" relationship between gains in strength and hypertrophy. It is very important to note that the process of hypertrophy is directly related to the *synthesis* (putting together) of cellular material. This is particularly true of actin and myosin protein filaments that constitute the functional contractile elements (sarcomeres) of muscle. The word "synthesis" implies that strength training is a positive, building process **(anabolic)**, as opposed to a negative, or **catabolic** (breaking down), process.

In my opinion, physiological evidence indicates that some breakdown of muscle will occur as an inevitable consequence of aggressive (proper intensity to maximize strength/hypertrophy gains) training. I believe it is an *improper* concept that muscle is "broken down" and then "repairs and grows stronger" as a *result* of muscle damage.

> **Key Point**
>
> The key stimulus for protein synthesis and neural adaptation is *proper overload*. Muscle damage does not, of itself, stimulate muscle to grow or the nervous system to adapt. However, muscle damage is often an invariable byproduct of hard training.

As an example, you can overstretch a muscle and create soreness, which is more accurately identified as muscle damage, or micro-trauma. However, damaging muscle in any training scenario does not represent the proper and specific overload stimulus to cause positive growth, and/or nervous system adaptations. Additionally, because of micro-trauma and related scarring in muscle tissue that is associated with muscle damage, and resultant lesser blood supply to the scarred area because of accumulated trauma, the fibers are more susceptible to recurrent injury.

Resistance training also increases local (local refers to the *specific* muscles trained) stores of ATP, CP and glycogen. Undoubtedly, this change in the biochemistry of muscle to favor anaerobic metabolism contributes to the rapid rate of anaerobic energy transfer required of this type of exercise. The increase in actin and myosin and energy-generating compounds (anaerobic enzymes, stored ATP, CP and glycogen) with "heavy" (8-12 repetitions to muscular fatigue) resistance training occurs *without* parallel increases in capillarization or in total volume of mitochondria or mitochondrial enzymes within muscle cells.

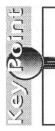

> A decrease in mitochondria and mitochondrial enzymes (important for aerobic metabolism) may be detrimental to endurance performance by decreasing the fiber's aerobic potential per unit of muscle mass.

Generally, this is of concern only to the most competitive and specialized athletes. Elite athletes usually try to optimize performance in only one of the body's energy systems. Most of your clients who cross-train with a variety of activities that challenge the basic components of fitness will realize both excellent cardiorespiratory and muscular strength and endurance gains. In most instances there is no measurable compromise of significance to improvement in any component of fitness, if viewed within a relationship to your client's health and fitness goals.

Gender Differences Related to Resistance Training

According to Sharkey (1990), at the ages of about 12-14, boys and girls are at similar strength levels. Males may gain an advantage when they enter puberty because of an increase in production of the predominantly male hormone testosterone. Men can have about 20-30 times as much testosterone as women, and testosterone is known to exert a very strong anabolic or tissue-building effect (McArdle et al., 1991). It should be noted that testosterone levels are on a continuum between men and women, with some females normally possessing high levels of this hormone (McArdle et al., 1991). There is a strong relationship between testosterone levels and increased muscle size and strength.

However, size of muscle is not the entire story. The issue, in terms of muscular force generation, is not as simple as it seems. For instance, how do you explain similar strength improvements in men and women, even though muscular hypertrophy is typically less in the female? In terms of gender differences, it seems clear that the main difference in response to resistance training between men and women seems to be only the degree of muscle hypertrophy (McArdle et al., 1991). And, a larger and stronger muscle is not necessarily more successful in sport or everyday tasks.

Studies indicate that college women tend to have about half the arm and shoulder strength, and about 30% less leg strength, than college men. The relationship between testosterone and strength could be incidental (that is, high levels of testosterone equate to high levels of strength and the ability to gain significant size), or strength differences could be due to other factors. Testosterone may make one more aggressive, and aggressive individuals train harder. A more likely possibility is body fat.

Women generally have more sex-specific body fat than men. When strength per pound of lean body weight (body weight minus fat weight) is considered, women have slightly stronger legs, while arm strength is still some 30% below men's values. Wilmore (1976) suggests that since women use their legs as men do, they are similar in strength. It may be that the typical woman's role in our society does not encourage her to challenge upper body strength. This may be the factor that is keeping women as a group from gaining in this category.

Generally, bigger muscles mean stronger muscles. The force a single muscle fiber generates is related to cross-sectional area of the fiber. Men, in many instances, are stronger in an absolute measure (they can lift more weight or exert more force) simply because they have *more* muscle tissue, not stronger muscle tissue. Naturally occurring high levels of testosterone favor greater muscle mass. Numerous physiology texts emphasize that there is no physiological difference between muscle fibers (muscle cells) in a male and a female. Fast-twitch (FT) and slow-twitch (ST) fibers are found in both females and males. Distribution of fiber types (% of FT to ST) and metabolic characteristics (contractile properties) are similar in men and women.

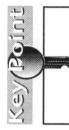

> The strength of a given cross-sectional area of a muscle fiber is the *same* for men and women. Gender may influence the *quantity* of muscle, but not the *quality* of it.

This information should answer the question, "Should women be trained differently than men?" The answer is an emphatic "No!" And, these facts simply indicate that there are other variables that influence different strength levels between men and women, as well as among *same* genders, that go well beyond the size of muscle.

Can You Really Control Results?

The degree of strength that can be gained by skeletal muscle hypertrophy and neural adaptations depends on a number of factors, which include:

- the characteristics of the training program
- the potential for muscle to increase in size

Progressive and intense resistance training stimulates an increase in the cross-sectional area of both slow-twitch (ST-Type I) and fast-twitch (FT-Type II) muscle fibers. Generally, a greater degree of hypertrophy occurs in Type II fibers. But, it should be emphasized that hypertrophy *does* occur in Type I fibers as well.

The greater degree of hypertrophy found in Type II fibers is probably the result of a greater involvement of these fibers with resistance training because of their metabolic and physical characteristics, which are conducive to gains in size and anaerobic metabolism. Likewise, the greatest amount of atrophy resulting from inactivity occurs in Type II fibers.

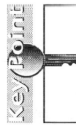

Since there are no studies that conclusively indicate that resistance training increases the *number* of Type II fibers relative to Type I, the potential for your client to increase muscle size and muscle strength may be genetically predetermined by the number of Type II fibers she possesses and by the resistance training program that you design.

It is clear from research that the ability to exert more muscular force after resistance training is not solely dependent on an increase in fiber size. Adaptations in the connective tissue harness and the nervous system serve as important contributors to total force production from muscles. In fact, many scientists argue that changes in connective tissue and the nervous system may be more important contributors to overall strength than muscle hypertrophy.

Muscle Soreness

After workouts, your clients may experience one of 3 types of muscle soreness. The first may be "soreness" that is felt while exercising (feeling the "burn" during high-intensity resistance training or cardiorespiratory conditioning) or immediately after intense exercise during the cool-down. This is usually a transient type of soreness related to lactic acid build-up during anaerobic effort. Lactic acid is usually cleared from the body in about 30-60 minutes.

McArdle et al. (1991) indicate that lactate buildup is not related to postexercise soreness and discomfort that occurs 24-48 hours after cessation of "normal" training. "Normal" training is in contrast to repeated high-intensity anaerobic training efforts over extended time periods. Remember, lactic acid is not a "waste" product, but simply a byproduct of anaerobic effort. When sufficient oxygen becomes available, lactate is metabolized and can be used as energy. However, you should be aware that any immediate soreness after exercise could be an injury related to micro-trauma (minor tears) to connective tissue or the muscle. Because of this possibility, monitor your clients with follow-up communication.

The second and third types of soreness may occur for an extended period of time following cessation of workouts. Your client may experience soreness and stiffness in the muscles and joints several hours after the workout, and then a residual, or **delayed-onset muscle soreness (DOMS)** may set in and last several days. DOMS can occur when (1) activity is resumed after a layoff, (2) participating in an unfamiliar activity, even if conditioned, and (3) intensity, frequency or duration is increased. DOMS is an indication that the body is adapting to demands of exercise to which it is unaccustomed.

The exact cause of DOMS is unknown. **Eccentric contractions,** and to some extent isometric contractions, generally cause the greatest amount of postexercise soreness (McArdle et al., 1991). This close relationship of DOMS to the eccentric, or "negative," phase of muscular contraction may occur because of the mechanics between actin and myosin protein filaments. During an eccentric effort, muscle is trying to shorten, or overcome external resistance. However, the outside force is greater than the force-producing capacity of muscles involved in the effort. This results in a lengthening of the muscle and associated connective tissue while the muscle develops tension.

This scenario leads to extremely high intramuscular forces and lends physiological credence to the most respected theories for muscle soreness and stiffness. These theories have the most experimental evidence to support an argument that points toward microscopic tears in muscle fiber, the musculo-tendon interface, and/or damage to the myofascial connective tissue surrounding muscle fibers and the muscle.

> New trainees should avoid activity that has a *concentration* of eccentric muscular effort. Activity that is unfamiliar to the seasoned client should be approached sensibly by using gradual progressions. And, if intensity, duration or frequency is being increased it should be done in a conservative and progressive manner.

Quick Index:

Chapter 9, effect of warm-up on muscle soreness

Implications for Resistance Training

In recognition of the need for a well-rounded training program to develop and maintain muscular as well as cardiorespiratory fitness, the American College of Sports Medicine (ACSM) revised its original Position Stand on "The Recommended Quantity and Quality of Exercise for Developing and Maintaining Fitness in Healthy Adults" to include a resistance-training component. ACSM recommends resistance training of a moderate to high intensity that is *sufficient to develop and maintain muscle mass*. Resistance training stands as an integral part of any adult fitness program. The recommended minimum: one set of 8-12 repetitions of 8-10 exercises that challenge the major muscle groups, at least 2 days per week.

ACSM bases these minimal standards for resistance training on at least 2 factors. First, the time it takes to complete a comprehensive, well-rounded program is important. Programs lasting more than 60-minutes per session are associated with higher dropout rates. Second, although greater frequencies of training and additional sets or combinations of sets and repetitions elicit greater strength gains, the magnitude of difference is usually small.

According to a review of research, Michael Pollock, Ph.D. (reported in the 1990 ACSM position stand) states that strength training 2 days per week, in accordance with these guidelines, confers 80% of the strength gains seen when training 3 days per week. When coupled with significant results, this lower frequency may encourage compliance.

In a study by Braith et al. (reported in the 1990 ACSM position stand), 2-days-per- week training was compared with 3-days-per-week training, over 18 weeks. The 2-days-per-week group showed a 21% increase in strength compared to 28% in the 3-days-per-week group. In other words, 75% of what could be attained in a 3-days-per-week program was realized in the 2-days-per-week program. Braith et al., and other researchers also found that programs using one set to fatigue showed a greater than 25% increase in strength. These results are favorable when compared to other more time-intensive programs that involve more total repetitions, sets and days of training. By training smart, you can effectively utilize your client's precious time investment to maximize her health and fitness.

Quick Index

Chapter 14, determining reps and loads for different goals

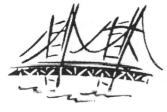

The Bridge

Effective resistance training results in wide-ranging health benefits and noticeable physical improvements for your clients. While an increase in muscle size is not necessarily a prerequisite for improving strength and/or power, it typically is a result. Hypertrophy seems to occur significantly after 6 weeks. Effectiveness means a program designed with an appropriate overload, or intensity. Both fast-twitch and slow-twitch muscle fibers need to be trained, and moderate and high intensity resistance training are desirable. Nonetheless, one set for beginners and 2 sets for average clients, done twice per week, is appropriate to realize significant strength gains. Eight to 10 exercises performed in a range of 8-20 repetitions, to fatigue, generally fits within strength improvement protocols.

CHAPTER 8

NEUROPHYSIOLOGY OF FLEXIBILITY

Too often clients fail to slow down and pause before rushing off to their scheduled and busy day. Yet by taking the time for flexibility training, you can give them a great opportunity to reflect on both short- and long-term accomplishments. Besides the important physical benefits, stretching creates an opportunity to increase one's sense of self-esteem by acknowledging what, for example, has just been accomplished during the most recent workout. Stretching can be a very enjoyable, relaxing part of a client's workout.

Once you have a clear understanding of the neurophysiology and physical properties of the tissues you are stretching, you can formulate a specific, safe and effective approach to stretching. There are many benefits for your clients. Improved flexibility can lead to:

• **Better posture**. Improved posture may help the client avoid chronic injuries due to poor postural alignment and muscular imbalances. Flexibility training can help realign skeletal structure that has adapted to habits of incorrect posture and poor exercise technique. Clients will find it easier to maintain proper posture throughout the day, and improved muscular balance will make the efforts of daily activities less strenuous and more efficient.

Furthermore, there is strong scientific evidence that the risk of incurring low-back pain and experiencing stress to the lumbar spine can be avoided with increased pelvic mobility (Plowman, 1992). This includes sufficient flexibility *and* strength in the hamstrings, gluteus minimus, medius, and maximus, hip flexors and low back musculature.

• **Increased range of motion (ROM) available at a joint or joints**. This can provide for greater mechanical efficiency and result in safer and more effective movement. A mobile joint moves more easily through a range of motion and requires less energy.

• **The development of functional or "usable" flexibility**. This entails challenging range of motion in a manner that closely mimics daily movement. Functional movement in daily activities and sports skills is often dynamic in nature.

• **Injury prevention**. Though there is insufficient scientific evidence to prove this assumption, most experts agree that increased ROM that is not excessive for a given joint decreases a tissue's resistance to stretch. Because of this, a person is less likely to incur injury because the maximum range (elastic limit) available to a tissue before soft tissue damage occurs will not likely be exceeded.

• **Increased blood supply, nutrients and joint synovial fluid**. Alternately holding and releasing sustained stretches increases tissue temperature (along with an adequate warm-up), circulation and nutrient delivery through the blood. Regular stretching decreases synovial fluid viscosity or thickness, which enables nutrients to be transported more readily to articular or hyaline cartilage. This change in qualitative aspects of synovial joint fluid may lead to a decrease in degenerative joint diseases and allow more freedom of movement at the joint.

• **Reduced muscular soreness**. Research indicates that slow, static stretching, performed after exercise, reduces or prevents delayed muscular soreness and enhances recovery from exercise (DeVries, 1961). Though the physiologic reason for this effect is far from clear, it may be partially attributed to the increase in muscle temperature, circulation, enhanced blood supply and nutrient delivery from the alternating tension and release experienced in the musculature during stretching activity.

• **Personal enjoyment, relaxation and reduced stress**. When conducted in the proper environment and with correct technique, stretching encourages muscular as well as mental relaxation. Though subjective, personal enjoyment and physical release through stretching can lead to a reduction in overall stress levels. Alternating tension and release on the muscle during stretching promotes optimal nutrition to the muscle, may decrease the accumulation of toxins in the muscles and reduces the likelihood of adaptive shortening or decreased flexibility in the muscle. It seems that these positive adaptations would lead to healthy, supple muscles that are more resistant to fatigue and injury.

The Anatomy of Flexibility

Flexibility is most easily introduced by defining it as the **range of motion (ROM)** available to a joint or joints. Healthy, or desired, flexibility should be viewed as a capacity to move freely in every *intended* direction. The movement should be confined to the joint's **functional range of motion (FROM)** or intended movement capabilities. This is different from the joint's normal ROM, because *normal* is not always healthy, nor adequate, for individual movement pattern needs.

Each joint in the body inherits an optimum FROM. For example, the knee joint was not intended to be used with circumduction (circular movement) movement patterns. Its natural movement pattern is characterized by a "hinge-like" action of about 135 degrees of knee flexion and zero to about 90 degrees of knee extension. However, this optimal range, at any joint, generally decreases with age, injuries and decreasing activity levels. Many of your clients may not be adequately addressing this important aspect of fitness in their workouts.

Connective tissues of the joint include cartilage, ligaments, tendons and muscle fascia or fascial sheath. **Cartilage** is often present between bony surfaces to present a degree of protection for bone surfaces by providing "padding" and shock absorption capabilities. The fibers in cartilage are more stretchable or "forgiving." This characteristic enhances its shock-absorbing capability.

Ligaments connect bone to bone and offer stability and integrity to joint structures in areas of the body such as the spine, knee and shoulder. **Tendons** connect muscles to bone. The force of muscle contraction is transferred via the tendinous attachment of the muscles to the skeletal system. This results in efficient bodily movement.

Muscle fascia is represented by 3 "layers" of fascia that "wrap" the muscle. **Endomysium** wraps individual muscle fibers or cells. The **perimysium** wraps groups or bundles of muscle fibers and the **epimysium** wraps the entire muscle. These various "layers" of fascia culminate in the tendons of the muscle. The muscle and its fascial layers are similar to the look of a twist-tied piece of candy. The candy's (muscle belly) wrappings (muscle fascia) culminate in twist ties (tendons), though it should be noted that neither the muscle's tendons or fibers are actually twisted. This image offers a good way to visualize the physical look of the muscle and connective tissue arrangement.

The physical properties of connective tissues determine flexibility at the joint. For example, ligaments and tendons are rich in the protein collagen. The fibers of these tissue are arranged in parallel and are closely "packed" together. This creates a high tensile strength and tissue that is designed to be non-stretchable or highly resistant to stretch.

Flexibility is **joint specific**: The degree of movement is specific to each joint. Being "flexible" in one joint does not influence flexibility in another joint. Johns and Wright (1962) identified specific limitations to degrees of motion about a joint. Joint shape (joint capsule) effectively limits motion by 47%. The joint cannot be altered unless injury occurs. The tendon limits motion by 10%, the muscle fascia limits it by 41% and the skin by 2%. However, connective or "soft" tissue can be altered long term. It is the elasticity, which means a measure of a soft tissue's *resistance* to stretch or *lack* of elasticity, that allows improvement in range of motion, or predisposes a client to injury if he engages in improper flexibility training.

Flexibility is influenced by a variety of factors, some of which may be changed, while others are unable to be altered, or if altered could lead to injury. These include:

- genetic inheritance
- the joint structure itself
- tension (partial contraction) in the muscle
- connective tissue elasticity within the muscles
- tendons
- ligaments
- skin surrounding the joint
- neuromuscular influence (from sensory organs such as the muscle spindle and Golgi tendon organ (GTO)

Flexibility is generally *limited* by 4 important factors:

1. The elastic limits of the ligaments and tendons crossing the joint.
2. The elasticity of the muscle fibers themselves and muscle fascia which "encases" single muscle fibers, groups of muscle fibers and the entire muscle.
3. The bone and joint structure.
4. The skin.

What Is Being Stretched During Flexibility Training?

Muscle fascia's *lack* of resistance to stretch makes it the most significant, changeable, limiting factor for gains in flexibility. It accounts for 41% (Johns and Wright, 1962) of the resistance to stretch or range of motion. Muscle fascia gives muscle the ability to change length. Muscle itself can be stretched to 150% of its length if relaxed and uninhibited by muscle fascia (McArdle et al., 1991).

For example, a muscle in its relaxed state of 10 inches in length could be stretched to 15 inches of length abruptly with no injurious effects. It should be noted that soft tissue components of a muscle begin to break down if the muscle is stretched beyond 160% of its normal length (Taylor et al., 1990). More is not better! The fascial sheath, which literally holds or wraps the muscle together, has both elastic—which consists of high and low degrees of elasticity—and inelastic properties (Kravitz et al., 1993). Based on these facts, it becomes apparent that the limitation to stretch is less affected by muscle fiber characteristics and inelastic fascial properties—and that elastic muscle fascia tissue greatly affects available range of motion.

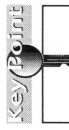

> The most modifiable and greatest improvement in flexibility seems to be related to the ability of your stretching program to target the muscle's fascial sheathes.

Muscle fascia's physical properties are not unlike that of candy taffy. When it is warm, it is "stretchable." When it is cold, it is brittle and breakable. Because of these physical characteristics, a participant should warm the body first and hold sustained stretches so that the muscle fascia can literally cool in a new and lengthened position. This is another excellent visualization that you can create for clients to help them better understand the goals of their stretching programs.

Vocabulary of Flexibility

For the sake of clarity, let's define several terms. **Distensibility** is a term that is used to describe stretchable, stretching or stretchability, as opposed to inextensible or non-stretchable. Muscle fascia is very distensible or stretchable as opposed to ligaments, which are not.

Elasticity is often confused with the term stretchable or distensible. Elasticity is a measure of a tissue's *resistance* to stretch. Ligaments and tendons have a high resistance to stretch and are characterized as having a high degree of elasticity. Muscle fascia, on the other hand, has a low-degree of elasticity, is distensible and easily stretched. Your ability to differentiate the term "elasticity" from "stretchable" is most important when reading and interpreting scientific literature.

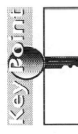

A tissue that has a high elasticity has a high resistance to stretch.

After the stretching force is removed during an **elastic** stretch, the tissue being stretched is able to recover or return to its original length. A **plastic** stretch is non-recoverable and results in "permanent" elongation of the soft tissue being stretched. **Elastic tissue** consists largely of muscle fibers, fascia, ligaments or cartilage. Muscle fibers, cartilage and ligaments will recover quickly from the force of a stretch or impact that does not exceed their elastic limit, while the plastic or permanent "deformation" of the connective tissue framework (muscle fascia) might remain with proper stretching. Whether this return to pre-stretched length is "good" or "bad" depends on what tissue is being stretched.

A tissue's **elastic limit** refers to the smallest amount of stress (stretching force) necessary to produce permanent or non-recoverable lengthening of a soft tissue. Once a tissue's elastic limit is exceeded, a return to its original length is not possible, even after the stretching force is removed.

Beyond the elastic limit, internal damage occurs in various soft-tissue protein arrangements. For example, exceeding the elastic limit of ligaments cause damage to their collagenous fibers. This is referred to as a **sprain**. Damage to muscle fibers or cells, caused by exceeding their elastic limit, is referred to as a muscle **strain**. There are varying degrees of sprains and strains that range from first degree or minor damage to the extreme of tissue rupture, or a complete tearing of the tissue involved.

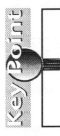

The results from exceeding the elastic limit of muscle fascia are entirely different from exceeding those of ligaments, tendons or muscles.

What determines if elongation of tissue is recoverable (elastic stretch) or non-recoverable (permanent or plastic stretch)? Five important factors influence the outcome:

1. type of force

2. mechanics of the stretch and exercise position

3. duration of the stretch

4. intensity of the stretch

5. temperature of the muscle during the stretch

Whether a stretch is productive and increases ROM without increasing risk for injury depends on the tissue being stretched, as influenced by proper or improper stretching procedure.

The Physiology Behind Stretch

Proprioception is a term that defines the normal, ongoing awareness of the position, balance and movement of one's body or any of its parts (Blakiston's Medical Dictionary). This sensory feedback is regulated by proprioceptors or sensory organs. **Sensory organs** relay information via the central nervous system, giving an individual a sense of body or limb position in space. This is also referred to as **kinesthetic awareness**. Sensory organs, for example, allow a person to predict the degree of elbow flexion or extension even if the individual does not have the advantage of visual feedback.

Two sensory organs, the muscle spindle and the Golgi tendon organ (GTO), have implications for flexibility training. The **muscle spindles** are located between the muscle fibers or muscle cells. They are sensitive to the resting length of the muscle, changes in the length of the muscle and the speed at which lengthening occurs. Muscle spindles help the body maintain tone and posture, and they present a defense mechanism, through the stretch reflex, that can help prevent muscle injury.

If the muscles are stretched too fast, the spindles initiate the **stretch reflex** (also known as myotatic stretch reflex). This causes the muscle group to reflexively shorten and protect itself from being overstretched. If an attempt is made to elongate muscle fascia while the muscle itself is shortening, the risk of injury to muscle fiber is obvious. The force produced by the stretch reflex is proportional to the force or speed of the stretch. Conversely, if the stretch is performed slowly and controlled, the stretch reflex may be avoided or be of low intensity.

The **Golgi tendon organs (GTOs),** located in the muscle tendon, or musculo-tendinous junction, are sensitive to force production and monitor tension in the muscle. When their thresholds are exceeded, their response causes the affected muscle(s) to relax. This is referred to as an inverse myotatic reflex or **inverse stretch reflex**. The force necessary to stimulate the GTOs is much greater than the force needed to activate a muscle spindle and resultant stretch reflex.

The GTOs' signal to relax overrides the muscle spindles' signal to contract, which relaxes the affected muscle group.

Reciprocal innervation is a reflex inhibition that involves agonist and antagonistic muscles. When a muscle group contracts, its opposing or antagonistic muscle group reflexively relaxes. Reciprocal innervation is a technique that can also be used in conjunction with stretching procedures, including PNF and active stretching, to promote muscle relaxation and optimal stretching conditions to increase ROM.

For example, if the goal is to stretch the hamstring group from a supine position, tightening the quadriceps would cause the hamstring muscles to relax because of reciprocal innervation. In general motor movement, reciprocal innervation is important because it allows for the occurrence of coordinated motor movement. During stretching, it is a reflex mechanism that can be taken advantage of to create a relaxed muscle. Potentially, this will allow for more effective stretching to take place.

Static Flexibility Compared to Dynamic Flexibility

Forces responsible for stretch can be broadly categorized as either active or passive. An **active** stretch occurs when an agonist muscle(s) moves a body part through a range of motion, and the force provided by the active contraction of musculature stretches the opposing (antagonist) muscles. For example, if the elbow is flexed, the contracting biceps actively stretches the opposing or triceps musculature.

Passive stretches occur when outside forces assist in the stretching process. Gravity, momentum or motion, a trainer applying passive force to another individual or force provided by some part of one's own body (pulling your leg forward into a hamstring stretch from a supine position) are examples of passive forces contributing to muscular and fascial elongation.

Two basic categories identify *how* flexibility is gained. **Static flexibility** generally refers to a combination of active and passive movements that lengthen the muscles and fascia in a *controlled* manner. Once lengthened, the position is sustained for at least several seconds.

Dynamic flexibility involves the use of momentum to gain an advantage in "overstretching" an area of the body. This is traditionally referred to as ballistic stretching. Though there is sufficient reasoning to justify this type of stretching in elite athletic participation, the risk versus effectiveness still should be carefully examined.

A professional tennis player needs sufficient dynamic flexibility in the shoulder to slam a tennis serve 120 mph. Likewise, a recreational exerciser and mother needs sufficient dynamic flexibility in various joints of the body to play softball on the weekends and care for her children. Normal ROM attained through static stretching may be sufficient to meet the "dynamic" needs of mom, whereas dynamic flexibility training may be required to meet the demands imposed on the body of a professional tennis player.

Hardy and Jones (1986) suggest that the use of dynamic flexibility is probably important in explosive speed events. This might include world-class gymnastics, a 100-meter track sprint, aerobics competitions, dance or diving. Hardy and Jones' study is not a confirmation that dynamic flexibility, and the associated ballistic movement, is the best method to improve flexibility. Rather, it is simply a recognition that ballistic movements are contained in these sports.

Hartley O'Brien (1980) defined active flexibility as the "maximum, unassisted range of movement." Thus, active flexibility can be improved by increasing the strength of the agonist and/or decreasing resistance to movement in the antagonist. Proprioceptive neuromuscular facilitation (PNF) stretching is a technique that can do this, which is why PNF stretching is very popular with athletes whose events require dynamic flexibility. PNF stretching is an advanced form of flexibility training that takes advantage of sensory organ response to facilitate flexibility gains. (See sidebar this chapter, Types of Stretching.)

However, it cannot be overemphasized that more aggressive attempts to increase dynamic flexibility should be met with careful scrutiny when being used with the general population. The risk of injury may greatly increase, while the gains for most clients will be about the same using sustained static stretching.

In fact, many experts suggest that abrupt stretching may lead to injury. That is why most fitness experts generally recommend static stretching programs that:

• gradually increase ROM, and

• hold stretching positions with static force (no bouncing) applied during the stretch.

Quick Index:

Chapter 17, PNF stretching and other techniques

Types of Stretching

There are 5 types of stretching techniques available:

1. Static Stretching.

Static stretching is defined as a controlled stretch, held at the point of mild tension for about 10-60 seconds. This places the muscle in a lengthened position.

2. Dynamic or Ballistic Stretching.

Dynamic or ballistic stretching uses bouncing, jerking or abrupt movements to gain momentum into the posture to facilitate overstretching.

3. Active Stretching.

Voluntary, unassisted movement which requires strength and muscular contraction of the agonist muscle (prime mover). For example, in a supine position the hip flexors can contract actively to draw the leg forward and the hip into flexion. The agonist is unassisted by external (passive) forces. The purpose of the stretch is to actively stretch the hamstring group by using only the muscular effort and strength provided by the agonist hip flexors.

4. Passive Stretching.

Passive stretching occurs when movements are accomplished through the use of an outside (external) force such as that provided by a partner, exerting pull on your own body part with another limb, gravity or momentum.

5. PNF Stretching.

PNF stretching works by first putting the targeted muscle on stretch and then generating a maximal force in the muscle being stretched. This procedure can activate a sensory organ called the Golgi tendon organ, which causes the affected muscle to relax. A relaxed muscle will more easily allow the muscle fascia to be elongated, thus creating a stretching environment where excellent gains in flexibility can be realized. PNF stretching can also involve a variation of the above methods.

Table 12. Types of Stretching

The types of stretching can further be categorized as to their relative risk. This table illustrates relative risk based on muscular force and tension produced with each approach.

Static	Low Force	Controlled Tension	Low Risk
Ballistic (dynamic)	High Force	High Tension	High Risk
Active	Low Force	Low Tension	Low Risk
Passive	Higher Potential Force	Higher Potential Tension	Higher Potential Risk
Controlled Passive	Low Force	Low Tension	Low Risk
PNF (high skill)	High Force	High Tension	High Risk

An excellent approach to stretching is to use a *combination* of active, controlled passive and static stretching techniques. Using this approach, an active contraction is initiated with agonist muscles. This begins the stretch process and defines an individual's active range of motion (AROM). Once the AROM is determined, this gives you a better idea of a client's elastic limit and associated constraints to safe movement. This step may, or may not, be followed by an application of an outside or passive force that is used to enhance movement through a greater ROM. And finally, a static and sustained stretch is held.

It should now be obvious—there is no one, best way to stretch. Using a variety of stretching methods improves flexibility. The goal of a client, current fitness level, individual limitations to ROM, the type of activity the participant is regularly active in and risk versus effectiveness must carefully be considered.

Flexibility Adaptations

Flexibility adaptations occur both immediately and over longer periods of time. That is because proper stretching involves sensory organs and connective tissue adaptations that may result in both elastic and plastic (permanent) changes.

Acute adaptations that can occur during stretching are the stretch reflex (muscle spindles), inverse stretch reflex (GTOs) and reciprocal innervation. A muscle spindle's effect can be neutralized during a stretch if the stretch is maintained. Over time, with repeated stretching, its threshold or point at which it is activated can be increased, making it less likely to "fire" and create tension in the muscle fibers.

Long-term adaptations or chronic changes relate more to plastic (permanent) elongation of muscle fascia. Constant application of appropriate force leads to progressive "creep" or change in length of fascia. This is a time-dependent mechanism that occurs as the muscle spindles' discharge is decreased. Permanent deformation of the muscle fascia (i.e., the candy taffy) occurs when the muscle and fascia are held in a lengthened position for sustained time periods. For permanent elongation, fascia responds best to low force, long duration holds and warm muscles.

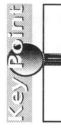

> It has been well established that increases in intramuscular temperature through a proper warm-up decrease viscosity, or a tissue's resistance to stretch (Sapega, 1981).

There is a multitude of circumstances that can add to or detract from the success of a flexibility training program. These include but are not limited to: age, exercise, inactivity, intramuscular temperature, body type and gender. According to Kravitz and Kosich (1993), there does not appear to be a body build that consistently represents "good flexibility."

Several authors report that females tend to be more flexible, in general, than males (Alter, 1988; and Holland, 1968 reported by Kravitz and Kosich, 1993). Though conclusive evidence is lacking, a female's tendency to be more flexible than most males in the pelvic region may be related to the female's role in childbearing. Beyond these issues, it seems that a regular commitment to exercise is the most influential variable that can affect flexibility gains or losses.

Age and Inactivity

Adults lose significant amounts of flexibility as they age. In many cases this loss of mobility is more related to inactivity than any "inevitable" aging process. Exercise contributes significantly to joint stability and flexibility maintenance (Spirduso, 1995). Spirduso reported that stretching and progressive resistance training exercise produced the same percentage of improvement in ROM of elderly subjects aged 63-88 years as it did in younger subjects, aged 15-19 years.

The greatest potential for increases in flexibility probably occurs between the ages of 7 and 12. Significant changes occur in connective tissue during the mid-20s that begin to affect the ease at which one maintains or gains ROM. Alter (1988) reported that aging increases both the diameter of collagen fibers and the number of intermolecular cross-links. This age-related change in connective tissues makes soft tissue more resistant to stretch or plastic deformation.

Because hydration of the musculature decreases as one ages, the delivery of nutrients and joint lubrication also decrease. This has the effect of creating musculature and soft tissue that is more susceptible to injury. However, the natural decrease in flexibility that occurs with aging is relatively small when compared to the influences of an inactive lifestyle. Functional ROM and movement options at all of the joints of the body can be readily preserved with a regular program of stretching and movement-related activities, including full ROM strength training.

The Bridge

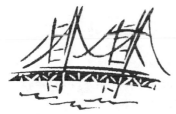

Stretching muscle fascia and protecting other connective tissue from injury is critical to an effective stretching program. When a client's goal is health and fitness, functional movement is the goal. There are 5 different types of stretching, and all must be evaluated for risk. Most clients will benefit from a combination of stretching methods.

References and Recommended Reading

Alter, M.J. (1988) *Science of Stretching*. Human Kinetics Publishers, Champaign, IL.

Alter, M.J. (1990) *Sport Stretch*. Human Kinetics Publishers, Champaign, IL.

Corbin, C.V. and Noble, L. (1980) Flexibility: a major component of physical fitness. *Journal of Physical Education and Recreation*, 51, (6).

DeVries, H.A. (1961) Electromyographic observations of the effects of static stretching upon muscular distress. *Research Quarterly for Exercise and Sport*, 32, pp. 468-79.

Etnyre, B.R. and Lee, E.J. (1987) Comments on proprioceptive neuromuscular facilitation stretching techniques. *Research Quarterly for Exercise and Sport*, 58, 184 8.

Francis, Peter, and Francis, L., (1988) *If it hurts, don't do it*. Prima Publishing, Rocklin, CA.

Hardy L. and Jones, D. (1986) Dynamic flexibility and proprioceptive neuromuscular facilitation. *Research Quarterly*, 57, pp. 105-153.

Hartley O'Brien, S.J. (1980) Six mobilization exercises for active range of hip flexion. *Research Quarterly*, 51 (4), pp. 625-35.

Holland, G.J. (1968) The physiology of flexibility: A review of the literature. *Kinesiology Review*.

Hutton, R.S. (1992) Neuromuscular Basis of Stretching Exercises. In P.V. Komi (ed.) *Strength and Power in Sport*, pp. 29-38. Blackwell Scientific Publications, Cambridge, MA.

Johns, R. J., and Wright, V. (1962) Relative importance of various tissues in joint stiffness. *Journal of Applied Physiology*, 17(5), 824-28.

Kravitz, Len, and Kosich, Daniel (1993) Flexibility: A comprehensive research review and program design guide. *IDEA Today*, June, pp. 42-49.

McAtee, Robert (1993) *Facilitated Stretching*. Human Kinetics Publishers, Champaign, IL.

Moore, M. and Hutton R. (1989) Electromyographic investigation of muscle stretching techniques. *Medicine and Science in Sports and Exercise*, 12 (5), pp. 322-29.

Murphy, R. D. (1991) A critical look at static stretching: Are we doing our patients harm? *Chiropractic Sports Medicine*, Vol. 5, 3, pp. 67-70.

Osternig, L.R. (1990) Differential responses to proprioceptive neuromuscular facilitation (PNF) stretch techniques. *Medicine and Science in Sports and Exercise*, 22, 1, pp. 106-11.

Plowman, Sharon (1992) Physical activity, physical fitness and low back pain, *Exercise and Sport Sciences Reviews*, vol. 20. pp. 221-42.

Sapega, A., et al. (1981) Biophysical factors in range of motion exercise. **Physician and Sportsmedicine,** 9 (12), pp. 57-64.

Siff, M.C. (1990) **The Science of Flexibility and Stretching.** Published: School of Mechanical Engineering, University of Witwatersrand, Johannesburg, South Africa.

Siff, M.C. (1992) **Proceedings at the International IDEA Research Symposium.**

Siff, M.C. (1993) **Super Training: A Textbook on the Biomechanics and Physiology of Strength Conditioning for Sport.** Published: School of Mechanical Engineering, University of Witwatersrand, Johannesburg, South Africa.

Smith, Bob (1993) **Advanced Fitness Teacher's Manual.** Published: Loughborough University- Ludoe Publications, pp. 22-30.

Spirduso, Waneen (1995) **Physical Dimensions of Aging.** Champaign, IL: Human Kinetics Publishers.

Stephens, R. (1992) **IDEA Educational Conference,** Fort Worth, TX.

Sullivan, M.G., Dejulia, J.J. and Worrell, T.W. (1992) Effect of pelvic position and stretching method on hamstring muscle flexibility, **Medicine and Science in Sports and Exercise,** 24, 12, pp. 1383-9.

Taylor, D. C. et al. (1990) Viscoelastic properties of muscle-tendon units: The biomechanical effects of stretching. **American Journal of Sports Medicine,** 18, 3, pp. 300-09.

Voss D., Ionta, M. and Myers, B., (1985) **Proprioceptive neuromuscular facilitation: Patterns and techniques,** 3rd edition, Harper and Row, Philadelphia, PA.

Wallin, D., Ekblom, B., Grahn, R. and Nordenberg, T. (1985) Improvement of muscle flexibility: A comparison between two techniques. **American Journal of Sports Medicine,** 13, pp. 263- 268.

CHAPTER 9

A PHYSIOLOGICAL BASIS FOR WARM-UP AND COOL-DOWN

Have you ever caught yourself paying less than sufficient attention to a client who is warming up or cooling down? The warm-up and cool-down are both important and productive parts of any workout.

Physiologically, the gentler, steady movements used in warm-up and cool-down prepare the client for successful activity, and allow for a comfortable return following the effort. Plus, warm-up and cool-down are productive times to effectively communicate and motivate your client. These quiet times are perfect for Step 2 of gathering information and Step 9 for success and adherence. While your client is training at lesser-intensity, you can update her on new health and fitness information, talk about exercise technique and discuss her diet, nutritional program and any other concerns or interests she might have.

Warm-up and cool-down are too often left out of client programs. Yet, resistance training and cardiorespiratory activities require *both*. Why are warm-ups and cool-downs so important to a safe and effective workout?

Quick Index:

Physiological Benefits of Warm-Ups

There are several possible mechanisms by which warm-up could improve performance as a result of increases in blood flow and increases in muscle and core temperature. (Sources: ACE Manual, 1991; ACSM, 1991; Giese, 1988; McArdle et al., 1991.) What can warm-up do?

1. Permit a gradual increase in metabolic requirements. This enhances cardiorespiratory performance and is less stressful to your client. Also, hemoglobin releases oxygen to the working muscles more readily at higher temperatures. This facilitates increased oxygen utilization (extraction) by the muscles, making physical performance more effective and efficient.

2. Prevent the premature onset of blood lactic acid accumulation and premature fatigue. A progressive warm-up prevents your clients from going too quickly from low intensity to high intensity by increasing blood flow through active tissues. For example, the working muscles represent active tissue, and as the specific or local vascular bed (capillaries serving the muscles in demand) dilates because of progressive increases in exercise intensity and the resultant increase in blood perfusion to the exercising muscle, the body can provide most of the energy requirements aerobically.

Blood flow increases because higher temperatures in the body's core and its musculature cause vasodilation (opening) of the blood vessels. During warm-up, blood travels from the body's core to the working muscles. More blood availability means more oxygen and nutrients to fuel exercise and muscle contraction, insignificant accumulations of blood lactate and efficient removal of metabolic byproduct production. This includes lactic acid (blood lactate), carbon dioxide and water.

3. Cause a gradual increase in muscle temperature. This reduces the likelihood of soft-tissue (muscle fascia or muscle) injury and increases the effectiveness of sustained stretching. Muscle tissue and fascia become more stretchable, and this reduces the risk of overstretching or tearing muscle fibers, tendons and connective tissues. This is especially important to your clients who are involved in activities that require greater range-of-motion demands.

Increased muscle temperature may also allow for greater mechanical efficiency because of lowered viscous resistance within the muscles. Viscosity (thickness) of the muscle protoplasm decreases, allowing the protein filaments (actin and myosin), which make up the muscle fibers, to contract easily without resistance. Warmed-up muscles move faster and generate force more effectively than "cold" muscles. Warm-up also facilitates joint lubrication, allowing for easier movement.

4. Enhance neural transmission for muscle contraction and motor-unit recruitment. Motor skills improve at higher temperatures because nerve impulses travel faster. This enhances the speed of muscle contraction and force generated, along with muscle relaxation. Sports and activities that require coordination, reaction time and agility benefit greatly from a warm-up.

5. Provide an "early alert" for screening potential musculoskeletal or cardiorespiratory problems. These may worsen at higher intensities of exercise.

It's obvious that warm-up accomplishes important changes in the body which may reduce the risk of injury. Graduated, low-level, aerobic exercise is essential for maximizing safe and efficient movement for most participants. The warm-up should progressively increase heart rate, blood pressure, oxygen consumption, the dilation of the blood vessels and *decrease* the elasticity (or the tissue's resistance to stretch) of the active muscles and fascial tissue. Warming up increases the temperature of the muscle and connective tissue, likely reducing the risk of soft-tissue injury, as well as facilitating flexibility gains. It may also reduce the stress placed on the heart and lessen the likelihood of heart attack in susceptible individuals. Warming up may make the exercise session seem more comfortable to your client and possibly more effective.

Since it is nearly impossible to design an experiment with participants to resolve whether warm-up definitively reduces the likelihood of injury or really improves subsequent performance, you won't find overwhelming scientific evidence to support warming up. Do not let this deter you.

⸺ A Physiological Basis for Warm-Up and Cool-Down ⸺

Engaging in some type of physical activity prior to vigorous exercise is generally accepted as a valid and useful procedure by scientists, coaches, athletes, personal trainers and the average person who is active.

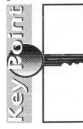

> Rather than demand substantial evidence to justify using a warm-up, the most prudent approach is to wait until there is substantial evidence justifying its elimination. A brief warm-up is certainly a comfortable and prudent way to lead up to more vigorous exercise.

Quick Index:

Psychological Considerations

Sports enthusiasts at all levels often consider some prior activity to prepare them mentally for their event or activity. Some evidence supports the contention that a warm-up specific to the activity itself improves the necessary skill and coordination. Consequently, sports that require accuracy, timing and precise movements generally benefit from some type of specific warm-up or "formal" preliminary practice.

There is also a feeling that prior exercise, especially before a strenuous effort, gradually prepares a person to go "all out" without fear of injury. Examples include: preparing yourself to run your fastest race and accelerating immediately to your race-pace off the starting line, the ritual warm-up throws of a baseball pitcher preparing to enter a game, the on-deck batter's swinging of a weighted bat, and a gymnast or aerobic competitor warming up away from the main event on apparatus specifically related to their soon-to-be maximal effort.

Warm-Up Theory Into Practice

A general warm-up may involve rhythmic and continuous movement, large-muscle group involvement and calisthenics exercises that are usually unrelated to the specific neuromuscular action of the activity that is to follow. A general warm-up will often precede an activity-specific warm-up. An **activity-specific warm-up**, which reflects the specificity principle, provides a skill rehearsal. Swinging a baseball bat or tennis racket are examples. Rehearsing resistance training movements with light resistance is another example of an activity-specific warm-up.

Passive warm-up techniques may use massage and heat applications. However, external techniques such as heat packs or sauna are less likely to warm deep muscles. In fact, they may be counterproductive. When surface temperature of the skin is increased, blood vessels near the skin surface dilate and divert large amounts of blood to the skin, rather than working muscles.

The warm-up should be gradual and of sufficient intensity to increase muscle and core temperature without causing fatigue or reducing energy stores. This consideration is highly individualized. Adequate warm-up for an Olympic athlete in a running event would totally exhaust the average recreational participant.

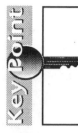

> **Gradual** means about 3-5 minutes, the time necessary for achieving steady-rate.

Warming up the body allows the cardiorespiratory system to adjust blood flow effectively from the abdominal area to the active muscles, where the need for oxygen is increasing in response to the exercise. This blood shunt is accomplished by vasoconstriction in arteries which supply blood to the viscera (gut) and vasodilation in arteries which deliver blood to the active muscles. If 3-5 minutes of gradual warm-up is not done, heart rate will quickly rise in an attempt to supply adequate oxygen. A near maximal heart rate may be reached if an intense pace is attempted too soon.

Increase **intensity** by elevating resting heart rates of 40-75 beats per minute (bpm) to about 90-120 bpm before moving on to higher intensity aerobic exercise. On the revised 10-point Borg scale for rating perceived exertion (RPE), a warm-up builds to 3, which indicates a "moderate" effort.

Thermal describes the temperature of working muscles, as heat is produced from energy production. Temperature of muscle tissue rises about 3.6 Fahrenheit degrees during the warm-up, which should produce sweating in about 3-5 minutes. However, monitoring sweat is an imprecise gauge, as many factors influence sweat response. These include individual sweat response, humidity and the temperature of the exercise environment.

Duration depends on the activity your client is participating in, the level and intensity (5K personal-best running effort or a moderate walk) of the activity and her current level of fitness. A *minimum* of 3-5 minutes is recommended for any activity. To reap the possible benefits from increased body temperature, it's ideal to begin activity within several minutes of the end of the warm-up. However, some benefit of warm-up may be retained for up to an hour.

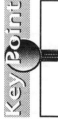

> Older exercisers, beginners, overweight individuals, pregnant women and cardiac patients may need a more gradual and longer 10- to 15-minute warm-up for a safe transition to more intense exercise.

The warm-up **activity** should move through an easy range of motion and never beyond a point of gentle tension or strain. Keep your client's movements fluid, rhythmic and controlled. This type of approach works well for resistance training warm-up, too. Attempt to use specific muscles in a way that mimics the anticipated activity and gradually brings about the range of motion (ROM) necessary for the ensuing activity.

An additional component of warm-up may be the addition of flexibility exercises *after* the progressive aerobic warm-up. Try to match the flexibility exercises to the demands of the upcoming activity. For example, extreme ranges of motion are not necessary prior to a fitness walking program. In this case, a warm-up without stretching will be adequate. However, if your client is going to perform a 5K race at her fastest walking or running pace or participate in an aggressive match of singles tennis, a more thorough warm-up and stretching segment may accommodate the energy demands, ROM and biomechanical stresses of high-intensity activity.

If the goal is to concentrate on flexibility gains, do so only after an extensive warm-up (15-20 minutes), or after warming up and participating in your client's chosen activity. Stretching may take place any time *after* your client is adequately warmed up.

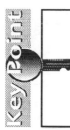

Stretching is *not* a good warm-up. Forcing range of motion when muscles are "cold" is less effective at increasing range of motion safely and can cause injury.

Quick Index:

Special Cases: Sudden Strenuous Exercise and Cardiovascular Response

Do you have clients who have heart disease or some other limitation related to the heart and vascular system? What about clients involved in occupations and sports requiring sudden bursts of high-intensity activity? Numerous studies (i.e., Barnard et al., 1973) have evaluated the effects of warm-up exercise on cardiovascular response to sudden and strenuous exercise. Remember, strenuous exercise is relative to an individual's fitness level. Walking at 3 mph may be strenuous for an unfit person.

Barnard and colleagues discovered that the adaptation of coronary blood flow to a sudden and vigorous cardiac workload is not instantaneous, and that transient myocardial ischemia (poor oxygen supply to the heart) may occur in apparently healthy and fit individuals. The effect of prior warm-up (at least 2 minutes of easy jogging for example) on the electrocardiogram (ECG) and blood pressure response appears to be significant in establishing a more favorable relationship between myocardial oxygen supply and demand.

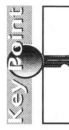

Warm-up is especially important for those who have cardiovascular problems that limit the heart's oxygen supply. Brief, prior exercise most likely provides for more optimal blood pressure and hormonal adjustment at the onset of strenuous exercise.

For clients with these circumstances, warm-up has the potential to:

• reduce the myocardial work load and thus the myocardial oxygen requirement.

• provide adequate coronary blood flow in sudden, high-intensity exercise that follows such a warm-up.

Your immediate thought might be, "But I don't work with high-risk clientele." However, regardless of how careful you may screen your clients, there is the possibility that one may have undiagnosed heart disease. There are a myriad of reasons for warming up. It's smart to add this one to your list!

Quick Index:

Chapter 3, heart disease

The Physiological Rationale for Cool-Down

The purpose of the **cool-down** is to slowly decrease heart rate and overall metabolism elevated during your client's workout. An adequate cool-down gives your client a psychological break to savor the great feelings of post-exercise accomplishment or "glow." What specifically can cool-down do?

1. Help in faster removal of lactic acid and lessen the *potential* for post-exercise muscle soreness. In normal exercise situations, lactic acid itself does not cause or contribute significantly to muscle soreness. Any soreness is probably a result of all-out or unaccustomed effort. In the presence of oxygen during recovery or lessened intensity, lactic acid becomes an energy source. But high-intensity exercise *associated* with lactic acid production often *does* create delayed-onset muscle soreness (DOMS). Soreness from DOMS is caused by actual damage to, or disruption of, the body's muscle-cell membranes.

Remember that delayed soreness usually occurs from micro-trauma of the tissues, dependent on the type and intensity of exercise. However, there is evidence that lactic acid may irritate tissue much like a piece of meat would deteriorate if suspended in a glass of carbonated beverage. Both situations represent very acidic environments and could contribute to breakdown of tissue (Smith, 1993). This finding may be especially relevant to an athlete's training program when she engages in, and repeats, high levels of anaerobic effort over a number of days, weeks and/or years.

2. Reduce any tendency toward post-exercise fainting and dizziness. The rhythmic "milking" action of muscular contraction and consequent compression of the veins is critical to ensure adequate venous return and reduce the likelihood of fainting or creating unnecessary stress to the heart. If blood is pooled in the lower extremities (**venous pooling**) from a sudden stop in exercise, the high hydrostatic forces cause a decreased venous return and blood pressure declines.

At the same time, the heart rate accelerates, which means the heart muscle needs more blood and oxygen at a time when its supply may be compromised. Having blood in the chambers of the heart does nothing in terms of supplying oxygen to the heart muscle. To nourish the heart muscle, blood must first be ejected from the left ventricle. With each heart beat, the driving force of the heart pushes a portion of blood out of the heart's left ventricle and into the coronary arteries. An adequate oxygen supply is critical for the myocardium, because unlike skeletal muscle, this tissue has an extremely limited ability to generate energy anaerobically.

3. May reduce the likelihood of some muscle soreness if stretching is added. By preventing muscle spasms or involuntary contractions of the muscles, soreness may be reduced.

4. Help lower blood levels of adrenaline. Adrenaline that lingers in the bloodstream can stress the heart. The continuation of mild exercise into recovery may minimize any possible negative effects on heart function because of elevated catecholamines epinephrine and norepinephrine. These adrenaline-like hormones affect the body's response to increasing quantity and intensity of exercise, and it is observed that their levels increase after exercise (McArdle et al., 1991; Dimsdale, 1987).

What happens if you do not cool down? After moderate or vigorous exercise, depending on your fitness level and body position:

- blood pressure decreases
- less blood returns to the heart (venous return)
- stroke volume decreases

Because of these physiologic adjustments, there is an increased chance that the heart or brain could be deprived of necessary oxygen, resulting in dizziness, fainting or a cardiac event. A **cardiac event** is associated with heart-attack symptoms that can include chest pains, angina or an actual heart attack (myocardial infarction, which means death of heart muscle tissue).

Quick Index:

Chapter 3, how the heart works
Chapter 7, delayed-onset muscle soreness

Applying Cool-Down Strategies

An **active cool-down** of moderate to mild exercise means that clients *continue* exercising at an intensity lower than they performed at during the main body of their cardiorespiratory conditioning workout. This level will facilitate blood flow through the vascular network (including the heart) during recovery. With a proper active cool-down, your heart will work less (fewer beats per minute) and require less oxygen. This situation is more likely to prevent an undiagnosed "cardiac event" or put unnecessary physiological or psychological stress on your client.

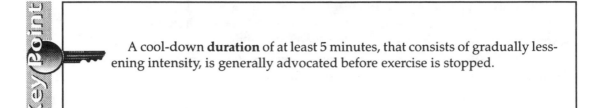

A cool-down **duration** of at least 5 minutes, that consists of gradually lessening intensity, is generally advocated before exercise is stopped.

This recommendation makes sense because it reduces the chances of abrupt physiologic alterations, especially those involving the heart. Any sudden cessation of activity is more likely to stress the cardiovascular system.

Using a low-level, rhythmic **activity** during the cool-down allows the body to reverse the blood shunt, or shift, that occurred as your client began her activity to help ensure adequate blood flow to the working muscles.

A "normal" reduction of exercise **intensity** will be reflected by the return of exercise heart rate—rather quickly—to lower levels and eventually to the individual's resting heart-rate level. When monitored accurately, heart rate is a very good indicator of her body's recovery status and is an excellent reflection of your client's current level of effort.

Encourage your client to attain a **recovery heart rate** of approximately 120 beats per minute (bpm) in about 3 minutes. After about 5 minutes, a heart rate of around 100 bpm should be attained. A "quick" recovery is dependent on your client's current fitness level, the intensity of effort for the preceding workout, and the appropriateness and intensity of the cool-down activity.

Quick Index:

Chapter 6, monitoring exercise intensity

Encouraging Compliance

A cool-down period is an effective time to ask your client to personally acknowledge the tangible and quite significant accomplishment(s) she has just achieved. It is also a good time to have your client ask, "How do I feel at this very instant?" Most feel at least "better" when compared to their feelings before the session began, and many "feel wonderful." A very few remain just outright ornery and combative!

Regardless, don't let your clients cheat their bodies and their "heads" (mental health) out of a cool-down. Too many times, your client's daily accomplishments can be lost because of a focus on long-term goals. Before she jumps back into a stressful and harried routine, give your client a chance to smile and say, "You know, that was a pretty good workout and I feel great!" Now, she can dive into the shower and tackle the day head on!

This is also your chance to assess each client's current feelings and to talk. If you always bring your discussions back to how your activities are important to the client's goals, there will be little resistance to your program design approach.

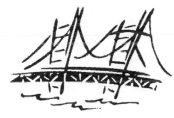

The Bridge

Warm-up and cool-down not only reduce the potential for premature fatigue and post-exercise fatigue, they reduce the risk of exercise-related injuries as well. A proper warm-up may also optimize performance and/or health and fitness gains. Because exercise may "feel" more comfortable and be less of a stress to the body after warming up and cooling down, both of these factors can contribute to high levels of client motivation and consequent exercise compliance.

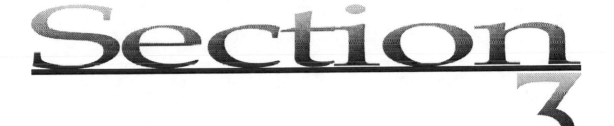

Section 3

Bridging Science Into Program Design

"Hitherto we have been taught to believe that present-day methods were all that could be desired, but the sooner we question this and discover something in advance, the better for all of us."

Arthur Newton (1949)

CHAPTER 10

PROGRAM PLANNING

The questions, "How much exercise is enough?" and "What type of exercise is best for developing and maintaining fitness?" are probably frequently asked by your clients. You might ask, "How can I devise a training program that improves the client's physiologic systems in a time-effective way?"

These are the questions you'll need to answer for Step 2 of program design—physical programming. This is where you look at your client's goals and integrate them with your knowledge. Your physical programming will determine if your client is successful and able to maintain a lifelong exercise program.

The training program of most of your clients is controlled by a balance between their "wants" and their "health and fitness needs." Your clients' "wants" can be identified by requests like, "I'd like to lose weight off my thighs," or "I'd like to feel better and knock off these love-handles." Maybe they tell you that they would like to exercise on a specific piece of exercise equipment, in a particular manner.

The first step will give you the information you need to understand your clients' goals, and really know who they are. In my observation, one of the biggest reasons trainers lose clients is because they fail to *actively listen* to each individual and customize the program to the clients' needs, and their stated "wants."

How you apply Steps 2 through 9 depends on your client's position on the continuum that ranges from health to elite performance. Your client's position on the continuum greatly influences your approach to program design for that particular individual. Step 10 is the consequence of your correct assessment of your client's current fitness status and personality, and reflects a personal understanding and sensitivity to your client.

The physical program will be based in the principles of cardiorespiratory, muscle strength and endurance and flexibility training. But, your *skill* is needed to overlay those principles with your knowledge of important program concepts:

- the continuum from fitness/health improvements to athletic performance
- rest and recovery
- specificity, progression and overload
- overtraining

When you put all of these together and *use* the principles derived from each step or concept, you are able to create successful programs that meet client "needs" and "wants."

Table 1. Ten Steps for Effective Program Design

Step 1: Information Gathering	Step 6: Active Rest
Step 2: Balanced Physical Programming	Step 7: Cross Training
Step 3: Cardiorespiratory Conditioning	Step 8: Special Needs for Healthy Populations
Step 4: Muscle Strength and Endurance	Step 9: Success and Adherence
Step 5: Flexibility Training	Step 10: The Reality Factor

Quick Index:

Chapter 1, overview of 10 effective steps to program design

Health or Fitness?

The American College of Sports Medicine (ACSM, 1991) recognizes that the term **physical fitness** is composed of a variety of characteristics, including the broad categories of cardiorespiratory fitness, body composition, muscular strength and endurance, and flexibility. **Fitness** is defined as the ability to perform moderate to vigorous levels of physical activity without undue fatigue. Fitness training should also encompass the capability and desire of your client to maintain such ability throughout his life. ACSM also states that the adaptive response to training is complex and individual. In other words, individual clients will most likely respond differently to exactly the same program. Because of this, it is important to record client progress, or lack thereof, so the appropriate changes can be made to create improvement or continued gains in their fitness.

Traditionally, fitness was often limited to a discussion regarding changes in max VO2, muscular strength and endurance, and body composition. The measurement of max VO2 is often used as an important indicator of fitness and referred to as the major criterion for measuring improvements in cardiorespiratory fitness. Recently, the benchmark of max VO2 has been re-evaluated. Is it really the best measure of fitness across a broad spectrum of issues, including health? Scientists are looking for new ways to best describe the quality, and capacity, of what we commonly refer to as aerobic fitness and its relationship to health and quality of life (Sharkey, 1991).

The 1990 ACSM recommendations for fitness were based on scientific literature examining the effects of controlled exercise training on physical fitness or enhanced exercise capacity, and were frequently measured by max VO2 improvements. In July 1993, ACSM and the Centers for Disease Control (CDC), in cooperation with the President's Council on Physical Fitness and Sports, released a statement announcing that a persuasive body of scientific evidence indicates that regular, moderate-intensity physical activity offers substantial **health benefits** to the public. Regular physical activity is an important preventive step with regard to diseases, especially coronary heart disease. In addition, regular activity may provide some degree of protection from other chronic diseases, including adult-onset diabetes (NIDDM), hypertension, some cancers, osteoporosis and depression.

The 1993 recommendations state that every adult should accumulate 30 minutes or more of moderate-intensity physical activity over the course of most days of the week (*Sports Medicine Bulletin*, 1993; ACSM and CDC, 1993). Pate et al. (1995) contend that performing a series of short bouts of exercise, of moderate intensity, lasting from about 8-10 minutes, with total duration being at least 30 minutes per day, will also provide significant health benefits. In other words, the *total amount of activity* is the key, not whether it is performed continuously. That is good news for someone who finds 30 minutes of continuous activity, of any kind, rather daunting.

The statement further recommends incorporating activity into daily routines. This is time efficient and non-intimidating. Examples of effective activity include walking stairs instead of riding elevators, gardening, raking leaves, shoveling snow, dancing, vigorously cleaning house and strolling. Planned exercise or recreational activity such as an aerobics class, tennis, swimming or strength training may also be used.

It is now clear that *lower* levels of physical activity than recommended by ACSM's 1990 position statement for improvements in max VO2 may reduce the risk for certain chronic degenerative diseases, and may or may not be of sufficient quantity and quality to improve max VO2. For the fitness professional, this is not an issue of "right" and "wrong," or easy, moderate or vigorous exercise, but an issue of appropriateness and encouraging a majority of the population to exercise effectively.

Moderate Exercise for Health

The relationship between physical activities that confer *health benefits* and inactivity as a risk factor for coronary artery disease (CAD) have been demonstrated in studies by Morris and Raffle (1954, London bus driver study); Zukel et al. (1959, North Dakota study); Paffenbarger and Hale (1975, longshoremen study); Paffenbarger et al. (1986, Harvard alumni study); Cooper (1976, showing aerobic fitness levels are inversely related to CAD); Blair and Kohl (1988, showing moderate levels of fitness may have the greatest impact on health); and Blair et al. (1989, showing significance of low levels of fitness on health). The American College of Sports Medicine (ACSM), the President's Council on Physical Fitness, and the Centers for Disease Control (CDC) still estimate that 250,000 deaths each year can be attributed to physical inactivity (Schardt, 1993). At least 43 studies have shown that those who are physically sedentary are at almost twice the risk for CHD as physically active individuals (*Sports Medicine Digest*, March 1994).

Some benefits can not be measured by longevity (epidemiological) studies. Higher levels of fitness may increase performance on the job and during leisure pursuits. Enhanced levels of muscular strength and flexibility may positively impact weight control and osteoporosis. The ongoing study of Harvard alumni suggested that individuals who exercise at, for example, a jogging pace of 6 or 7 mph (10-8.5 minutes per mile) or walking at 4-5 mph (15-12 minutes per mile) were likely to live longer (*ACE Fitness Matters*, July-August 1995).

Despite the fact that people recognize the value of physical activity, statistics indicate that a low percentage of people are participating. According to one report, 24% of adult Americans are completely sedentary, while 54% are inadequately active. All would benefit from regular physical activity. Why do so few choose to participate? Possibly it relates to the public's belief that high-intensity, continuous activity is the only way to gain health benefits.

Briskly walking as little as 2 miles is an example of how to meet the 1993 ACSM/CDC recommendations. As you can see, most of your clients could identify with this standard of exercise and say, "Yes, I could do that!"

An interview (Schardt, 1993) with leading researchers may give you additional confidence and scientific support for how moderate exercise can really affect your clients. This information is exciting and motivating because the potential health benefits are outstanding, while client time investment and effort are minimized.

• Stephen Blair, P.E.D., director of epidemiology at the Institute for Aerobics Research, reports that a moderate amount of exercise increases HDL cholesterol, lowers blood pressure, helps control weight, increases insulin sensitivity in muscles and decreases the risk for blood-clot formation.

• Laurie Hoffman-Goetz, an expert on cancer, reports that there is consistent and strong epidemiological evidence that suggests moderate exercise is associated with a lower rate of colon cancer, and possibly breast cancer in humans (Schardt, 1993).

• Barbara Drinkwater, Ph.D., an expert in the area of osteoporosis, says that for women to most effectively build up their bones, exercise is necessary for extended periods of time. While regular aerobic exercise coupled with strength training may increase bone density by 6-8%, the real issue is avoiding bone loss. Women are encouraged, at a minimum, to engage in some weight-bearing activity that they really enjoy, like walking (Schardt, 1993).

• Andrea Kriska, an epidemiologist, states that studies suggest that more active people are less likely to develop non-insulin-dependent diabetes (NIDDM), formerly called adult-onset diabetes. Moderate activity increases the muscle cell's sensitivity to insulin, so it helps control and lower both blood sugar and insulin levels. Kriska says that the kind of activity that works best is movement that requires the body to use large muscle groups, and is something that can be done on a regular basis. Walking, cycling and dancing are good examples. Those at greatest risk of diabetes are overweight, sedentary, middle-aged and older adults (Schardt, 1993).

• Abby King, senior scientist at the Stanford Center for Research in Disease Prevention, emphasizes the importance of exercise in combination with eating fewer calories. It is the combination of these 2 approaches that helps maintain weight loss. Activity can provide a double payoff, according to King. Activity burns calories, of course, and it can increase muscle tissue, which can raise metabolism (Schardt, 1993).

• David Nieman, an immunity expert, claims that physically fit people get fewer colds and upper respiratory-tract infections than people who are unfit. Scientists think that moderate exercise increases the circulation of T-cells or "natural killer cells" and immunoglobulins that protect the body against foreign invaders. Exercise seems to offer this protection for only a few hours after exercise, but apparently it is enough to ward off a few infections. An accumulation of 30-45 minutes of exercise *throughout the day* may provide this benefit. On the other hand, too much exercise can suppress the immune system and make your clients more susceptible to colds (Schardt, 1993).

• Jim Hagberg, a professor of medicine at the University of Pittsburgh, says that 45 studies have looked at the effects of exercise on mild or moderate hypertension. Many of the studies show that low-intensity, rhythmic, repetitive exercise like walking can reduce blood pressure as effectively as higher-intensity exercise. The results are the same for young or old. And major weight loss, which itself lowers blood pressure, does not seem to be necessary for a decrease in blood pressure to occur (Schardt, 1993).

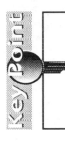

For most inactive individuals, the message is simply "get moving, do something." If you are already fit "keep it up!"

Intensity Levels for Fitness and Health

When you have a full understanding of exercise recommendations for health and max VO2 improvements, you realize there is nothing "wrong" with fitness guidelines presented by ACSM (1990 Guidelines for Cardiorespiratory Fitness, Body Composition and Muscular Strength and Endurance). These recommendations from ACSM are thoroughly researched formulas that target healthy adults. The emphasis is on fitness improvements in healthy, active adults, as gauged by increases in an objective measure—max VO2. These exercise recommendations of frequency, duration and especially intensity best influence various physiologic thresholds associated with improvements in max VO2.

Improvement in max VO2 is directly related to frequency, intensity and duration of training. Depending upon the quantity (duration, frequency) and quality (intensity) of training, improvement of max VO2 can range from 5-30%. Most studies show that a minimum increase in max VO2 of 15% is generally attained in programs that meet stated guidelines (ACSM, 1991) for frequency, intensity and duration.

The **minimum training intensity** threshold for improvement in max VO2 is approximately 60% of maximum heart rate (MHR), which is equivalent to about 50% of max VO2 or heart rate reserve (HRR). It is interesting to note that 50% of HRR represents a heart rate of approximately 135 beats per minute (bpm) in a young person, aged 20, with a resting heart rate of 70. As a result of age-related change in MHR (it goes down with age), the absolute heart rate needed to achieve this threshold can be as low as 105-115 bpm. This example gives you a clear picture of what "moderately intense" efforts actually correlate to with regard to a specific measure of heart rate. Moderate levels of exercise are easily attainable by most adults.

Intensity and duration of training are interrelated, with *total amount of work* accomplished being an important factor in improvement in fitness. According to ACSM (although more inquiry is necessary), present evidence suggests that when exercise is performed *below the minimum intensity* threshold of 60% of MHR, the total amount of work accomplished is an increasingly important factor in *fitness* development and maintenance. Improvement will be similar for activities performed at lower intensity/longer duration, when compared to those performed at higher intensity/shorter duration, if the total energy costs of the activities are similar. This principle holds for improving general fitness, but the quality (intensity) of exercise remains an important factor for training in specific activities where *performance* is a concern.

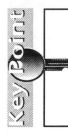

> There are potential health benefits if exercise is performed (1) more frequently, (2) for longer durations and (3) at lower intensities than often advocated.

Initial level of fitness is another important consideration in planning exercise and establishing goals. The client with a low fitness level can achieve a significant training effect with a sustained training heart rate lower than 40-50% of HRR, or about 50-60% of MHR, while clients with higher fitness levels require a higher training stimulus for continued improvements and/or maintenance of fitness.

Table 13. Moderate Exercise Works

Encourage your clients to "just go and do...something!"

• Any exercise is better than no exercise, whether formal, recreational or functional. For example, take the stairs instead of the elevator.

• Accumulate 30 minutes of moderate activity most days of the week.

Moderate exercise, engaged in on a regular basis can:

• Lower the risk of coronary heart disease (CHD).

• Lower insulin levels by increasing the muscle's sensitivity to insulin, thus decreasing the likelihood of non-insulin-dependent diabetes.

• Lower blood pressure.

• Increase resistance to colds and upper respiratory-tract infections.

• Help control and keep weight off.

• Lower the risk of colon cancer and possibly breast cancer.

• Reduce or relieve depression.

00000000000000000000000

Incorporating Rest and Recovery Time

The recovery-building process is as important as the exercise phase in program design. It helps clients avoid an overuse injury and can elicit a strong and regular effort from your clients. Regardless of fitness level, it's a good idea to thread the concept of **active rest** throughout the fitness routines. The active rest concept utilizes well-thought-out sequencing of chosen exercises to structure a workout. I find that this approach optimizes time availability and accommodates the fitness level of the individual.

A large amount of time in traditional fitness programs involves recovery from work performed. Sometimes long recoveries are appropriate for sport-specific applications with highly trained athletes. The science behind recovery time periods usually supports the need for a specific energy system of the body to recover fully before another optimal effort can be performed in a safe manner. This is especially relevant to strength training. However, the majority of your clients are probably not at this level of competition and do not have available to them the required time investment that goes along with this type of training.

There are several ways to minimize nonproductive recovery time, or to eliminate it:

1. Use perceived exertion and intervals (work, recovery) to keep your client in motion during cardiorespiratory conditioning.

2. Sequence resistance training exercises so that they alternate from muscle group to muscle group, or from upper to lower body to the trunk.

3. If a muscle group is targeted for consecutive multiple sets, the recovery phase(s), if of sufficient length, can be utilized for flexibility training.

For the trainer looking to maximize results with minimal client time investment, active rest is a great way to optimize the finite time you have available with the typical client. Your programs should differentiate between training for athletic performance and creating functional health improvements. The approaches and time investments are entirely different in these 2 distinct areas. Where does your client fit?

Quick Index:

Specificity, Progression and Overload

Specificity. This is the principle that takes the guesswork out of training. Your client's body adapts to the specific type of training you choose. When applied to training, **specificity** refers to adaptations in the body's metabolic and physiologic systems specific to an activity. Since specific exercise elicits specific adaptations, you should be able to effectively manipulate the results you desire with the training program you develop.

Adaptations, or training effects, that occur depend on the type of overload imposed. It is known that a specific exercise stress, such as power strength training or plyometrics, causes specific strength/power adaptations. Specific aerobic or cardiovascular exercise elicits specific endurance training adaptations. And, there is essentially no relationship between strength and aerobic training because these goals are on the opposite ends of the training continuum. Furthermore, aerobic fitness is best developed for a particular activity, like swimming, running or bicycling, by participating in that specific activity.

Progression. Proper progression is tied very closely to the occurrence, or non-occurrence, of overuse injuries and overtraining. Challenge the body's abilities gradually. Injuries occur from piling on too much, too soon. To help alleviate the potential for improper progression:

1. Allow about 2 weeks for your client to adapt to any new overload *before* making the workout any harder or longer.

2. Before you add additional work, the client should have no residual soreness and the last workout should have been easily accomplished.

3. When adding on additional minutes (duration) or resistance, consider increasing the time or current resistance by about 5%. This guideline helps keep you from adding on too much, too fast and risking injury to the soft tissues of the body.

4. For typical clients, progression can probably *not* occur too slowly. If in doubt, err on the side of conservative progression. Your client has hopefully made a lifetime commitment to exercise, so patience is the rule.

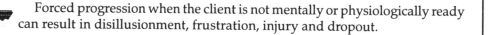

Forced progression when the client is not mentally or physiologically ready can result in disillusionment, frustration, injury and dropout.

Overload. The concept of individualized and progressive overload applies to the athlete, the sedentary client, the physically challenged and even the cardiac or high-risk client. Different activities, depending on duration and intensity, require the activation of specific energy systems. Overload is accomplished by increasing the frequency, duration and/or intensity of the established level of exercise—in other words, working harder than the client is accustomed. Another way to add overload is with periodization. Periodization occurs when you change frequency, duration and/or intensity over set time periods. By exercising at a level above normal, a variety of training adaptations enables the body to function more efficiently.

Another, often overlooked, way to vary overload for strength training is by using different activities or body positions. Absolute effort (resistance lifted) may stay the same, but the body will respond with different muscle recruitment patterns. This will stimulate an adaptive response by the body because of the introduction of this movement to which your client's body is not accustomed, even though the resistance may not be increased.

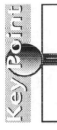

Overload your client's current fitness levels with no more than 5% increments above his present ability.

When changing any variable in your programs, it is important not to manipulate more than one at a time. For instance, if your client has been jogging for several weeks, 30 minutes per session, successfully and pain free, you might increase his duration about 2 minutes or a 5% increase. However, it is not advised to simultaneously increase his speed (intensity). Introducing 2 new variables increases the likelihood of injury.

Though these guidelines are very conservative, why risk the possibility of an injury? It pays to build intensity, duration and frequency very slowly. The ultimate goal is lifelong exercise that is enjoyable. Why create an avoidable setback?

Quick Index:

Chapters 5 and 7, for specific cardiorespiratory and strength adaptations
Chapters 4 and 12, how to overload each energy system
Chapter 13, explains overloads and active rest cycling
Chapter 14, strength training overloads and rest

Case Studies: Applying the Principles

Let's look at 2 very different clients and see how the principles of moderation, specificity and overload apply to their programs.

Client One: Danielle. Danielle is new to fitness but a sophisticated, well-read consumer. She is also confused, and a bit overwhelmed, as she enters into the "land of health and fitness." She has heard that if you cannot attain 20 minutes of continuous exercise there is no real benefit. She says to you, "You know, the magic number is 20. I hear that you can't burn fat or get much benefit out of the activity unless it's 20 minutes or longer." Furthermore, Danielle characterizes her exercise experience as "never been active," "hate to exercise" and "never felt accomplished or successful in sports or any movement pursuit."

Client Two: Merrilee. Merrilee is a highly trained runner who rarely takes days off for recovery and seldom changes activity. She has never heard of the concepts of cross training and active recovery. She believes in "discipline," never missing a run and never deleting even a tenth of a mile of a planned run once it is logged in her training diary. She perseveres through annoying discomfort that often borders on pain and believes in "slogging out the miles." She says, "It's part of discipline and made me the runner I am today." Her 5K (3.1 miles) best is 19 minutes and "change" (a few seconds), while her 10K best is 39 minutes and 56 seconds. She is obviously an accomplished runner.

How would you apply training concepts to each of these clients?

We know that the 20-minute fat-burning rule is a myth. Fat is burned at and during low-intensity exercise. Therefore, it is obvious that 20-minutes is *not* a magic, fat-burning threshold that must be crossed to utilize fat for energy expenditure.

Most exercise physiologists believe you can end up in almost the same place, in terms of health, if you work at moderate intensity for either one 30-minute session, or shorter sessions that total 30 minutes. Scientists have found that even a series of 5-10 minute aerobic exercise bouts can improve cardiovascular fitness and help clients lose weight. The focus should be on total amount of exercise accomplished, which determines total calories burned. This approach is especially useful and motivating for a person who is new to exercise, like Danielle.

This kind of information may be just the boost that Danielle needs to help her embrace her program with hope and enthusiasm. Twenty-minute aerobic sessions are certainly not a requisite for her current program design and health needs.

On the other hand, researchers are finding that to *optimize* fitness gains, 20-minute sessions may be too short. The point at which exercise starts to produce considerably greater gains in *maximum* aerobic capacity is after 20 minutes. To boost stamina, fitness and performance, you may want to gradually increase duration but you also need to consider intensity. When you take the next step and begin thinking about running a competitive race or optimizing your fitness return, how *hard* you train, not necessarily how long or often, is the key. If you work for less time but at a higher intensity, say 80-95% of your maximum heart rate, your competitive fitness will improve much more, as compared to going longer at lesser intensities.

Now, Merrilee would jump at this chance to further "discipline" her training and to increasingly "pound" her body into submission. However, you can emphasize the right combination of less total work, and intense, quality efforts. Total training needs to be balanced with cross training, adequate recovery time and easier workouts to balance the more intense efforts.

Your clients' different fitness goals and psychological makeup offer you a variety of opportunities to encourage optimism and adherence to regular exercise, or to change programs so that they meet the needs of your client in the safest and most effective way. As the cases of Merrilee and Danielle demonstrate, every individual has unique needs. Some need to be told to temper their workouts. They may need to focus on quality workouts and allow for recovery. This will keep the results coming without inviting overuse syndrome into the training picture. Others, like Danielle, need to be assured that "some activity is better than none." The more knowledge you accumulate, the fewer limits you will have in approaching this problem-solving puzzle called program design.

Programming for Life

No program or exercise guideline is written in stone. Err on the side of conservatism. Intensity is relative to the individual. You must know your client's physical limits and *his* perception of what is too much. Do not join the ranks of many trainers who create programs that are too hard for their clients. If you do not injure them, you surely will defeat them.

Recommendations should be used in the context of your clients' needs, goals and initial abilities. A *sliding scale* allows you to individualize the amount of time, training frequency and intensity of effort for each client. This flexible approach is important for the cardiorespiratory, muscular strength and endurance, and flexibility components of the program.

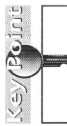

Design a program that provides the proper amount of physical activity to attain maximal benefit at the lowest risk of injury, with minimal time investment.

Your ultimate goal, as a personal trainer, is to help in maintaining your client's newly acquired level of health and fitness, throughout his lifetime. Maintaining, for example, fitness level and desired percentage of body fat is a self-acknowledgment of his happiness with his current physical self and state of health. This is a positive phase that will hopefully last a lifetime.

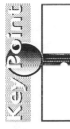

Maintenance is not regression. Maintenance is the health or fitness level you have identified with your client that allows him to be comfortable with the changes in his physical self and lifestyle. After any amount of sustained training (several months or more), a slow-down in training benefits is inevitable. Prepare your client in advance of this inevitable physiologic phenomenon so that he experiences it in a positive manner.

Depending on a client's willingness to commit more time or to "exercise harder," this exercise plateau with regard to gains in strength, cardiorespiratory fitness or flexibility may, or may not, be permanent. Plateaus are an *opportunity* to reevaluate goals, set new ones and most important, find out where your client wants to go with his exercise programming. A plateau is certainly not characterized by a time of doing nothing, boredom or a seeming dead-end. Instead, it may lead to further gains in fitness through a revised program. And at the very least, it requires a continual effort on your part, and your client's, to *sustain* this level of health and fitness. Accomplish this by motivating your client to exercise regularly and with variety. At some point, *maintenance* of health and fitness will become the most important, rewarding and exciting time of the rest of your client's life!

Quick Index:

Chapter 11, maintenance levels and detraining

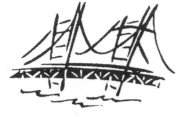

The Bridge

Differentiate between training programs for athletic performance and fitness/health improvements. Health benefits occur if exercise is performed (1) more frequently, (2) for longer durations and (3) at lower intensities than often advocated. Short 8- to 10-minute bouts of exercise, of moderate intensity totaling 30 minutes per day, will provide significant health benefits. Increase intensity or duration by about 5%, changing only one variable at a time.

SPECIAL SECTION
HOW TO RECOGNIZE AND RECOVER FROM OVERTRAINING

A basic principle of training is to stress, or overload, the physiologic system. Positive overloads cause the body to respond with, for example, increases in strength, muscular endurance and/or cardiorespiratory capacity. Because of this basic training principle—progressive increases in overload—there is a risk of overtraining. **Overtraining** is a combination of stress that is experienced through work, home, social interactions and training load. It can lead to staleness, exhaustion and injury.

Susceptibility to overtraining can result from a lethal combination of a zealous, hard-driving trainer and a client who is extremely motivated. Attempting to perform his best during every training session, and being motivated to extend this effort by a well-meaning trainer, invites injury or emotional burnout. Nothing will shut down the training process and compliance more quickly than this scenario. It can also cause a trainer to lose the confidence of the client, possibly losing him as a client, or making him hesitant to refer other individuals.

The underlying causes of overtraining, or staleness (mental and physical), are a combination of emotional and physical factors. Hans Selye (1956) in his book, *The Stress of Life*, noted that a breakdown in tolerance of stress can occur as often from a sudden increase in anxiety as from an increase in physical distress. The emotional demands of life, family pressures, a personal desire to excel at every undertaking and the expectations of significant others can be sources of intolerable emotional stress. In addition to the stress of exercise and training, environmental factors such as heat stress and improper nutrition may also lead to overtraining symptoms.

When planning programs, consider the *total* stress your clients are under. For example, during tax season an accountant may be more susceptible to overtraining. The ability to design a training regimen that provides the level of stress needed for optimal physiological improvement without exceeding your clients' tolerance is a difficult task. Much like heart disease, which develops insidiously, overtraining exhibits no preliminary symptoms to warn you that your clients are approaching the edge of becoming overtrained. By the time you realize that you have pushed clients too hard, the damage is already done.

Though the symptoms of overtraining may vary greatly from one individual to another, the most common are feelings of "heaviness" and the inability to perform well and concentrate. Working out is no longer a joy. It has turned into a struggle. If you feel this situation exists, it is time to make some immediate changes in the program. Remember, do not hesitate to ask your client!

Table 14. Overtraining Warning List

Signs of Overtraining in Your Client's Health
- Elevated resting heart rate, blood pressure or both
- Generalized body aches and pain
- Head colds (especially if chronic), allergic reactions, or both
- Body weight loss with decreased appetite
- Occasional nausea

Signs of Overtraining in Your Client's Life
- Personal problems, increased tension, anger, irritability
- No interest in activities they usually enjoy
- Sleep disturbances (loss of sleep)

Signs of Overtraining in Your Client's Training
- Loss of motivation to train, or staleness
- Cutting sessions short: "An hour seems too long!"
- Performance going down
- Unusual muscle soreness and tenderness after training
- Fatigue lingers during workout and through the day
- Recovery takes longer immediately after the workout

Idiosyncratic personality variables, as well as mood swings, can be distinguished from overtraining by simply verbalizing your observations to your client. Also, day-to-day variations in the *sensations* of fatigue should not be confused with overtraining. It is okay for your client to feel tired or challenged from a workout. It is not uncommon for your client to feel "heavy" after a day of hard training. These are often short-lived sensations that dissipate before the next training session. Coupled with rest, a light day or no training after the hard session and proper nutrition, these symptoms are usually relieved. By keeping track of these general indicators and erring on the side of caution, you can prevent most cases of overtraining.

If you're a veteran trainer reading the Overtraining Warning List, I imagine that a smile is spreading across your face! Head colds, general body aches and pains, personal problems and loss of motivation are often challenges that you deal with every day, 365 days per year, with certain clients. It might even lead you to the tongue-in-cheek conclusion that your client may have been and will continue to be in a perpetual state of overtraining! All joking aside, signs of overtraining warrant a sincere and objective investigation.

Physiological Indicators of Overtraining
In an effort to objectively diagnose overtraining, several researchers have used various physiological measurements. Examples include measurements of blood enzymes, resting levels of blood lactate, observation of muscle damage, white blood- cell count, alterations in blood plasma and study of electrocardiograph (ECG) tracings. Despite these various attempts to objectively diagnose overtraining, no single physiological measurement has proved 100% causative. In a

practical sense, these variables would be of no use to you anyway, as most trainers do not have access to sophisticated testing.

It is not surprising that overtraining has a dramatic effect on the energy demands for a given, submaximal exercise bout (Wilmore and Costill, 1988). When your client shows symptoms of overtraining, you will find that his heart rate for a given effort is significantly higher, and often, oxygen cost of the activity is greater. For instance, if your client's heart rate (HR) for a workload of 5 mph on a treadmill is normally 135 beats per minute (bpm), this same level of effort might increase to 145 bpm if your client was approaching, or already in a state of, being overtrained.

The reasons for this increase in HR are not totally clear. Your client is not losing his aerobic fitness, but his skill, form and efficiency may be deteriorating. This means he is less efficient mechanically and physiologically, which translates to increased heart rates and energy expenditure for given workloads when compared to a trained state where overtraining has not occurred.

The best and most practical way for personal trainers to monitor overtraining is by observing heart response during rest or during activity.

Using Heart Rate to Indicate Overtraining

This method is effective during activity:

1. Record your client's heart rate (HR) at a fixed pace and load, on any piece of "aerobic" equipment at the *onset* of training, or *prior* to a new phase in your client's program. This is called the untrained heart rate response (UT).

2. Record your client's HR at the same given pace and load, and on the same piece of equipment, anytime *after* significant and progressive training. This is called the trained heart rate response (TR).

3. Record your client's HR at the same fixed pace and overload, and on the same piece of equipment during any period when he demonstrates symptoms of being overtrained. This is called the overtrained heart rate response (OT).

When these HR measurements are compared, you would probably find the UT heart rate to be highest, followed by the OT and finally TR heart rate. These results would indicate that the TR heart rate was most efficient for the above-given pace and overload, on a particular piece of equipment. The OT heart rate was higher than the TR rate because of overtraining, but was still lower or more efficient than the initial untrained state (UT). Based on heart rate response to given workloads, you can objectively monitor the direction of training so that it remains beneficial. This kind of data and observation may provide a warning signal for overtraining.

If your client's **resting heart rate** (RHR) is 10% above normal, it indicates he may be overtrained.

Recovery From Overtraining

Relief from overtraining usually comes from a significant reduction in training intensity, a change of activity or complete rest. Many coaches and trainers generally suggest a "few days of easy training," using the same activity. Many experts, to the contrary, observe that participants recover faster when they rest completely, or engage in some other form of low-intensity exercise.

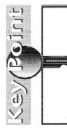

> If you suspect overtraining, encourage your client to take a day off from training, introduce variety (cross train) or at least cut back in volume and intensity of overload.

If your client's RHR is 20% above normal, encourage him to avoid training that day, or significantly alter the planned workout. For example, an emphasis on stretch and relaxation may be appropriate.

It appears that the intensity (e.g., speed of running or amount of weight lifted) is *potentially* more stressful than volume of training (reps, more days, duration of each session). However, excess in either, or simultaneous increases in intensity and volume, may lead to overuse injuries and overtraining.

Prevention is always preferable to the challenge of attempting to remedy the psychological and physiological state of an overtrained or injured client. An excellent way to minimize the risk of overstressing is to follow cyclic (periodization) training procedures. Periodization alternates easy, moderate and harder periods of training over specific time frames (Chapter 13). As a general rule, one or 2 days of hard training should be followed by an equal number of easy days.

The importance of variety, cross training, active recovery and actual days of rest for the mind and body cannot be overemphasized. Simply by utilizing a different activity and a different exercise stress, your clients' bodies will likely respond positively to the workout challenges. The optimal adaptive response often occurs when the training you present is mixed with new activities and recovery.

CHAPTER 11

MAINTAINING GAINS IN FITNESS

"What happens if I travel or get sick?"

"What is the most efficient way to keep fit?"

"Is there a way to maintain my gains in fitness when I don't have the time to work out the way I'd like to?"

Many of your clients want to know how easily they can lose, or regain, their hard-won training benefits. The familiar answer is, "You can't store exercise." Detraining starts to occur fairly rapidly once you stop exercising. Though there is a significant difference in the *rate* at which various components of fitness and their associated fitness levels are lost, generally, after only one or 2 weeks of complete inactivity, reductions in muscular strength and endurance, flexibility and cardiorespiratory fitness can be measured.

The positive side is that fitness gains may not be lost as quickly as you might think. And, additional good news is that it may take *less* exercise than you think to *maintain* fitness levels. A philosophy I like to instill in my clients is, "Why lose it when it's so easy to keep?"

Much of the scientific literature about physical **detraining,** or the **reversibility principle,** comes from studies of athletes or clinical research with patients who have been forced to be inactive as a result of injury or surgery (Wilmore and Costill, 1988, 1994). Additional information has been gained from aerospace research because the lack of gravity removes a number of physiological stresses (overload) which stimulate normal body functions and adaptations. Some of this information can be applied to your clients' questions.

It has been well established that the effects associated with physical training are indeed transient and reversible if regular training is not possible. On the other hand, recent studies have made it clear that a few days of rest, or a *reduction* in training, will not negatively affect the training process and performance—and may even enhance it (Wilmore and Costill, 1994). This is especially true for highly trained athletes and is probably related to the importance of recovery in optimizing the adaptation response, and in avoiding overtraining.

You may be thinking, "The *last* thing my clients need is encouragement to reduce their training." Nonetheless, regardless of fitness level, a reduction or change in training volume, intensity or type of activity over specific time periods is probably a good idea. Ultimately, *too much* recovery or irregular training is not in the interest of your average client or an athlete because, at some point, a decrease or cessation of activity will produce a deterioration in fitness and/or performance.

Quick Index:

Maintaining Cardiorespiratory Fitness

The heart is not unlike other muscles in the body. If it is not conditioned by large muscle, rhythmic activity that simultaneously increases heart rate and a large volume of blood back to the heart, it becomes deconditioned and less efficient at delivering blood and oxygen. A lack of endurance training on a regular basis can significantly compromise the cardiovascular system. There has been a good amount of study centered on cardiorespiratory fitness, and it's possible to generalize some of the results to the average fitness client.

In one study, 21 days of complete bed rest caused a significant *increase* in submaximal heart rate for given workloads when compared to the trained state before bed rest. Submaximal stroke volume and maximal cardiac output both *decreased* by 25%. A 27% *decrease* was seen in maximal oxygen consumption. Complete bed rest corresponded to about a 1% decrease in physiologic function each day (McArdle et al., 1991; Wilmore and Costill, 1994).

These changes may be caused by dramatic decreases in heart volume, total blood and plasma volume, and ventricular contractility (Wilmore and Costill, 1994). Recent studies confirm that a reduction in blood volume occurs after only a few weeks of detraining and significantly reduces stroke volume of the heart, thus compromising cardiovascular function (Coyle et al., 1986, as reported in Wilmore and Costill, 1994).

Complete bed rest is quite drastic and it must be pointed out that bed rest is *very different* from not exercising while still carrying on day-to-day activities. Minimal activity—whether formal workout or simply being busy with daily routine—is an important contribution to maintenance of fitness gains.

It is interesting that in the bed-rest study, untrained subjects experienced a smaller decrease in max VO2 than trained subjects, and regained their initial fitness levels in less time. In fact, it took only 10 days of reconditioning for the untrained, versus 40 days for trained, subjects to attain full recovery. This demonstrates that a highly trained athlete has more to lose in terms of fitness, and takes significantly longer to regain peak performance/conditioning levels.

This observation has important implications for sports conditioning specificity for your competitive clients. They need a year-round training program that includes maintenance phases so significant levels of fitness are not lost. For your clients who are not as competitive and tend to have lower absolute levels of fitness, it will be easier to regain their previous fitness level.

The heart, like all muscles in the body, strengthens itself in proportion to the force it must contract against. Because of this, periods of inactivity lead to substantial cardiovascular deconditioning.

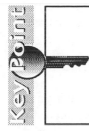

> Even *limited* activity provides considerable conditioning for the heart.

Day-to-day activity provides some maintenance of key cardiovascular functions because the heart must contract forcefully enough to circulate the blood against the demands of gravity. It is important to reemphasize that there is a significant difference between complete inactivity (bed rest) and cessation of training because of travel or sickness that occurs while your client can still participate in her normal daily routine.

Minimum Quantities of Cardiorespiratory Exercise

Your clients are sure to ask about the optimal frequency, duration and level of exercise intensity required to maintain aerobic improvements attained through training.

Early studies (Brynteson and Sinning, 1973, as reported in Wilmore and Costill, 1988 and 1994) found that cardiovascular fitness, as measured by max VO2, was maintained by exercising 3 times per week. Significant losses in endurance conditioning, as measured by changes in max VO2, were observed in subjects when they exercised only once or twice per week. Duration and intensity were held constant.

A series of studies by Hickson et al. (1985) have shown that in addition to frequency and duration, training *intensity* plays a principal role in maintaining aerobic power or max VO2 during periods of reduced training. Their data suggest that the intensity of training must be at least 70% of max VO2 (approximately 75-80% of maximum heart rate) to maintain the training-induced improvements in max VO2. As little as a one-third (33%) reduction in training intensity for 15 weeks produced a significant decline in max VO2 in subjects who were previously trained for 10 weeks at a one-third higher intensity. Frequency and duration were held constant (Wilmore and Costill, 1994).

Studies by Hickson et al. (1985) also found that a reduced *frequency* resulted in significant losses in aerobic capacity only when training frequency was reduced by greater than two-thirds of the regular training load. For example, dropping from 6 workouts initially to a frequency of 4 (about one-third reduction) and 2 (about two-thirds reduction) times per week had little effect on cardiorespiratory training benefits. The same intensity and duration were maintained.

The effect of reduced training *duration* on the maintenance of improved aerobic fitness has also been studied by Hickson. In this study, the original training duration was reduced from 40-minute sessions to either 26 (about one-third reduction) or 13 minutes (about two-thirds reduction) per day (reported in McArdle et al., 1991). Almost all of the cardiorespiratory benefits were maintained despite this reduction in training duration by as much as two thirds. Intensity and frequency were held constant.

Probably the key variable that Hickson identified, in regard to a maintenance effect on max VO2, was the degree of effort, or intensity. A closer look at Hickson's study reveals that he left frequency (6 days per week) and duration (40 minutes) constant, and had the subjects cut back only their intensity. One group trained at 67% effort and another group trained at 33% effort. In both groups max VO2 and performance faltered. Thus, as little as one-third reduction (this occurs at about 67% effort) in intensity resulted in significant decreases in max VO2.

> **Key Point**
>
> Intensity of training is the primary factor in maintaining the trained state. To maintain cardiorespiratory fitness, as measured by max VO2, generally requires at least 3 training sessions per week at a training intensity of at least 70% of max VO2.

The results of these studies should not be interpreted to mean that exercise performed less than 3 times per week at 70% of max VO2 is not valuable. Health gains can be realized with much less exercise and lower intensities. Furthermore, health gains do not necessarily require improvement in, or maintenance of, max VO2. Individual goals and initial fitness levels must be considered. If previous exercise intensity is maintained during a period of lesser training, regardless of a client's absolute fitness level, the frequency and duration of physical activity required to *maintain* this specific level of aerobic fitness is *less* than that required to improve it (McArdle et al., 1991).

This information can easily be applied to a client's current fitness status. Everyone has a percentage of max VO2, that corresponds to a steady rate or lower, that they can easily work at. A deconditioned client may barely sustain a 2- to 3-mph (30-20 minutes per mile) walk. A highly conditioned client may be able to sustain a 10 mph (6 minutes per mile) running pace. Regardless of the fitness level, if either of these specific intensities is reduced by about one-third or greater, a decrease in aerobic conditioning will occur. However, if intensity is kept constant and no more than a two-thirds reduction in frequency and duration occurs, any physiologic adaptations or health and fitness gains realized by this client will probably be maintained.

For a client who is vacationing, recreating or on business travel for around 10 days and is "normally" active or involved in some type of training on a regular basis, a decrease in structured activity will have little impact on overall health and fitness. It is very encouraging for clients to understand that most of their cardiorespiratory training benefits can be kept by maintaining their current level of effort while simultaneously reducing frequency and duration of effort by as much as two-thirds.

Quick Index:

Do Less Without Reducing Effort

In Ken McAlpine's article "The Minimalist's Maxim" (*Outside Magazine*, April 1993), the author asserts that many athletes and fitness enthusiasts would be better off using less time and more effort. He is supported by Dr. Robert Hickson, whom I have already cited. Hickson completed a series of 3 studies that led him (Hickson) to a conclusion that "Individuals who have reached a pretty good level of fitness can maintain their fitness fairly easily."

The argument for less is relevant to both health-oriented clients and athletes in regard to (1) increased performance, (2) the same or possibly less time commitment, (3) a reduced risk of injury from overtraining, and (4) less chance of personal burnout. Your client may be training as hard as she ever has and notices that her fitness gains, or performance, are falling off. Of course, as you become more fit, fitness gains are harder to come by. But at some point your client may wonder, "Why keep working so hard if it's not doing me any good and isn't that fun?"

McAlpine reported that a top-ranked athlete thought just this, and proceeded to cut back his training drastically. Guess what? His training *improved* drastically. Part of his initial gains might have been attributed to rest and recovery, which allowed for positive training adaptations to take place in response to the hard efforts. However, the gains continued until his retirement 4 years later. What was the other "secret" ingredient? Intensity!

Here's the concern. Most exercisers across the world need not worry about doing too much, or working too hard. Most simply need to *start* an exercise program on a regular and moderate basis! Your clients can maintain any level of fitness with reduced duration and frequency if intensity is maintained. The key is to first attain an acceptable level of fitness. After this, you can worry about maintaining it and manipulating the various variables of frequency, intensity and duration to best fit into your client's schedule. Until your client actually "gets in shape," you won't get far thinking about minimums, and if intensity is focused on before proper increases in duration and frequency, there is a higher risk of injury and non-compliance.

McAlpine points out that once you attain a desired level of fitness, you can maintain and even improve on your fitness with surprisingly little training. Though you will not become a world-class competitor on 30 minutes a day, you do not need to worry about a few missed workouts, either.

Key Point

McAlpine calls it "Training's corollary of compromise: Less is *not* more, but less is often enough! Sometimes you have to give up what you know for what works."

It could not be said more perfectly and it proves there is some justice in regard to gaining, losing and maintaining training effect, after all!

Maintaining Muscular Endurance, Strength and Power

If your client is following a regular strength-conditioning program of 3 sessions a week and misses a workout or so, does her strength greatly decline? Or, if your client temporarily needs to cut down on the number of workouts per week, is the result going to be disastrous? Most people have an innate fear that muscular strength and endurance gained through training will be lost after a brief period of time off from their regular training effort. "Not to worry," say most researchers! Compared to cardiorespiratory conditioning, strength is kept over a much longer period of time after detraining begins.

Wilmore and Costill (1994) report that no loss of strength is noted 6 weeks after cessation of a 3-week training program. They also noted that only 45% of the original strength gained from a 12-week training program was lost by the time the subjects, who participated in no additional training, were reevaluated one year later. Similar results have been found for muscular endurance (reported in Wilmore and Costill, 1988).

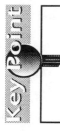

While levels of strength, power and muscular endurance are reduced once you stop training, these changes are relatively small during the first few months following the cessation of training.

Muscular Endurance

Muscular endurance can be described as the ability to sustain repeated muscular contractions over time, without undue fatigue. It is not known whether changes in muscular endurance occur because of changes in the muscle, changes in aerobic capacity or changes in both (Wilmore and Costill, 1994). The type of overload (for example, resistance training performed in a range of 1-20 repetitions to fatigue) will greatly influence the training effect and energy system adaptations. Though there is a continuum for muscular endurance from minutes to hours, do not confuse cardiorespiratory fitness with muscular endurance gained from traditional resistance training workouts.

After as little as 2 weeks of inactivity, significant *decreases* in muscular endurance occur. After one or 2 weeks of *complete* immobilization, a decrease in oxidative enzymes of 40-60% can occur. Coyle et al. (1984, as reported in Wilmore and Costill, 1994) observed a nearly 60% decrease in oxidative enzymes, whereas glycolytic enzymes (important for anaerobic energy production) showed no change in activity for up to 84 days of detraining. As little as 2 weeks of detraining can affect longer-duration performance, whereas 4 weeks or more of inactivity may not affect, for example, sprint event times.

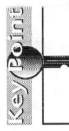

The muscle's capacity for *anaerobic* performance is much easier to maintain, based on the changes noted in localized muscular adaptations, than the muscle's capacity for maintaining aerobic conditioning or muscular endurance (Wilmore and Costill, 1994).

Costill et al. (1985, reported in Wilmore and Costill, 1994) reported that endurance trained muscles tend to store more glycogen. However, as little as 4 weeks of detraining decreased muscle glycogen levels by 40% and returned them to a level that equaled that of untrained subjects.

Another factor that affects muscular endurance is related to *blood lactate levels*. Following 4 weeks of detraining, participants in one study (Wilmore and Costill, 1994) showed very small changes in blood lactate levels after the first few weeks of inactivity when tested with a given workload. By the fourth week, blood lactate levels changed significantly. The same workload elicited much higher lactate levels, and the buffering capacity for lactate also decreased. During detraining blood flow may also be compromised as a result of a decrease in capillary supply. Though research findings are not conclusive regarding decreased capillarization, this would certainly impair oxygen delivery to the muscles and thus the ability to tolerate and efficiently clear or oxidize lactate.

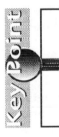

The muscle's oxidative and anaerobic energy systems change relatively slowly. A few days of recovery, or missed workouts, will probably have little effect. A week, or two, of complete inactivity starts to impact these systems, with anaerobic performance being much easier to maintain.

Development of muscular strength requires an anaerobic effort, and it has been shown that maintenance of strength levels requires fairly little time investment compared to maintaining aerobic or muscular endurance capacity.

Quick Index:
Chapter 14, the fitness continuum from endurance to strength

Muscular Strength and Power

When an individual breaks an arm or a leg and the broken limb is placed in a rigid cast to immobilize it, changes immediately start taking place in both the bone and surrounding muscles. It is now clearly understood that skeletal muscles will undergo substantial decreases in size (atrophy) with complete inactivity. Accompanying this decrease in size is a considerable loss in strength and power (Wilmore and Costill, 1994).

The physiologic mechanisms responsible for this decline in muscle strength with immobilization are not clearly understood. One thought reported by Costill (1994) is that muscle disuse also reduces the frequency of neurological stimulation and normal pathways for the recruitment of muscle fibers (motor units). Part of the strength loss that is associated with detraining may be produced by an inability to activate previously active motor units. This makes sense because part of the reason for *increases* in strength is related to increased motor-unit recruitment of previously dormant units. Thus, the importance of neural contributions to strength loss are essential to consider during periods of reduced activity.

While total inactivity will lead to very rapid losses in both strength and power, periods of *reduced* activity may lead to gradual losses that become significant only as the changes accumulate over long periods of time. Just as in cardiorespiratory conditioning, being active with daily tasks and reducing training has much less impact on muscle and bone loss than being confined to a bed or immobilized by a cast.

Costill (*Sports Medicine Digest*, May 1988) reports that muscle strength and power gained during training can be kept for up to 6 weeks of *inactivity*. In addition, Costill states that about 50% of the strength gained with training can be maintained for up to a year following the end of the training program. And, other studies have shown that it takes less effort to regain lost strength than it does to gain it (*Physician and Sportsmedicine*, 1985). This is welcome news for any training schedule that is interrupted by "life's events."

But more exciting than facing the proposition of regaining strength, research appears to confirm that *maintenance* of strength gains can be prolonged for long periods of time with minimal stimulation. It appears that intensity rather than exercise duration is the key stimulus for increases in strength. Single-set training seems to be as effective as multiple-set training.

> By working out once every 10-14 days, clients can maintain the strength, power and muscular endurance that was gained through more frequent and longer resistance training sessions, if *intensity* is maintained (*Sports Medicine Digest*, May 1988).

When reducing the number of workouts, for example, from 3 to 1 or 2, strength can be maintained. Researcher Dr. Graves explains, "If you want to maintain your strength when you are working out less often, you must make sure that your workout is just as difficult as the workout you conduct when you are training more frequently." (Reported in *IDEA Today*, July-August 1989).

Evidently, a muscle requires only a minimal stimulus to retain its strength, power and size. This has exciting implications for an injured participant and can be a powerful motivator for those clients who have attained a muscular strength and endurance level they would like to maintain, but no longer can invest the same time that was necessary to achieve this fitness level.

Maintaining Flexibility Gains

Even though flexibility is gained quickly, it is lost rather quickly during inactivity.

Flexibility is sometimes not a program focus because your client's body has the capacity to attain significant flexibility gains at any age, and stretching results often seem less significant to your clients when compared to cardiorespiratory conditioning or resistance training. Your clients may view the results of flexibility training as less important than a decreased heart rate for a given workload, or the ability to lift more weight and have aesthetically pleasing muscles.

Because of this prevailing attitude, balanced fitness is a key point to emphasize along with the benefits of flexibility training. While flexibility can be attained in a relatively short period of time, it is in the best interest of your clients to maintain functional levels of flexibility on a consistent basis. There is the possibility that reduced flexibility may leave them more susceptible to injury and can affect their actual performance and enjoyment of physical activity. Besides all of this, it feels good!

Retraining: Regaining Fitness

Many studies support the idea that regaining previous fitness levels requires far less effort than they took to first acquire. This is motivating news, and though I am not in dispute with this thought, I contend that it is far easier to *maintain* some semblance of training and general activity. When clients yo-yo between low and high levels of fitness, they risk lack of compliance to their exercise program and possible injury.

It is very disheartening, to say the least, to attain a new level of fitness and health, and for various reasons, lose a majority of the gained benefits. As life straightens out, your client will resolve once again to "get on the perfect program." Do your clients a favor and help them realize that "no such beast exists." These expectations often occur because many people have been set up with a philosophy of "all or none" in terms of their approach to an exercise program, and life in general. This learned attitude emboldens the philosophy that if you cannot embrace the training regime with optimal time investment and consistency, "Why do it?" This is the perfection scheme that sets many clients up for personal failure with regard to their exercise and nutrition program. With the research presented previously, it is obvious that some of something is better than nothing. Moderation is in! It is effective and supported by research. Also, it is quite easy to maintain, or regain, fitness levels with smart and sensible training. Support and encourage your clients along this path.

The warning with regard to injury is obvious. If your client stops exercising for 2 weeks or longer, do not encourage her to pick up where she left off. Start at a lower intensity, for instance less resistance, slower speeds and shorter durations. The odds are that she will regain her previous levels of fitness fairly quickly if you allow for this progressive adaptation to the "new" stresses you are placing on her body. Your role as a trainer is to temper your client's enthusiasm for starting out too intensely, based on your knowledge of the body's physical needs and how it adapts to overload.

Maintaining the Training Effect

To maintain the training effect, exercise must be continued on a regular basis and be of sufficient intensity. The American College of Sports Medicine (ACSM) sums up the maintenance of cardiorespiratory and strength gains in its position statement (1990):

• A significant reduction in **cardiorespiratory fitness** occurs after 2 weeks of detraining.

• Clients may return to near pre-training levels of cardiorespiratory fitness after 10 weeks to 8 months of detraining.

• A loss of 50% of their initial improvement in max VO2 has been shown after 4-12 weeks of detraining. However, many individuals who have undergone years of continuous training maintain some benefits for longer periods of detraining. While complete cessation of training shows dramatic reductions in max VO2, reduced training shows modest to no reductions for periods of 5-15 weeks.

• To maintain cardiorespiratory fitness, workout 3 times per week and utilize proper intensity.

• When **strength training** exercise is reduced from 2-3 days per week to one day per week, strength can be maintained for 12 weeks of reduced training. Intensity is maintained during the reduced frequency (reported in the 1990 ACSM position statement in reference to Hickson's research).

• Maintenance: 2-3 workouts per week for muscular strength and endurance fitness, though research indicates that one resistance workout performed every 10-14 days, one set per exercise, can maintain gains if proper intensity is used. Proper intensity is especially important when reducing frequency and duration of training effort.

The Bridge

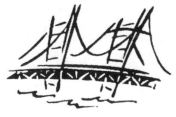

It appears that missing an exercise session periodically will not greatly affect current levels of fitness. Regardless of fitness level and component of fitness being trained, intensity of effort is the key factor to optimizing training effects and creating results-oriented use of time. Reducing training frequency and duration will not drastically affect fitness as long as training intensity is maintained. Minimal activity—whether formal workout or simply being busy with daily routine—is an important contribution to maintenance of fitness gains.

CHAPTER 12

What do an athlete in a competitive tennis match, your client running to the gate to catch an airplane and a grandmother climbing a hill during her afternoon walk have in common? All are using an **effort interval**, working a little harder than steady-rate or what is comfortable. This acceleration in level of effort is then followed by a moderate **recovery interval** or time period, where activity returns to an easily sustainable level of effort. Nordic skiing over typically undulating terrain, bursts of intense activity in team sports, and daily tasks are common examples of the body's responding to "interval" demands that are placed on it throughout any given day.

If a simple definition of interval is "varying the pace of an activity above what is routine," then the natural rhythm of life of active people is, by definition, a series of intervals. The beauty of an interval conditioning program is that the physiological requirements demanded of the body are very similar to movement experiences of everyday life.

Fitness interval conditioning can be engaged in by almost every one of your clients. There is no focus on strictly structured or extremely high-intensity effort intervals, and the client controls his own intensity level. This built-in flexibility allows for a successful and effective experience. Interval *conditioning* used for general health and fitness gains may allow your clients to experience some of the same benefits that highly trained athletes experience from interval *training*. These may include:

1. Expending more Calories.

2. Increasing endurance capacity by increasing max VO2, and/or increasing the ability to work at a higher percentage of max VO2, which is closely linked to increasing maximum steady-rate exercise level.

3. Increasing tolerance to lactic acid production when exercising intensely, and decreasing lactic acid production for given work loads.

By simply varying the pace of an activity, exercise may be performed for a longer duration at higher efforts, when compared to continuous exercise performed at a vigorous pace. Also, most clients exercise in the same time frame each day and do not have an infinite amount of time available for workouts. Interval conditioning can allow for a more efficient workout in a given time frame.

The thought of exercising hard or even continuously for 20-60 minutes is overwhelming to many of your clients. However, it is quite motivating for your client to successfully complete several to 60 minutes of cumulative interval conditioning that challenges his ability to exercise at higher intensity levels, on an intermittent basis. Accomplishments like this lead to high rates of compliance, as this type of quality effort is manageable and successful for most clients.

Research suggests that interval training may be done all at once or at different times during the day, with similar fitness results for selected populations (Haskell, 1994). This is good news for the client in a time crunch or who perceives smaller doses of exercise as attainable and non-intimidating. Because interval conditioning requires clients to "tune in" to how they feel and changes the level of effort required at any given moment, this helps exercise time go by quickly and enjoyably.

What's in an Interval?

Performance interval training has been used for many years by competitive athletes. In **performance training,** intervals often involve periods of maximal or near-maximal effort followed by short periods of rest. Efforts may range as high as 85-110% of max VO2. Such a method of training leads to significant performance benefits, in great measure due to an increased tolerance to the buildup, removal and lower production rate of lactic acid, and resultant increases in max VO2. Additional adaptations include enhanced levels of glycogen and glycolytic enzymes. Improvements may also be attributed to improved motivation and tolerance to high levels of "discomfort" associated with high-intensity cardiorespiratory exercise. Only well-trained athletes should participate in performance intervals. Because of the high-intensity nature of this type of training, an untrained client is at an increased risk for injury, not to mention quick fatigue, if performance intervals are attempted.

On the other hand, you can encourage your clients to perform fitness intervals. In **fitness interval conditioning,** the client periodically increases intensity throughout a workout and recovers or "catches his breath" before initiating another higher-intensity bout. Fitness intervals can vary in terms of *duration* of the effort interval and recovery from the effort, though there are specific recommendations. However, *intensity* is usually controlled by the client. This is in contrast to performance interval training where there are specific guidelines associated for both duration and intensity of effort.

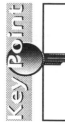

> Interval *training* is different from interval *conditioning*. The concept of interval conditioning serves a broader spectrum of fitness levels and needs, while simultaneously preserving the classic, high-intensity approach to intervals, referred to as performance interval training.

By targeting specific client goals, needs and current fitness levels, interval training *principles* can be used by the less fit individual, higher risk or special need clients that include multiple sclerosis and pregnancy, the fitness enthusiast, those clients looking for health benefits, or the performance athlete. *How* and *why* the effort interval is varied—as well as how the recovery interval duration and intensity is manipulated—is dependent on individual client goals.

Interval Conditioning for the Highly-conditioned and Less-fit Client

This is how interval conditioning might graphically look in performance and fitness training applications. The less-fit client uses an extended warm-up and steady-rate preparation period and recovers from his effort intervals below his steady-rate threshold. Note the difference between the steady-rate thresholds (80% versus 40% of max VO2) of the conditioned and less-fit clients. After reaching peak intensity, the highly conditioned client returns quickly to steady-rate and utilizes a shorter recovery time period. Intensity of effort (vertical axis) is paired with duration (horizontal axis) of effort and recovery. Figure 4 illustrates how interval conditioning can be applied to a wide range of clients, and can optimize a workout regardless of current fitness level.

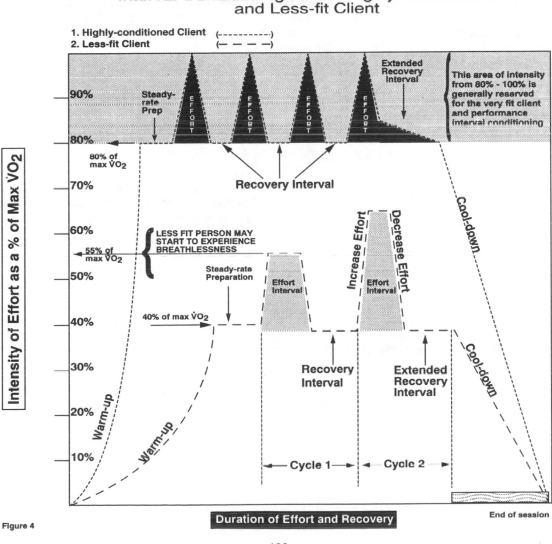

Interval Conditioning for the Highly-conditioned and Less-fit Client

Figure 4

Benefits of Interval Conditioning

There is very little research data dealing with interval *conditioning* for general populations. It seems that the potential physiological benefits may closely parallel those of athletes who utilize interval *training*. Research suggests that both interval training and continuous training have similar effects on aerobic endurance (Haskell, 1994; Cunningham et al. 1979; Edy et al. 1979; Gregory, 1979). Currently, there is not enough evidence to specify superiority of one system over another in improving aerobic capacity. Each method results in success. The most-effective programs will utilize both approaches, since optimal cardiorespiratory fitness is comprised of *both* aerobic and anaerobic conditioning.

Interval conditioning can increase a client's ability to exercise longer at the limits of aerobic metabolism. This is greater than what can be accomplished with continuous training (Lamb, 1984). Because of this, fitness levels and total caloric expenditure may improve greatly. Interval conditioning may be more effective in reducing body fat than continuous training for some individuals (Tremblay, 1994). Interval conditioning can train the body's aerobic processes to increase cellular capacity to sustain higher rates of aerobic energy transfer in relation to higher intensity efforts (McArdle et al. 1991).

Interval conditioning can help the nervous system adapt to movement patterns, making the particular movement more economical (Sleamaker, 1989). This type of adaptation can occur if the interval movement speed and mechanics are specific to the movement speed and mechanics used in a particular activity. This is potentially very important to athletes.

Proper and appropriate interval conditioning can raise a deconditioned, or a very fit, participant's blood lactate threshold. This resultant change in blood lactate threshold allows an individual to work at increasingly intense paces, and for longer durations. Overall, for a given time period, more total exercise effort is accumulated during a workout. For your clients who have limited time to exercise, this allows them to burn more total calories and fat, and become more fit in a given exercise time period. Interval conditioning makes more effective use of a client's time, whether deconditioned or highly fit.

Maximum VO2, along with the ability to sustain a high percentage of max VO2, determines performance capabilities and an ability to optimize fitness gains. Anaerobic intervals increase your client's ability to sustain a higher percentage of max VO2. This means he can work increasingly harder and longer, and still predominate with aerobic energy production. This level of effort that your client can sustain is referred to as **maximum steady-rate (MSR)**. Increasing your client's anaerobic threshold or MSR, is directly dependent on high-intensity anaerobic interval conditioning that is relative to current fitness level.

> The use of interval conditioning has important implications for optimizing fitness gains, performance, interest, compliance and results. Interval conditioning can optimize results in a deconditioned or highly trained person. The key is to ensure that the training intensity is relative to the individual's current state of fitness.

Interval Conditioning Benefits

1. **Increased Cardiorespiratory Fitness and Aerobic Endurance From Increases in:**
   - Maximum VO2 or aerobic capacity
   - An ability to work at a higher percentage of maximum VO2
   - Maximum steady-rate (MSR) threshold. An increased MSR can push back the onset of blood lactate threshold (OBLA), respiratory threshold, anaerobic threshold and lactate threshold
   - Lactate tolerance

2. **Increased Endurance of Muscle Fibers From:**
   - Increased endurance of fast-twitch, especially type IIa, muscle fibers (motor units)
   - Increased ability to use blood glucose during exercise, which spares glycogen

3. **Increased Total Calorie Utilization per Session and Increased Total Fat Utilization**

4. **Increased Exercise Compliance as a Direct Result of:**
   - Participant fun and enjoyment
   - Exercise variety
   - New and challenging physiological overload
   - Decreased overuse injury potential
   - Client concentration and focus
   - Client being mentally engaged, causing an impression that workout time passes quickly

5. **Increased Work Effort in Manageable Doses**

6. **Client Maximizes Time Usage**
   - Client realizes more total work (intensity) and caloric expenditure within given time frames. This results in more effective use of your client's finite time availability.

7. **Creates Client Perceptions of Confidence and Feelings of Accomplishment**

How Intervals Compare to Circuits and Continuous Training

Optimal **interval conditioning** results require that a cardiorespiratory recovery interval be performed after the effort interval. Effort intervals and recovery intervals *both* consist of cardiorespiratory activity. Some **circuit training** formats substitute another fitness component such as strength training for the recovery interval. This is not considered interval conditioning.

A circuit is generally characterized by your client performing physical activity at a variety of work stations. Your client may move from one station to another or perform the circuit in unison at one versatile station. Traditional circuits often contain work "stations" that are composed of: (1) entirely cardiorespiratory activity, (2) entirely muscular strength and endurance activity, or (3) a combination of both types of physical training.

In a circuit that has at least one station that represents cardiorespiratory activity, interval conditioning can be an *option* within that cardio station. Interval conditioning may be a part of cardiorespiratory circuit training or a tool used at a particular cardiorespiratory circuit station, but is not circuit training itself.

Continuous training is characterized by efforts longer than 5 minutes, but more commonly from 10-20 minutes and longer. Continuous training is a submaximal effort than can be maintained comfortably for extended periods of time and is performed at either low, moderate or high aerobic intensity (40-85% max VO2 or HRR). Continuous activity can be maintained at a specific percentage of max VO2 and is dependent on your client's level of fitness.

Continuous training produces significant aerobic adaptations in both the central circulation (heart and blood vessels) and peripheral tissues (muscles). During continuous exercise, effort or overload is generally increased by extending the exercise duration, though intensity may be manipulated as well (McArdle et al. 1991). More commonly, the intensity or work rate progresses naturally as training improvements are gained and duration is added to the effort. Training adaptations allow your client to work at increasingly higher levels of intensity, without necessarily increasing his perceived level of exertion.

Quick Index:

Chapters 4 and 5, steady-rate conditioning and oxygen utilization

The Science Behind Interval Programs

Interval conditioning involves both aerobic and anaerobic processes. An important point to reemphasize is that energy needs of the body's musculature are not switched on or off. Any time exercise intensity (increase or decrease) or duration (longer or shorter) changes, there will be an appropriate shift to either more or less involvement of a particular energy system(s), depending on the nature of the change. For example, as your client's cardiorespiratory workout lasts longer than about 3-4 minutes, the aerobic system supplies a large percentage of the required energy to the working muscles. During high-intensity cardio activity up to about 3 minutes, anaerobic energy sources are the significant contributing factor. It is important to train the aerobic and anaerobic systems because cardiorespiratory fitness is comprised of both.

For a healthy, untrained client, lactic acid begins to accumulate and rise quickly at about 50-55% of maximal aerobic capacity, max VO2, or HRR (60-65% of max HR). In a conditioned client, this may not occur until 80-85% of max VO2. The increase in lactic acid becomes exponentially pronounced as the activity becomes more intense relative to current fitness levels.

At some point, whether at 50%, 85% or some other percentage of maximal aerobic capacity, your client will reach a threshold, or a limiting factor, that does not allow him to continue performance at that particular level of intensity. Generally, a deconditioned client will begin to accumulate lactic acid in significant amounts at about 55% of maximal aerobic capacity. This point of lactate accumulation is commonly termed **anaerobic threshold,** but more precisely labeled **blood lactate thresh-**

old. For practical purposes, these terms are used similarly.

Steady-rate, which is often referred to as steady-state, is a balance between energy demands by the muscle and aerobic metabolism. It occurs when the pace of activity is easily maintained for a sustained duration; for example, longer than 5 minutes. During steady-rate activity, any lactic acid production and accumulation is minimal.

Maximum steady-rate levels and lactate threshold vary from one individual to the next, depending primarily on a person's ability to deliver and utilize oxygen. This, of course, is dependent on individual genetics and conditioning level. For a sedentary client, going from rest to slow walking, about 3 mph or a 20-minute-per-mile pace, may push his needs for energy (ATP) by the muscle into anaerobic metabolism. His maximum steady-rate exists at very low intensity levels of activity. Contrast this to a highly conditioned client, where the energy balance can be maintained aerobically at very intense levels of exercise. For example, in a highly conditioned and genetically blessed marathon runner, steady-rate aerobic metabolism can be maintained at an average pace near 5-minutes-per-mile, for 26 miles!

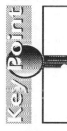

> Steady-rate exercise is the highest exercise intensity your client can maintain for prolonged periods of time. The long-term energy system predominates if steady-rate is maintained.

Quick Index:

Chapter 4, relationship between the aerobic and anaerobic energy systems
Chapter 5, adaptations in the cardiorespiratory (C-R) system to training

Muscle Fiber Type and Firing Patterns

To understand interval conditioning more fully as it relates to maximizing conditioning benefits, muscle fiber type must be taken into account. Muscles are predominantly composed of a certain percentage of 2 muscle fiber types: slow twitch (ST or type I) and fast twitch (FT type IIa and IIb). The ratio of ST to FT muscle fibers is generally believed to be (1) genetically determined, (2) variable between individuals and (3) unchangeable. However, the results of an extensive review of scientific literature concludes that *extreme* and *prolonged* training may produce skeletal muscle fiber type conversion (Abnerthy et al. 1990; reported in Wilmore and Costill, 1994).

Regardless of a participant's percentage of ST to FT fibers, with proper intensity, both can be trained to (1) produce more energy, (2) recover more quickly after engaging in challenging interval conditioning, and (3) help the body move faster. When exercise is at a low to moderate intensity, the activity involves ST fibers. The ST fibers' primary role is to sustain continuous, endurance, steady-rate type of activity. As the exercise intensity increases, progressively more FT muscle fibers are recruited, especially the FT-IIa. The FT-IIa muscle fiber is highly modifiable to either high-intensity interval conditioning or strength training. Maximal effort will call into play ST and both types of FT motor units. If only low to moderate intensity efforts are performed, the ST fibers (motor units) will predominantly be trained. Ultimately this type of training will limit training benefits.

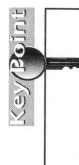

As FT motor units (especially Type IIa) become more accustomed to the demands of repeated interval efforts, the muscles produce lower amounts of lactic acid and the musculature is better able to handle (clear) and tolerate (buffer) high levels of lactate. These adaptations lead to an increased lactate threshold and increased aerobic capacity. The body becomes better able to deliver and utilize oxygen more efficiently. And, more calories can be expended in a given time frame, since these adaptations may allow a greater intensity and total exercise duration to be maintained.

Quick Index:

Chapter 7, detailed description of muscle fibers (Fig. 2) and order of motor unit recruitment patterns (Fig. 3)
Chapter 14, choosing resistance training intensity levels to activate different types of muscle fibers (fast-twitch or slow-twitch motor units)

Interval Conditioning Terminology Summary

1. Interval Conditioning

A form of training that utilizes repeated cardiorespiratory effort intervals that are often performed above intensities achieved during continuous training, and reflects a level of effort to which your clients are *not* accustomed. Interval efforts are followed by cardiorespiratory recovery intervals.

2. Effort Interval

The time period when your client is working harder than during either steady-rate or continuous training.

3. Recovery Interval

The time following an effort interval. A recovery interval consists of cardiorespiratory activity that is performed at relatively low intensities, such as steady-rate or slightly lower.

4. Cycle

An effort interval followed by a recovery interval.

5. Set

A new set occurs when either the duration of the previous effort interval or recovery interval changes.

Source: Brooks et al. (1995) Reebok Interval Program

Interval Program Concepts

Interval conditioning utilizes repeated cardiorespiratory **effort intervals** that are often performed *above* intensities that participants are used to working at, such as that which occurs during steady-rate effort or continuous training. In order to sustain these higher intensities, the effort intervals are followed by cardiorespiratory **recovery intervals** that are performed at a steady-rate or lower intensity. An effort interval followed by a recovery interval is termed a **cycle.** One or more cycles performed consecutively are called a **set.** A new set begins when one to several cycles are followed by an effort or recovery interval that is *different in length* than the previous effort or recovery interval(s). Generally, it is simpler to focus on the number of cycles completed, versus number of sets.

For example, you may choose to initiate a series of aerobic interval cycles using 3 minutes for the effort interval and 3 minutes for the recovery interval. This is called a 1:1 effort interval-to-recovery interval ratio. After the third effort interval is completed, you might choose to extend the recovery interval to 5 minutes instead of 3. This *change* in recovery interval duration marks the end of the first set of interval conditioning.

After the extended 5-minute recovery interval, you begin a new set of aerobic intervals using, once again, 3 minutes of effort interval followed by 3 minutes of recovery interval. After 2 cycles you decide that your client will immediately go into an anaerobic interval effort with 60 seconds of effort followed by 3 minutes of recovery interval. In this scenario the recovery interval actually stayed the same but the effort interval changed, identifying the beginning of a third set.

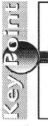

Any change in either the effort or recovery interval, whether increasing or decreasing duration, marks the beginning of a new set. However, the most important trainer focus should be the total number of interval conditioning cycles (frequency) that are completed during each workout.

Though it is variable, some scientific literature classifies interval efforts as **intermittent exercise** that can last from one to 6 minutes and continuous exercise is defined as an effort longer than 6 minutes (Shephard, 1992). The Reebok Interval Program (Brooks et al. 1995) uses the term **interval conditioning,** which includes aerobic and anaerobic intervals. Interval conditioning involves interval activity that lasts up to 5 minutes. **Continuous exercise** constitutes efforts longer than 5 minutes.

There are 3 types of interval conditioning defined by the Reebok Interval Program:

1. Spontaneous intervals
2. Fitness intervals
3. Performance intervals

When working with general populations, the very structured guidelines of *performance intervals* and the somewhat structured guidelines of *fitness intervals* should not be looked at as rigid and inflexible. In both performance and fitness intervals, determining the ratio of effort interval to recovery interval is probably more of an art than a science. A skilled and sensitive trainer will know when to adjust effort intervals and recovery intervals based on client feedback. However, the Reebok Interval Program recommendations are very good parameters to start and/or stay within to ensure safe progression and excellent participant results.

Though spontaneous intervals, which are less structured accelerations in intensity and often referred to as "speed play," and fitness intervals are not exclusive to the deconditioned or average fitness enthusiast, their application to these types of clients is very appropriate. Performance intervals are more appropriate for your "athlete" clients who have identified high performance goals. This chapter will focus on *fitness intervals*, which have a broad and clear application to most of your clients.

Aerobic interval conditioning involves training just below, at or slightly above lactate or maximum steady-rate (MSR) threshold. Though some anaerobic metabolism occurs to supply the energy need in this type of effort, especially if above MSR, it is predominantly aerobic. On the other hand, **anaerobic interval conditioning** involves training significantly *above*, and recovering at or below lactate or MSR threshold. This type of training requires a predominance of anaerobic energy metabolism.

Anaerobic interval conditioning enables the participant to "push back" the point (anaerobic threshold) at which lactate accumulates significantly. This happens because of the specific training adaptations that occur in response to this type of higher intensity overload. These adaptations occur, in part, because of enhanced levels of glycogen and glycolytic enzymes, lower levels and higher tolerance to lactate production, improved motivation and increased mental tolerance to fatiguing exercise. These adaptations translate into an ability to sustain higher-intensity aerobic efforts, greater overall endurance gains, increased performance and more total calories used.

In discussing aerobic and anaerobic interval conditioning, it is somewhat unfortunate that the terms aerobic and anaerobic are used in physiology, because they imply energy production with or without oxygen. More accurately, these terms represent energy production with or without *sufficient* oxygen. The type, intensity and duration of the activity, relative to level of fitness, will determine which system(s) contributes the most to energy production.

Quick Index:

Chapter 4, the energy spectrum

Structuring Effort and Recovery Intervals

No appreciable lactic acid accumulates with either steady-rate aerobic exercise, or brief 5- to 10-second bouts of all-out exercise. (However, brief, 5- to 10-second maximal efforts are very strenuous and not applicable to average clients. Because of this, the training models that follow do not exemplify this type of specialized and high-intensity training.) Because the accumulation of lactate during steady-rate activity is minimal, recovery is rapid. Additional exercise can begin again without the lingering effects of lactic acid-induced fatigue. *Aerobic intervals* performed at an intensity that a participant normally works at, or even *slightly* higher, represent this type of effort and allow for a quick recovery.

Periods of **anaerobic interval conditioning** are performed at the expense of lactate buildup in the exercising muscles and blood. Recovery from this type of activity takes longer and is reflected by the ratios of effort and recovery durations.

Recovery of proper duration and intensity after effort intervals is more crucial than for continuous or steady-rate training. Recovery allows specific adaptations to occur after intermittent, high-intensity cardiorespiratory effort. For example, stroke volume may be at its greatest during recovery efforts, as opposed to during the effort interval. This has important implications for associated training adaptations. And, recovery is important to expeditiously clear ("flush") lactic acid through oxidative processes.

Procedures for speeding recovery from effort intervals can generally be labeled as either **active** or **passive**. In **active recovery,** submaximal exercise (usually steady-rate or lower) is performed in the belief that this continued movement prevents muscle cramps, stiffness and facilitates the recovery process. With **passive recovery,** the person usually lies down or is totally inactive, with the hope that complete inactivity may reduce the resting energy requirements and thus "free up" oxygen for the recovery process. Remember, oxidative processes of the aerobic energy system are necessary for the complete recovery from activity that results in the use of anaerobic energy production.

Lactic acid removal is accelerated by **active aerobic recovery** exercise and clearly is more effective in facilitating lactate removal compared to passive recovery (McArdle et al., 1991). Though the reasons are not clear, it is speculated that the facilitated removal of lactate may be the result of an increased circulation of blood through "lactate using" organs like the liver and heart. Easy aerobic exercise may facilitate the removal of lactate by flushing organs that use lactate, like the liver and heart, with increased blood flow. Increased availability of blood flow and oxygen to the muscle, at moderate levels of exercise, would also allow the lactate to be oxidized within the muscle cell mitochondria, via the Krebs cycle. Both "flushing" and low-level exercise enhance removal and utilization of lactate (McArdle et al. 1991).

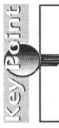

Low-level, active recovery will be the rule for most interval recoveries when the interval effort is above 55-60% of max VO2, HRR or an individual's lactate threshold.

An exception to this general recovery rule may be extremely high-end, sport specific, brief bouts of maximal effort. As pointed out, increased blood flow through the muscles in active recovery would certainly enhance lactic acid removal because muscle tissue can use this substrate lactate, and oxidize it via the Krebs cycle, which is an aerobic energy pathway for energy metabolism. However, if the exercise during recovery is too intense and above the lactate threshold, it may prolong recovery by increasing lactic acid formation.

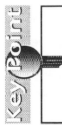

During recovery intervals, maintain an intensity of steady-rate or lower, and a duration that equals or exceeds the effort interval duration. Active recovery is of great importance when recovering from intervals that produce appreciable levels of lactic acid.

If clients are left to their intuition, most will naturally select an optimal-recovery exercise intensity. This will be at a level:

• Just below their lactate-accumulation threshold; in other words, at a level of exercise intensity that they can easily maintain.

• Where your client is not breathless and can speak 3 or 4 words at a time without gasping.

• Where his muscles are not "burning" or uncomfortable from lactic acid accumulation.

• That corresponds to a "somewhat easy" or "moderate" level of exertion.

Quick Index:

Chapter 4, dynamics of oxygen debt, or more accurately recovery oxygen consumption

Working at the Right Level of Effort

Heart rate is a relatively accurate means of monitoring exercise intensity. An appropriate range of training that accommodates most levels of fitness is from 40-85% of max VO2 or HRR. To calculate the appropriate target heart rate (THR) for interval conditioning, it is desirable to calculate heart rate reserve (HRR) according to Karvonen's formula.

An easy and practical way to monitor the intensity of effort and recovery intervals is with **rating perceived exertion (RPE)**. Using a manual heart rate count to monitor exercise intensity during interval conditioning is often difficult, distracting and inappropriate for high-risk populations. Because there is a high correlation between the participant's heart rate response to exercise and perceived exertion, RPE is a means for the participant to "check in" with how he is feeling at any given moment. RPE is often referred to as the "talk test." Once the relationship has been established between exercise heart rate and his own RPE, perceived exertion can be used in place of, or better yet, with heart rate monitoring.

The **training sensitive zone** based on a heart rate reserve (HRR) of 40-85% (equivalent to about 50-90% of maximal heart rate), corresponds to an RPE of 3-7 on the revised Borg scale. A rating of 3-7 classifies the exercise intensity as "moderate" to "very hard." Generally, a perceived exertion of 3-7 for most personal training clients is safe and effective. Anaerobic intervals may use ratings as high as 7-10 ("very hard," to "very, very hard").

As a client's fitness level increases, the *intensity* of activity that he engages in continuously will increase, if continued improvements are expected. In this case, after training adaptations occur, to elicit a similar RPE will require an increase in aerobic exercise intensity. If intensity is simply maintained, as opposed to being progressively increased over time, a phase of maintenance will be entered (see Chapter 6, Measuring Exercise Intensity).

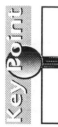

Even though your client will have a *similar RPE*, the actual intensity of exercise needed to elicit this same RPE will increase as his fitness progresses.

Fitness Intervals

Utilizing fitness intervals in any of your clients' programs is an excellent idea. Remember, intensity is controlled by the client, and you are simply encouraging him to work a little harder than that to which he is accustomed.

For less-conditioned participants, it may make more sense to begin interval conditioning with **spontaneous intervals** or "speed play." In this type of training you simply ask your client to in-

Table 9. Modified Borg Scale

The **C-R Conditioning** (interval conditioning) column represents recommended exertion levels for recovery (2-3), aerobic interval training (4-6) and anaerobic intervals (7-10). These ratings, and their association with the numerical rating of the Borg scale, are found by looking horizontally across the scale. The **Trainer Exertion Cues** represent language that may be more practical to use by the trainer, as opposed to the original language suggested by Borg and found in the middle column.

C-R Conditioning (Interval Conditioning)	Borg Scale Numerical Rating: 0 - 10	Instructor Exertion Cues
	0 Nothing	
	0.5 Very, very weak	Very, very easy
	1 Very weak	Very easy
Recovery Effort	2 Weak	Somewhat easy
Recovery Effort	3 Moderate	Moderate
Aerobic Effort	4 Somewhat strong	Somewhat hard
Aerobic Effort	5 Strong	Hard
	6	
Anaerobic Effort	7 Very Strong	Very hard
Anaerobic Effort	8	
Anaerobic Effort	9	
Anaerobic Effort	10 Very, very strong	Very, very hard

Source: Borg, G. (1982). *Psychological Bases of Perceived Exertion, Medicine and Science in Sports and Exercise,* 14:377-387.

crease cardiorespiratory effort intensity for various amounts of time and follow this with adequate recovery. For example, you might encourage a client who is running or walking outdoors to "speed up a little" until he reaches the stop sign that is several hundred yards away.

Fitness intervals are more structured than spontaneous or "speed play" intervals. They allow participants to select an individualized exercise intensity while the duration and frequency of each interval is controlled by the trainer. Because participants engaging in fitness intervals determine their own level of exertion, it is *not* necessary that they have a moderate to high level of fitness to participate.

Fitness intervals focus on completing preset *durations* of the effort interval and recovery interval as opposed to exercising at a preset *intensity*, such as a percent of heart rate reserve (HRR) or max VO2. Effort is based on how the participant feels, or rating of perceived exertion (RPE). The goal is to have participants work from "somewhat hard" to "very hard." Remember, the level of intensity for the effort interval should be greater than that to which your client is normally accustomed.

Fitness intervals can be performed using an aerobic or an anaerobic model. An important advantage interval conditioning has over continuous training is that it can challenge *both* the aerobic and anaerobic systems. This, of course, leads to optimal cardiorespiratory conditioning. However, proper intensity and duration must be observed to effectively achieve this goal.

It is recommended that **aerobic fitness intervals** utilize a 1:1 effort-to-recovery ratio. In scientific literature this ratio is referred to as the "work-to-rest" ratio. This ratio implies that there is an equal amount of effort to recovery in each interval cycle. It does *not* mean that one minute of effort is always followed by one minute of recovery. For example, using a 1:1 effort-to-recovery ratio, a 3-minute effort interval is followed by a 3-minute recovery interval.

During **anaerobic fitness intervals** a 1:3 effort-to-recovery ratio is used. Using this ratio, a one-minute effort interval will be followed by a 3-minute recovery interval. Generally, it is best to perform anaerobic effort intervals for a duration of 90 seconds or less. If effort intervals are performed at proper intensity, a 90-second or less duration ensures that the anaerobic system will receive a conditioning challenge.

Table 15. Fitness Interval Models

- Frequency and duration are fixed, set by the trainer.
- Intensity is not fixed, set by client.
- Assumes a moderate to high level of fitness for *anaerobic* effort intervals.
- Use RPE (rating perceived exertion) and/or heart rate to monitor effort and recovery intervals.

Model	Effort Intervals	Recovery Intervals
Aerobic	4-6 on RPE scale	2-3 on RPE scale
Anaerobic	7-10 on RPE scale	2-3 on RPE scale

Aerobic Fitness Model

Ratio:	1:1 effort to recovery (work-to-rest ratio)
Duration:	3-5 minutes for effort interval
	3-5 minutes for recovery interval
Intensity:	Participant controlled
Frequency:	Number of cycles accomplished is dependent on time availability and client fitness level.

Minutes of effort/recovery may vary from 3-5 minutes as long as the 1:1 ratio of effort to recovery is observed for each cycle.

Anaerobic Fitness Model

Ratio:	1:3 effort to recovery
Duration:	30-90 seconds of effort interval
	1.5 to 4.5 minutes for recovery interval
Intensity:	Participant controlled
Frequency:	Number of cycles accomplished is dependent on time availability and client fitness level.

Each effort interval may vary from 30-90 seconds, while each recovery interval may vary from 1.5-4.5 minutes. However, the 1:3 ratio of effort to recovery is observed for each cycle.

Source: Brooks et al. 1995 Reebok Interval Program

Performance Intervals

You might have a client who is a competitive triathlete, race-walker or runner who desires to increase his speed. Or, you might have a client who is superbly conditioned, a little bored, looking for a challenge and more results, and wants to take his level of cardiorespiratory fitness to the next level. Performance intervals are an excellent training technique to enhance higher levels of cardiorespiratory fitness and/or performance. The most structured of the interval formulas, this particular model for performance intervals is an example of classic, high-intensity performance interval training. Before you use it, make sure your client is highly conditioned, properly motivated and ready to train in the structured and physically intense environment of performance interval training.

Performance intervals require the use of precise, high-intensity work periods that are interspersed with specific recovery periods. Training focus is on *intensity* of effort for specific effort intervals and durations. Effort and recovery intervals should not be randomly manipulated if specific performance training goals have been identified and are desired. To follow these guidelines, the client must be highly fit and extremely motivated.

During performance intervals, heart rate monitoring with wireless telemetry (for example, Polar heart rate monitors) is recommended. Perceived exertion (RPE) works well for clients who understand the relationship between heart rate response and breathing rate, but this relationship needs to be established through accurate heart rate monitoring that is associated with an RPE. This feedback helps a participant to accurately rate his own perceived exertion as it relates to the Borg scale and training heart rate range.

Table 16. Performance Interval Models

- Intensity, duration and frequency are *fixed* according to specific performance goals.
- Monitor heart rates with electronic (wireless telemetry) heart rate monitors.
- Assumes a high level of fitness.
- Use RPE and heart rate to monitor effort and recovery intervals.

Model	Effort Intervals	Effort Intervals/RPE Rating	Recovery Intervals
Aerobic	80-85% of HRR	4-6 on RPE scale	2-3 on RPE scale
Anaerobic 1	85-90% of HRR	5-8 on RPE scale	2-3 on RPE scale
Anaerobic 2	90% or > of HRR	8-10 RPE scale	2-3 on RPE scale

Aerobic Performance Model

Ratio:	1:1 effort/recovery
Duration:	3-5 minutes of effort interval
	3-5 minutes of recovery interval
Intensity:	80-85% of HRR or max VO2
Frequency:	Number of cycles accomplished is dependent on time availability and client fitness level.

Effort/recovery intervals may vary from 3-5 minutes each as long as the 1:1 ratio of effort to recovery is observed for each cycle.

Table 16. Performance Interval Models(continued)

Anaerobic Performance Model #1

Ratio:	1:3 effort/recovery
Duration:	30-90 seconds of effort interval
	90-270 seconds (1.5-4.5 minutes) of recovery interval
Intensity:	85-90% of HRR or max VO2
Frequency:	Number of cycles accomplished is dependent on time availability and client fitness level.

Effort intervals may vary from 30-90 seconds, while each recovery interval may vary from 1.5-4.5 minutes. However, the 1:3 ratio of effort to recovery must be observed for each cycle.

Anaerobic Performance Model #2

Ratio:	1:2 effort/recovery
Duration:	30-90 seconds of effort interval
	60-180 seconds (1-3 minutes) of recovery interval
Intensity:	Greater than 90% of HRR or max VO2
Frequency:	Number of cycles accomplished is dependent on time availability and client fitness level.

Effort intervals may vary from 30-90 seconds, while each recovery interval may vary from 60-180 seconds. However, the 1:2 ratio of effort to recovery must be observed for each cycle.

Source: Brooks et al. 1995 Reebok Interval Program

Total Caloric Expenditure and Fat Utilization

There is a lot of confusion surrounding the concepts of "fat-burning" versus "carbohydrate-burning." There is no such exercise that can be defined as *only* "fat-burning" or *only* "carbohydrate-burning." This is especially true within the context of large muscle, rhythmic, continuous activity. Besides, to optimize caloric expenditure and fat utilization, such a distinction is not necessary. At rest, each Calorie that is utilized to sustain various metabolic functions comes from *both* fat and carbohydrate being "burned" or metabolized. In an average individual about 60% fat and 40% carbohydrate are being used for *each Calorie* of energy that is expended to meet the body's resting energy needs. At rest, about 1.5 kilocalories (kcal) or Calories of energy is expended per minute (McArdle et al. 1991).

Many of your clients believe that it is necessary to exercise for at least 20 minutes and work at a low exercise intensity to utilize fat. First, let's dispel the 20-minute myth. "Rest" is certainly an exercise intensity that requires a VO2 or submaximal consumption of a specific volume of oxygen. An individual is very "aerobic" at rest and is using fat to meet resting energy requirements, though it is a relatively low energy output (about 1.5 kcal/minute). It is clear that it is not essential to exercise a minimum of 20 minutes to begin using fat as an energy source, since 50-60% of each calorie used at low levels of intensity comes from fat. Admittedly, "rest" is not a very effective level of effort to expend a large number of calories. But, it is evident that fat is an important energy source, even at rest.

Next, let's clear the confusion surrounding the "best" level of effort to maximize fat utilization. Here's the big question: For your client's weight-loss goals, is the more important issue maximal fat utilization or total caloric utilization?

During prolonged low-intensity exercise, which includes levels of effort from rest to 50% of maximal aerobic capacity or max VO2, there is no question that fat supplies a large part of the energy requirements. However, at this relatively low intensity both fat and carbohydrate are used at a fairly slow rate of 3-5 Calories per minute. Contrast this to higher-intensity aerobic activity, which may use a smaller percentage of fat per Calorie burned, but results in a greater total caloric expenditure of 7-9 Calories per minute.

As activity is increased above resting level, it is a well-established physiological fact that *more* carbohydrate and *less* fat is burned *per single Calorie expended*. This seems to support the premise that as exercise becomes increasingly more intense, *less total* fat is burned. Indeed, physiological data related to fat and carbohydrate utilization for given time periods, supports the fact that as exercise becomes increasingly intense, less fat is burned per *each Calorie* expended, but more *total* fat and Calories are burned overall. Misinterpretation of this information often leads to inaccurate conclusions regarding optimal exercise intensity for maximizing total caloric and fat expenditure.

Another factor needs to be considered to understand the "big picture." As an individual exercises *harder*, more oxygen is breathed in and utilized. Each liter of oxygen consumed equates to 5 Calories being used or "burned."

Let's review what we have so far and tie in the oxygen factor. While it is true that when exercise intensity is *increased, a smaller percentage of fat* from each Calorie burned is utilized, at the end of the more-intense exercise effort, more total oxygen will have been consumed during a given amount of time. More oxygen consumed equates with *more total Calories* burned, because for every liter of oxygen taken in, 5 Calories are expended. Therefore, a smaller percentage of fat used per Calorie, multiplied by more total Calories expended, equates to more total fat being used.

Let's answer the question, "Is total fat expenditure or total caloric expenditure more important?" In terms of fat loss, most experts feel it is not important what percentage of fat or carbohydrate is burned per Calorie during activity. Instead, what's important is the total number of Calories expended in activity (Kaminsky et al. 1993; Ballor, 1990).

This whole discussion of fat utilization comes down to these concepts:

1. It is not necessary to slow down exercise intensity if your client can maintain the pace for the desired period of time. Exercising as hard as your client comfortably can will *optimize* total Calories and fat utilized.

2. If the intensity of exercise is too high and cuts short the goal amount of time your client would like to spend exercising, or the level of intensity is not easily tolerable, then it's appropriate to slow down and go longer.

Case Study of Fat Utilization

The following numerical data supports the conclusion that a smaller percentage of fat used per Calorie, multiplied by more total Calories expended, equates to more total fat being used. (Stanforth et al. 1989).

Subject: John

- exercise duration: 30 minutes
- has a max VO2 of 32 milliliters (ml) of oxygen (O2) per kilogram (kg)

of body weight per minute

- weighs 200lb or 91kg
- conversion of ml to liters (L)

    32 ml of O2 X 91kg = 2912 ml/1000= 2.9L or about 3L

It is not necessary to understand the conversion of milliliters to liters. However, using 3 liters creates an easy reference because it is known that one liter of oxygen equals 5 Calories burned. When ml/O2 per kg of body weight is not converted to liters, the numbers are difficult to interpret in a usable manner.

Example 1: John's max VO2 is 3 liters and he is exercising for 30 minutes at 50% of his max VO2, which is equal to 1.5 liters (L) of oxygen per minute. Most clients exercising at 50% of their max VO2 feel like they are working at a level that is "somewhat easy" to "moderate."

- 50% of John's max VO2 = 1.5L of O2 per minute
- 1.5L X 5.0 Calories per minute X 30 minutes = approximately *225 total Calories* expended

Example 2: John is exercising at 70% of his max VO2, which is equal to 2.1 liters of oxygen per minute. Most people exercising at 70% of their max VO2 feel like they are working at a level that is "somewhat hard" to "hard."

- 70% of John's max VO2 = 2.1L of O2 per minute
- 2.1L X 5.0 Calories per minute X 30 minutes = approximately *315 total Calories* expended

Examples 1 and 2 demonstrate that working at higher intensities for the same amount of time consumes more oxygen—2.1L per minute versus 1.5L per minute—and results in the utilization of more Calories—225 versus 315—for a *given* time period.

It is obvious that working harder in a given time frame expends more total Calories. But is more *total* fat burned?

Example 3: When working at the lesser intensity of 50% of max VO2, approximately 50% of the total Calories expended come from fat.

- Total Calories expended   = 225
- 50% of 220   = 113 Calories expended from fat

Example 4: When working at a higher intensity of effort, in this case 70% of John's max VO2, approximately 40% of the total Calories expended come from fat.

- Total Calories expended   = 315
- 40% of 315   = 126 Calories expended from fat

In these examples, a lesser exercise intensity burns 50% of its Calories from fat, whereas a higher intensity burns "only" 40% of its Calories from fat. However, 40% (a smaller piece) of a larger pie (315 total Calories burned) equals more total fat Calories burned at the higher intensity and most importantly, the higher intensity burns more *total* Calories than the lower-intensity exercise. This data convincingly illustrates that a smaller piece (less percentage of fat burned per Calorie) of a huge pie (more total Calories burned) can be better than a large piece (greater percentage of fat burned per Calorie) of a small pie (fewer total Calories burned).

Table 17. Fat Utilization Summary

Exercise Intensity	50% of max VO2	70% of max VO2
Total Calories Utilized	225 (50% from fat)	315 (40% from fat)
Total Fat Calories Utilized	113	126

Using Interval Conditioning to Utilize Fat

Many traditional workouts are designed to accommodate about 30-45 minutes of *continuous* cardiorespiratory training. If the participant's goal is to lose weight, the individual would be better off working at 80% of his max VO2 or HRR. However, even though 80% of HRR would maximize Calorie and fat utilization compared to a lesser level of intensity, it is a much more difficult workout. A more realistic exertion level would be about 70% of HRR, or about 75% of maximum heart rate, for a fairly fit person. This intensity level is more likely to be maintained over 30-45 minutes, and this level of effort still uses plenty of Calories.

But, some of your clients may have difficulty maintaining high, or even moderate, levels of continuous cardiorespiratory effort. Interval conditioning allows participants to accumulate more total exercise, performed at higher intensities, and in tolerable doses of duration. For most clients it is much easier to endure relatively short durations of higher intensity work.

What if your client is deconditioned? This individual should probably exercise at a level of intensity he can *maintain* to optimize fat and Calorie burning. Since intensity of effort is controlled by the exercising client in fitness intervals, accumulated yet manageable effort intervals of *slightly* higher intensity than that to which the client is accustomed, might be appropriate.

If the less-fit client was working out with a continuous training format at an intensity of 50% of HRR, and this limited desired duration or was perceived as uncomfortable, you could encourage the individual to slow down and go longer—probably at an intensity of about 40% of his max VO2. Or, and possibly more effective, have this client work at a perceived exertion level (RPE) that allows him to carry on a conversation while exercising. This would create an exercise environment that keeps the client exercising long enough to burn significant amounts of fat and calories. In addition, based on this successful experience, there is a good likelihood that the client would return for another session and evolve into a committed exerciser for a lifetime!

Interval Programs for Health and Fitness

The type of interval conditioning, length, intensity level of the exercise and recovery periods are dependent on the goal of the client and his current level of conditioning. For those wishing to enhance aerobic fitness, longer work periods are required. For those desiring improved anaerobic cardiorespiratory performance, shorter work periods performed above lactate threshold and/or near max VO2 are necessary.

It is important to consider that maximum steady-rate (MSR) threshold is relative to current fitness level. A deconditioned client's MSR exercise level may be at 40% of his max VO2, whereas a conditioned client's MSR exercise level may be at 75% of his max VO2. To elicit an MSR at 40% of max VO2 from a deconditioned client may require going only from a slow walk to a quick shuffle. To elicit an MSR at 75% of max VO2 in a conditioned client might require timed and significant increases in running, biking or walking paces.

These guidelines will help you adapt interval conditioning principles for your clients' health and fitness workouts:

1. As with any type of fitness activity, precede the workout with a warm-up of at least 5- to 10-minutes and follow it with a cardiorespiratory cool-down of at least 5 minutes. After the cool-down participants should feel like their heart rate and respiration are back to pre-exercise levels.

2. Remember that interval conditioning, in its simplest form, can be as easy as varying the intensity of the cardiorespiratory activity up and down once, or several times. The effort interval is followed by a duration of less-intense activity called the recovery interval.

3. The need for *exacting* structure and precision for exercise intensity and duration is unnecessary for fitness intervals. However, fitness intervals do provide guidelines and a starting point for structuring intervals with regard to duration and frequency. Intensity is controlled by the client.

4. When compared to an elite athlete in training, the intensity and the number of cycles completed by fitness enthusiasts is usually less. Also, the recovery intervals of the fitness enthusiast might be longer and would be more dependent on perceived exertion as opposed to preset recovery heart rates or durations (Figure 4).

5. Beginning exercisers, should not participate in *anaerobic* interval conditioning.

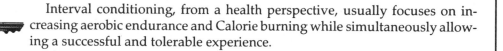

Interval conditioning, from a health perspective, usually focuses on increasing aerobic endurance and Calorie burning while simultaneously allowing a successful and tolerable experience.

6. Fitness interval intensity levels may be performed in a broad range. An approximate range for the average client would include working from 40-80% of heart rate reserve (HRR) or max VO2. This intensity level range is broad enough to challenge most fitness levels, yet it is low enough to allow for a fairly complete recovery of the energy systems challenged. A complete recovery from interval efforts above maximum steady-rate keeps lactate levels from progressively rising during the workout. This keeps the workout tolerable and effective.

7. Carefully monitor clients. Exhaustion is not the goal. Interval conditioning should be enjoyable, and though challenging, should not create post-exercise exhaustion or a negative experience.

8. The duration and increase (acceleration) in intensity of the effort interval need not be precise in fitness interval conditioning. Generally, after a proper warm-up, it is best to accelerate quickly to the desired RPE and/or heart rate during the effort interval. However, less conditioned participants may *slowly* increase their level of effort to an RPE of "moderate" to "somewhat hard." This slow acceleration simply limits the amount of time they will spend exercising at a theoretical, "optimal" exercise intensity.

9. Remember, individual effort level is controlled by your client. During the next effort interval or as your client becomes more fit, he may choose to use a faster acceleration to desired RPE or heart rate. A more fit individual may always accelerate sharply to or above his anaerobic threshold, depending on whether an aerobic or anaerobic interval is being performed.

10. If a client who wants to gain the benefits associated with interval conditioning is able to continue exercising at the same intensity level during recovery as he did during the effort interval, an increase in the level of intensity during the effort interval is appropriate.

When working with **special populations** that include the physically challenged, cardiac rehabilitation patients, diabetics, asthmatics, perinatal clients, youth, seniors, Parkinsonism or multiple sclerosis patients, interval conditioning may be the best choice of conditioning to optimize aerobic benefits. However, the program needs to be carefully planned with each client's physician.

In many cases heat buildup is a major concern of the exercising client with special concerns. This may be true for the client who is pregnant, has multiple sclerosis or anyone who has a sensitivity, whether temporary or permanent, to core temperature buildup. In any of these instances, interval conditioning at the right intensity may keep the core temperature from rising as dramatically as in continuous aerobic training.

The Bridge

Interval conditioning has many benefits, whether the client is deconditioned or an elite athlete. The key is to be flexible in effort/recovery ratios, focusing on appropriate duration and client controlled intensity. Most clients will naturally discover the appropriate recovery interval, while you can guide the effort interval. Interval conditioning can maximize fat burning because clients can complete more work and burn more Calories in a given time period. Plus, creating intervals is interesting for you and the client.

References and Recommended Reading

Anderson, Owen (1989). *Understanding the 10K, **Running Research News (RRN)**, Vol. 5, No. 6,* (517) 393-3150.

Ballor, Douglas L., et al. (1990). *Exercise intensity does not affect the composition of diet and exercise-induced body mass loss. **American Journal of Clinical Nutrition,** Vol. 51: 142-146.*

Barstow, Thomas (1994). *Characterization of VO2 Kinetics During Heavy Exercise. **Medicine and***

Science in Sports and Exercise. Vol. 26, No. 11, pp. 1327-1334.

Borg, G. (1982). *Psychological Bases of Perceived Exertion,* **Medicine and Science in Sports and Exercise,** 14:377-387.

Bouchard, Claude, et al. (1992). *Genetics of Aerobic and Anaerobic Performances.* **Exercise and Sport Science Reviews,** Vol. 20.

Brooks, Douglas, et al. (1995). *Reebok Interval Program. Stoughton, MA.*

Brooks, Douglas (1994). **Your Client's First 10K and Beyond.** *IDEA Personal Trainer Magazine, September.*

Brooks, George A. (1986). *The Lactate Shuttle During Exercise and Recovery.* **Medicine and Science In Sports and Exercise,** Vol. 18, No. 3, pp. 360-368.

Cunningham, D.A., et al. (1979). *Cardiovascular response to interval and continuous training in women.* **European Journal of Applied Physiology.** Vol. 41: 187-197.

Daniels, Jack (1992). *Making the most of your available training time,* **RRN,** Vol. 8, No. 5.

Daniels, Jack (1989). *Training Distance Runners: A Primer.* **Sports Science Exchange,** Vol. 1, No. 11, Publisher: Gatorade Sport Science Institute.

Ebbeling, C.B., Ward, A., and Rippe, J.M. (1991). **Comparison between palpated heart rates and heart rates observed using the Polar Favor heart rate monitor during an aerobics exercise class,** *Exercise Physiology and Nutrition Laboratory, University of Massachusetts Medical School, Worcester, MA.*

Edy, D. O., et al. (1979). *The effects of continuous and interval training in women and men.* **European Journal of Applied Physiology.** Vol. 37: 83-92.

Gaesser, Glenn (1994). *Influence of Endurance Training and Catecholamines on Exercise VO2 Response.* **Medicine and Science in Sports and Exercise.** Vol. 26, No. 11, pp. 1341-1346.

Gregory, L. W. (1979). *The development of aerobic capacity: A comparison of continuous and interval training.* **Research Quarterly.** Vol. 50: 199-206.

Janssen, Peter (1987). **Training Lactate Pulse-Rate.** *Published by Polar Electro Oy.*

Kaminsky, L. and Mitchell W. (1993). *Effect of Interval-Type Exercise on Excess Postexercise Oxygen Consumption (EPOC) in Obese and Normal-Weight Women.* **Med. Exerc. Nutr. Health;** *Vol. 2, pp. 106-111*

LaForge, Ralph, and Kosich, Daniel (1994). **Interval Exercise.** *IDEA Personal Trainer Magazine, November/December.*

Lamb, David (1984). **Physiology of Exercise: Responses and Adaptations,** *New York, NY: Macmillan Publishing Company.*

McArdle, W., Katch, F. and Katch, V. (1991). **Exercise Physiology - Energy, Nutrition, and Human Performance.** *3rd edition. Malvern, PA: Lea and Febiger.*

Myers, Jonathan, et al. (1994). *Increase in Blood Lactate During Ramp Exercise: Comparison of Continuous and Threshold Models.* **Medicine and Science in Sports and Exercise.** Vol. 26, No. 11, pp. 1413-1419.

Plisk, Steven S. (1991). *Anaerobic Metabolic Conditioning: A Brief Review of Theory, Strategy and Practical Application.* **Journal of Applied Sport Science Research,** Vol. 5, No. 1, pp. 22-34.

Poole, David (1994). *Role of Exercising Muscle in Slow Component of VO2.* **Medicine and Science in Sports and Exercise.** Vol. 26, No. 11, pp. 1335-1340.

Poole, David, et al. (1994). *VO2 Slow Component: Physiological and Functional Significance.* **Medicine and Science in Sports and Exercise.** Vol. 26, no. 11, pp. 1354-1358.

Rontoyannis, George P. (1988). *Lactate Elimination From the Blood During Active Recovery.* **The Journal of Sports Medicine and Physical Fitness,** Vol. 28, pp. 115-123.

Shephard, Roy, and Astrand, P. O., editors (1992). **Endurance in Sport.** Boston, MA: Blackwell Scientific Publications.

Sleamaker, Rob (1989). **Serious Training For Serious Athletes.** Champaign, IL: Human Kinetics Publishers.

Stanforth, Dixie, and Buono, Michael (1989). *The Fat Burning Concept: Implications for Aerobic Dance,* **International Symposium on the Scientific and Medical Aspects of Aerobic Dance—Exercise Manual.**

Tremblay, Angelo, et al. (1994). *Impact of Exercise Intensity on Body Fatness and Skeletal Muscle Metabolism.* **Metabolism,** Vol. 43, No. 7, July, pp. 814-818.

Wells, C. and Pate, R. (1988). *Training for Performance of Prolonged Exercise, in* **Prolonged Exercise,** Vol. 1 (Chapter 8). Edited by D. Lamb and R. Murray. Indianapolis, IN: Benchmark Press.

Whipp, Brian (1994). *The Slow Component of O2 Uptake Kinetics During Heavy Exercise.* **Medicine and Science in Sports and Exercise.** Vol. 26, No. 11, pp. 1319-1326.

Willis, Wayne, et al. (1994). *Mitochondrial Function During Heavy Exercise.* **Medicine and Science in Sports and Exercise.** Vol. 26, No. 11, pp. 1347-1354.

Wilmore, J. H., and Costill, D.L. (1994). **Physiology of Sport and Exercise.** Champaign, IL: Human Kinetics Publishers.

Wilmore, J. H., and Costill, D. L. (1988) **Training for Sport and Activity,** Dubuque, IA: Wm. C. Brown publishers.

CHAPTER 13

Despite how often we see that word "periodization," is it really clear how it applies to fitness?

Scientists define periodization as the overall, long-term, cyclic structuring of training and practice to maximize performance. Many articles mention that periodization should be incorporated into every program-planning process. While there is quite a bit of information in reference to periodization training developed for elite athletes, these programs are very technical, highly specific, focus on "peaking" for athletic performance, and are often confusing since there is no one, standard approach. However, very few formulas exist for trainers that explain how to incorporate a periodized program into the fitness routines of their clients. Furthermore, the whole process must be time-efficient for the busy trainer.

Fortunately, when these existing models of periodization for athletics are carefully studied, it's possible to identify common characteristics that you can use to bridge seemingly ambiguous and complex training principles into fitness. Periodization is probably most simply defined as "planned results." By manipulating volume of work and intensity of effort, and by strategically placing rest, maintenance and recovery phases in the overall periodization plan, you can transfer the concepts of periodization to fitness goals such as weight management, increased muscle strength and improvement in cardiorespiratory fitness.

For your clients, this approach has the potential to:

- Promote optimal response to the training stimulus or work effort.
- Decrease the potential for overuse injuries.
- Keep your clients fresh and progressing toward their ultimate training goal(s).
- Optimize your clients' personal efforts.
- Enhance client compliance.

Periodization Principles

Periodization is a method to organize training. It cycles volume (reps, sets, minutes, distance, duration) and intensity (load, force, weight lifted, speed) over specific time periods.

Periodization may be viewed from 2 perspectives:

1. The use of an activity or sport by itself to develop fitness or enhance health improvements.

2. The use of a sport, specific movement skills and cross training activities to develop fitness or health improvements and to keep the training progressing.

Considerable scientific research and experience shows the second system—using sport movement and supplementary training that includes a *variety* of cardiorespiratory, muscular strength and endurance, and flexibility conditioning—is far more effective than training with activity skills or sport alone (Siff, 1993). Regardless of which approach is used, the underlying science is related to *optimal stress or intensity* and *restoration or recovery*. Of these key aspects—intensity and recovery—one is not better than the other. Each must be given equal emphasis and preferential time.

From Athlete to Fitness Client

Periodization attempts to provide for adequate recovery while simultaneously preventing detraining or overtraining. By using known physiological training principles such as progressive overload, progressive adaptation and training effect, as well as what is known about maintaining fitness gains, avoiding overuse injuries, peaking for performance and training for health gains, an identifiable formula for periodization emerges for fitness. An important step in creating a periodized program is to develop:

- **short-term microcycles**, which deal with the daily and weekly variation in volume, intensity, loading and exercise selection.

- **mid-term mesocycles**, which usually begin with a high-volume phase and end with a high-intensity peaking phase.

- **long-term macrocycles**, each of which is generally composed of several mesocycles.

Volume refers to repetitions, sets, minutes, distance and duration. **Intensity** refers to load, force, weight lifted and speed.

For elite athletes a microcycle typically lasts 5-10 days; a mesocycle lasts 1-4 months; and a macrocycle lasts 10-12 months. Three major phases of training are recognized during a year (macrocycle) and these same phases can be recognized within a several-month time period that I call a "mini" macrocycle. The phases include: (1) preparation, (2) competition and (3) post-competition.

The most obvious difference between elite athletes and most fitness participants is that the need to "peak" for performance is minimal or nonexistent for the latter. For the athlete, maximal performance generally coincides with important competitions (Siff, 1993). Thus, the change from one phase of training to another will be more subtle for fitness training than for the high-level athlete. For the average client, macrocycle phases translate to (1) preparation or buildup, (2) goal attainment and (3) restoration/recovery. Within the preparation or goal-attainment phases, specific energy and physiologic system manipulations may be accomplished to attain goals that include muscle hypertrophy and increased oxygen uptake. For most active people who have achieved a desirable level of fitness, the goal may be variety of activity, solidifying current fitness levels and establishing commitment to exercise on a regular basis.

A well-planned periodized program looks at short-term, mid-term and long-term needs of the client. Such a planning process considers:

1. Daily workouts

2. An agenda that accounts for 3-4 weeks of training

3. An overall annual scheme, or at least several months of planning

That is the essence of periodization: training with variety of activity; training with varied, progressive intensities; training with 3- to 4-week mesocycles of progressive overload—always following a concentrated effort of progressive overload with at least several workouts of active recovery. **Active recovery**, or active "rest," is usually performed at lower intensities of effort and duration than previous exercise levels. Also, you should consider using different activities, at least part of the time, for this recovery and restoration time period.

When planned results are achieved, the intensity of effort or load is determined for the next phase. Generally, unless entering into a restoration phase or ending a mesocycle of 3-4 weeks, the sequence of the preceding workouts is repeated at higher intensity levels. This cyclic process will determine the contents and organization of the programming process.

Quick Index:

Applying Periodization to Fitness

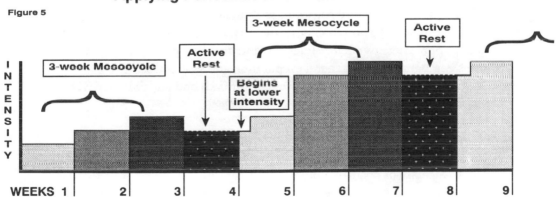

Figure 5

Reprinted with permission. Goss, Keller, Martinez Design: Del Mar, California, 1996.

Applying Periodization to Fitness

Figure 5 illustrates a progressive overload pattern using active rest after each 3- to 4-week mesocycle. The beginning of each new mesocycle should be started at a lower intensity than used in the last week of the previous mesocycle.

Periodization Model for Health and Fitness

To the average client, periodization means varying workouts over set time periods to optimize performance and fitness gains. Follow these steps to plan a progressive, goal-oriented training program that achieves superb results.

Step 1: Set the Goal(s)
- Cardiorespiratory
- Muscular strength and endurance
- Flexibility
- Other

Step 2: Determine How to Achieve the Goal(s)
- Assess time availability.
- Identify types (mode) of activity.
- Match training to goals.
- Choose activities that your client likes.

Step 3: Identify Training Phases

1. *Training Phases*
- Develop 3- to 10-day short-term planning (microcycle).
- Develop a 3- to 4-week training plan (mesocycle).
- Develop a yearly organizational training plan (macrocycle), or at least 3-4 months of mesocycles.
- Plan a general preparation phase of 3-4 weeks (one mesocycle), which may repeat several times.

2. *Exercise Plan*
- Manipulate frequency, intensity and duration of each activity for specific results in the body's energy and physiologic systems.
- Apply appropriate frequency, intensity and duration principles to each fitness component in the general preparation and goal phase.
- Control results by proper intensity of effort (load) and adequate recovery (restoration).

Step 4: Plan Volume and Intensity (overload)

1. *Vary volume and overload on a cyclic basis.*
- Change every 3-4 weeks at least, and possibly within a 3- to 10-day microcycle.
- Plan to increase or decrease volume and intensity.
- Use lower intensities and less duration during restoration (active rest).
- Start the new mesocycle after active recovery at a slightly lower intensity than the previous cycle (Figure 5).

2. *Allow for the Restoration/Recovery Process.*
   - Generally, do not increase progressive overload for more than 3 continuous weeks.
   - Follow any sustained, progressive overload of about 3 weeks with at least several days of active recovery activity at lower intensity. (The effort is less intense when compared to the last overload phase in which the client participated.)
   - After active recovery, start the new mesocycle at a slightly lower intensity than the previous cycle (Fig. 5).
   - Break every 3- to 4-week progressive increase in overload (mesocycle) with active recovery at a lower intensity (Fig. 5). The key to optimal results is *not* a steady, relentless increase in intensity over long periods of time.

Step 5: Regularly Evaluate the Periodization Planning Process
   - Monitor results and progress.
   - Use fitness assessment (optional).
   - Recognize goal achievement.
   - Maintain an ongoing dialogue with the client.
   - Observe client compliance and enthusiasm toward the program.

Case Study: From Theory to Client Program

Let's apply these principles to the program of a hypothetical client. Jenna is a new exerciser and her goals are weight loss, weight management and "increased energy level." Jenna understands that a long-term plan (macrocycle) will focus on important fitness components that will help her realize her training goals.

1. Set the Goals.

An *optional* first step in creating a periodized program is to assess Jenna's current fitness levels in categories related to her goals of weight loss, weight management and increased energy. Fitness testing will establish a reference point for comparing fitness improvements over time. This is one way to evaluate the effectiveness of a planning program.

Jenna chose to have a percent body-fat analysis performed with skinfold calipers and to have a submaximal cardiorespiratory assessment.

2. Determine How to Achieve the Goals.

Improvements in cardiorespiratory fitness and muscular strength and endurance will be very important to help Jenna attain her goals. She understands the important contribution cardiorespiratory fitness gives to calorie burning and that if she becomes more fit, she will be able to burn more calories and fat. She also will develop greater endurance, which could lead to a feeling of "more energy."

Strength training will enhance Jenna's feelings of personal power and control. Because gains in muscle strength increase muscle endurance, she will have new energy and strength at the end of the day. Also, increases in lean muscle mass will "reshape" her body and increase her resting metabolic rate, which will help her lose body fat and maintain her new, desirable weight.

Part of the solution to attaining goals is to create an environment where your client has a sense of ownership (a feeling that "this is what I want to do") and personal responsibility, and an understanding of why a specific approach is being organized and planned. This feeling of ownership and responsibility can be realized only through communication and education.

After talking about her goals, it became clear that Jenna wanted to accomplish her goals with a multi-activity approach.

3. Identify Training Phases.

It is usually unrealistic to plan an entire year and expect typical clients to stick to this. Instead, stay focused on microcycles and mesocycles. This will save valuable time when one of "life's events" inevitably necessitates a major change in your client's training program or schedule.

• Over a **3- to 10-day microcycle**, plan a menu of workouts that fit into the session.

• Extend the microcycle to a planned **3- to 4-week mesocycle**.

• A "mini" **macrocycle of 3- to 4-months** (long-term planning) is the next step.

Since Jenna is new to fitness and her goals are set, her first 3- to 10-day microcycle will focus on a preparation phase that reflects the goals of increased overall endurance ("energy") and weight management. Her program looks like this:

• A series of 6 or 7 microcycles (about 2 months) emphasizing a basic, but progressive, resistance and cardiorespiratory program. This series of microcycles is equivalent to 2 mesocycles. (Each mesocycle is about 3-4 weeks in length.)

• After the first mesocycle (3-4 weeks), active "rest" should be used for about 3-5 workouts.

• A second mesocycle will emphasize continued, progressive increases in intensity. If Jenna is ready, exercise variety will be introduced within each fitness component.

4. Plan Volume and Intensity.

After the preparation phase is well established (in about 8 weeks), the third mesocycle begins and progresses to the goal phase. This cycle emphasizes a hypertrophy phase for strength and continued challenges in duration and intensity of effort for cardiorespiratory conditioning. For example, Jenna may have progressed from a 12-20 repetition overload to fatigue, to an 8-12 repetition overload to fatigue. Since the first 2 mesocycles built the base of aerobic endurance, the third mesocycle will incorporate intervals, and intensity, duration and frequency will be manipulated.

The goal of these specific time periods is to provide an overload that is challenging, progressive and appropriate to Jenna's new fitness gains. Micro- and mesocycles also create goals that are reasonable, and most important, attainable in short time frames. This keeps the participant motivated, compliant and physiologically fresh.

After the completion of this third mesocycle, active rest will be used, including a variety of cross training activities. Jenna will experience different cardio conditioning activities, will change strength exercises or will switch to entirely different (non-related) activity during this active recovery.

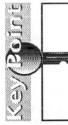

Remember, active recovery is performed at lower intensities of effort (and usually with less quantity or duration) than in previous micro or mesocycle time periods. Active recovery allows for physical recovery and enhancement of the adaptation process. Effort is 50% of the training equation, and recovery/restoration is the other important half!

5. Evaluate the Program

Reassessment of Jenna's goals, results, her interest and enthusiasm can never happen too often. This keeps an open and fresh communication with Jenna's needs and wants, and continues to ask the question, "Where should we, as a team, go from here?"

Quick Index:

Table 18. Applying Periodization to Fitness Results

1. Determine and select goal(s).

2. Determine and assess starting fitness level (optional).

3. Develop a 3- to 10-day menu (microcycle) of daily workouts.

4. Develop a 3- to 4-week menu (mesocycle) of daily workouts.

5. Develop a 4-month menu (modified macrocycle) of workouts.

6. Develop at least four mesocycles (12-16 weeks of workouts). Four mesocycles could be considered as a "mini" macrocycle.

7. Reevaluate goals, progress and effectiveness of the program after each daily workout, and especially after each 3- to 4-week mesocycle.

8. Plan and organize a recovery or restoration phase, consisting of at least several workouts, after every mesocycle (3-4 weeks). Utilize the concept of active rest. Active rest encourages the participant to engage in different activities, preferably at lower intensities. This "unloading" phase is critical to optimizing results and minimizing injury potential.

9. Make sure the client exercises at the right intensity or level of effort for each fitness component. Intensity should reflect personal fitness level and personal goals.

10. Develop an individual exercise plan. When developing meso- or macrocycles, make sure that all necessary fitness components are included in the planning process and emphasized in the right amounts (frequency, duration) and appropiate intensity to move the client toward the accomplishment of her goals.

Implementing Periodized Fitness

The key to successful periodization is the ability to create challenges to the body with new activities and progressive overload (intensity). If your client's body is constantly challenged, it will keep responding, her mind will stay inspired and her risk of overuse injury will go down. Just as her body experiences the peak benefits of one mesocycle of planned workouts and starts to adapt to it, she moves into a whole new 3- to 4-week cycle that offers an entirely new set of challenges.

Management and organization of a client's program involves your awareness of what drives the client's motivation and personality. Ralph Laforge, MS, points out that within a 24-hour period, a person's perceptions of his or her fatigue, strength and motivation may vary, so it is helpful to be aware of influences on your client that will challenge you to adapt your planning.

There are several ways you can track a periodization program. One idea is to label a manila folder with each mesocycle and keep the client's workout card in the file. You may have 4 manila file folders hanging inside one Pendaflex® for each client. You can organize the same system on your computer by creating a file for each mesocycle and placing programs in it. "The Periodization Planning Worksheet" is a model that you may want to follow as you develop your own record-keeping system (see sidebar).

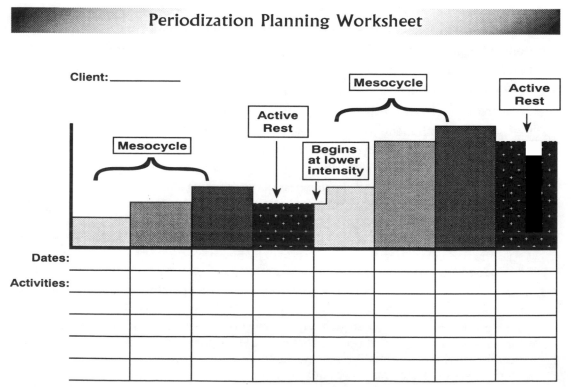

Periodization Planning Worksheet

Reprinted with permission. Goss, Keller, Martinez Design: Del Mar, California, 1996

A comprehensive, accurate planning process will draw heavily on your practical experience and knowledge of the scientific theory behind training. It is obvious that periodization, planning and program organization are not inherently complex. However, planning does require considerable forethought and time investment. On the other hand, it is well worth that investment, since periodization makes both the trainer and client accountable for results. Because the process involves management, planning and organization, it is "results oriented." And, everybody wins!

The Bridge

For fitness results, client compliance and variety, periodization works. Determine the client's goals, identify the training phases and include recovery time. Training phases include short microcycles, month-long mesocycles and annual macrocycles. Manipulate volume and intensity within the cycles, changing one element at a time. Keep careful records to maintain the cycling, and enable evaluation of the program and results.

References and Recommended Reading

Bompa, T. (1983). *Theory and methodology of training.* Dubuque, IL: Kendall-Hunt.

Bruner, R. et al. (1992). *Soviet training and recovery methods.* Pleasant Hill, CA: Sport Focus Publishing.

Metveyev, L. (1981). *Fundamentals of sports training.* Moscow: Progress Publishers.

Ozolin, N. (1971). *The athlete's training system for competition.* Moscow: Fizkultura i Sport Publication.

Siff, Mel et al. (1993). *Super training: special strength training for sporting excellence.* South Africa: School of Mechanical Engineering, University of the Witwatersrand.

Vorobyev, A. (1978). *A textbook on weight lifting.* Budapest: International Weightlifting Federation.

Yessis, M. (1987). *The secret of soviet sports fitness and training.* Published: Arbor House.

CHAPTER 14

REPS, SETS AND LOADS

Much of the folklore surrounding resistance training originates from competitive sports such as body building, power lifting and Olympic lifting. Athletes and coaches generated a large body of empirical (based on observation or experience only) evidence about training in these and other sports. As resistance training for general fitness became popular, enthusiasts looked to these individuals for expertise in designing their exercise programs. Unfortunately the "experts" often did not know how to separate the very *specific* objectives of resistance sports like body building or Olympic lifting from the very different needs for general fitness.

Certainly this is not a critique of these excellent sports, but simply a documentation of the evolution of many programs in use today. It is also where the principle of **specificity** comes in—training for the requirements of a specific activity. For example, body builders have exacting and demanding programs to meet the requirements of their sport. They also spend a great deal of their lives developing their physical training base and their competitive natures. These "weight competitors" have years of background and experience, and commit endless hours to their goal of being competitive. How appropriate is this specific type of training for novice weight trainers?

Do not make the mistake of blindly adopting a program simply because it was used by a successful weight-trained athlete. Do not jump on the bandwagon because "everyone is doing it." Make sure the training system you choose meets your client's needs and current situation. All resistance-training systems or programs can be understood and appropriately planned once you utilize the following guidelines.

Six Types of Resistance Training

All resistance training programs rely on 6 *types* of resistance training (Fleck and Kraemer, 1987). Three of these are named by type of muscle contraction.

1. Isometric Training

With **isometric** or static force development, there is no change in muscle length during force production. (Technically, as is true for eccentric movement, a "contraction" does not occur since no *shortening* of the muscle occurs during the isometric hold or eccentric movement.) During isometric force production, the muscle does not generate enough force to move the object that is resisting it; for example, when pressing against an immovable object such as a wall, or when using free weights or a machine that is loaded beyond your client's maximal concentric strength. Typically, a weak muscle works against a stronger muscle to elicit an isometric contraction. For example, try to flex your right elbow and resist this movement by pressing down with your opposite hand. The stronger triceps can effectively resist the weaker biceps of the right arm.

2. Concentric Training

Concentric muscle contraction (also referred to as positive resistance training, or the positive phase) causes *shortening* of the muscle during force production (Fig. 2, Chapter 7). This can occur when you lift weight or pull, push or press against another form of resistance. Dynamic constant- or variable-resistance exercises generally require concentric contractions as part of the movement.

3. Eccentric Training

Eccentric muscle training (also referred to as negative resistance training, or the negative phase) results in *lengthening* of the muscle during force production. This type of contraction is common to activities in daily life. For example, walking down a hill or section of steps requires the quadriceps and hip extensor muscles to perform eccentric contractions. And resistance that is lowered, such as during strength exercises using resistive equipment, requires eccentric contractions.

An eccentric muscle contraction can generate up to 30% more force than a concentric contraction (Wilmore and Costill, 1994). However, general scientific consensus is of the opinion that eccentric contractions are no more—or no less—effective in producing strength gains for typical clients when compared to isometric and concentric training. But, they have a tendency to be associated with delayed onset muscle soreness (DOMS).

Don't overemphasize eccentric contractions with new trainees or deconditioned clients. Also, before you conclude that eccentric muscular contraction is an excellent way to train your clients for functional strength, remember that the eccentric contractions performed "naturally" as a part of everyday living are submaximal, or in other words, a very high RM (repetition maximum).

4. Dynamic Constant Resistance

A typical example of **dynamic constant resistance** is lifting a dumbbell. The force generated by the muscle is "dynamic" and changing through a given range of motion (ROM). The force changes are represented by a **strength curve** that varies for each muscle as the position of the joint changes.

Dynamic constant resistance is often incorrectly labeled "isotonic." Iso means "same" and tonic refers to "tension." The term isotonic implies that the same tension is generated by the musculature through a given exercise range of motion. As is well documented, the same tension is *not* exerted through an entire ROM due to leverage variations that change with mechanical advantage, or disadvantage, of the involved joint. This is dictated by anatomical factors such as muscle attachment points. What remains "constant" is the external resistance, force or weight. An example is the weight of a dumbbell through a given ROM.

5. Dynamic Variable Resistance

A simple example of **dynamic variable resistance** is elastic tubing, which provides more resistance as it is stretched. A more sophisticated approach involves variable-resistance equipment that changes the amount of resistance being lifted through a lever arm, cam or pulley arrangement.

The "dynamic" aspect of this type of training relates to the muscle's capacity to generate different forces throughout the ROM. The resistance is made "variable" in an attempt to match the increases and decreases of the strength curve exhibited by the muscle. In theory, this matching of strength to overload would result in the muscle being required to exert maximal effort throughout the entire ROM. (Even if this could be accomplished, research seems to indicate that there may be no real advantage in terms of strength gains.) Ideally, there would be no part of the ROM that would be "too easy" or "too hard."

Unfortunately, due to the unique variations in each person's limb length, muscle attachment points and body size, it is impossible to envision one mechanical arrangement of lever arms, pulleys or cams that can accommodate each and every strength curve. This is not "good" or "bad," but a point to be aware of.

6. Isokinetic Training (Isokinetics)

Isokinetic training involves either a concentric or eccentric production of force where limb-movement velocity is held constant. Isokinetic equipment offers no preset resistance: Any force applied against this type of machinery results in an equal reaction force supplied by the machine. Theoretically, this makes it possible for the muscle(s) to exert a continual, maximal force production throughout a given ROM, and at a constant speed of movement.

Proponents of this type of training, which requires fairly expensive equipment, *feel* that movement speeds that mimic athletic performance can be challenged more effectively, and they *believe* that the ability to exert maximal force throughout a full ROM leads to optimal strength increases. But, this question needs to be asked: "Optimal strength increases for what?" The requirement for maximal force exertion through an entire ROM is absent from most daily activities and athletic performances. Also, studies seem to indicate that there is no clear superiority of isokinetic training over other types of training (Fleck and Kraemer, 1987).

Resistance Training Model

Resistance training program design (RTPD) is crucial to a well-rounded fitness program and the overall health of your clients. (The term resistance training is used to cover all types of "strength" or "weight training.") However, the best model to follow is often very difficult to identify because there are so many training systems to choose from. **Training systems** can be defined as *any* combination of sets, repetitions and loads. Every imaginable kind of training system exists. At least 27 different systems are listed by Fleck and Kraemer (1987), and this is not an exhaustive list.

Which type of training gets the best results? In various research reviews (for example, Fleck and Kraemer, 1987) it is documented that there is *no one best way to train.* Any of these methods or types of training can result in significant strength training improvements. The real trick in designing your client's resistance training program is determining the unique needs and interests of the individual. Develop the goals of the program first.

There are certainly some definable parameters that most scientists would agree on in terms of effective RTPD, but the most effective approach is probably a combination of science and art. Most systems or combinations of reps, sets and loads will produce results, sometimes in spite of their design! The body will adapt to any load to which it is not accustomed.

The defining variable is probably not how often you train, but how you arrange or **periodize** the order and number of sets and repetitions (volume), and loads (intensity). Of these, intensity is probably most important. Extensive reviews of existing scientific literature indicate that for significant strength improvement, the *optimal* number of repetitions ranges from 2-10 RM and the *optimum* number of sets varies from 2-5 (Fleck and Kraemer, 1987).

A diversity of methods and the use of periodization will ensure the "best" results, when driven by the goals of each client.

Quick Index:

Chapter 7, explains muscles' response to overloads
Chapter 13, how to periodize programs

Steps for Designing Resistance Training Programming

Since the client's needs and current conditioning level are critical to the success of a program, use this process to ensure you are addressing them. The first step is a needs analysis, the second is matching needs to the training system and the third is determining the appropriate overload.

Step 1: Analyze client's needs.

The answers to these questions will largely determine your programming approach.

• *What are the goals of your client?*

Common goals include muscular hypertrophy, increasing maximal lifts, increased performance in a particular sport, decreased body fat, feeling stronger, personal physical independence and increased self-esteem. Listen to what your client thinks he wants to accomplish through your program, and act on what you hear.

• *What are the requirements of the activities or sports your client participates in?*

Your client's goals will require a training scenario that emphasizes general health and fitness, functional strength and balance, and/or training for a competitive sport such as body building, race walking or volleyball. Analyze the activity to determine its requirements for muscular strength and/or endurance, sport specificity, movement patterns and special training requirements such as plyometrics. It is necessary to weigh all of these considerations against the current fitness and experience base of the client.

• *Is training dictated by the needs of the individual or the requirements of a sport?*

The answer to this question greatly affects the approach. For competition, an athlete trains to excel at the particular sport, oftentimes at any cost. For example, Olympic lifting requires a full squat. The rules of the sport command its execution regardless of the risk to the athlete. However, if the needs and desires of an individual are health, fitness and well-being and there is no aspiration to participate in a competitive sport, there is considerable flexibility in the approach to program design.

• *How much time will the client have available?*

It is impossible to create an effective approach to RTPD without knowing the client's time commitment. Part of your responsibility is to let your client know what kind of time investment is required to attain the goals identified in steps one, 2 and 3. General strength goals can usually be accomplished with an approach that simultaneously addresses cardiorespiratory fitness and flexibility training. Regardless of the client's time commitment, try to make it your personal challenge to accommodate and optimize any amount of time. One way to do this is to plan workouts that the client must complete on his own.

Step 2: Match goals to system (reps, sets and loads design).

All systems fit into Table 19, Specificity Chart (this chapter), which you can use to match your client's goals to work loads. The **goal range** (number of repetitions) is determined by a variety of factors that include: the client's current fitness level specific to resistance training, current exercise history and stated resistance-training goals—whether muscular endurance, strength and/or hypertrophy.

The focus of early workouts is *not* to create muscle failure, but to *work on correct exercise technique* and allow the tissues of the body to adapt progressively to new challenges. Most of the early improvements in a person's ability to work against more resistance are the result of nervous system adaptations, not changes in the muscle fiber structure.

Step 3: Identify the appropriate overload.

Choose a safe starting resistance. For most clients, this amount of resistance allows completion of at least 12-20 repetitions. This intensity (12 reps or greater) equates to less than 70% of one repetition maximum (one RM). Research indicates that a 10 RM lift equates to about 75% of a person's maximum lifting capacity for any given lift. A 10 RM intensity seems necessary to *optimize* muscular strength and hypertrophy gains, but it may be reached in a progressive manner.

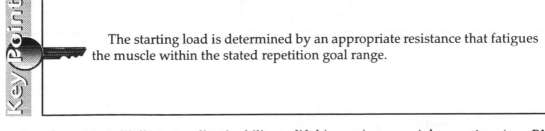

The starting load is determined by an appropriate resistance that fatigues the muscle within the stated repetition goal range.

I prefer not to initially test a client's ability to lift his maximum weight one time (one RM) and then calculate a percentage of this maximum lift to determine starting weight. The contradiction is obvious. Why put the client in a high-risk, maximal-performance situation he is not prepared for? This situation totally ignores the progressive adaptation principle. Err on the side of using too little weight rather than too much weight to determine starting points. If too many reps are being performed, the number of reps can easily be brought down by increasing resistance.

For continued increases in strength, you'll need to plan a *progressive* increase in resistance over time that challenges all of the major muscle groups to the point of muscular exhaustion (in about 30-90 seconds).

Sets, Reps. Recent ACSM guidelines (1990) suggest that a basic program can maintain both muscular strength and endurance and balanced strength between agonist and antagonist muscles. The program's effectiveness is based on performing 8-12 repetitions, at least 2 times a week, for each major muscle group of the body (8-10 exercises). Remember to begin with 12-20 reps and progress to 8-12 reps to fatigue. At least one set of exercise should be performed for each exercise. And naturally, as an individual gains strength, it makes sense that he will be able to perform more reps at a given weight (reflective of increased muscular endurance) and increase the weight lifted (reflective of increased strength).

Load (Intensity). Results depend on proper intensity. If, in the repetition schemes suggested (8-20 reps), you can bring the muscle near fatigue ("I have one or 2 reps left in me with good form."), exceptional results will occur for most clients. You must present the exercising muscle with sufficient challenge or intensity to cause muscular fatigue. The key is *not* how much absolute weight or resistance is used. More important are the questions, "Is the overload relative to the individual's current strength levels? Can you fatigue the muscle in the suggested rep framework?"

Quick Index:

Chapter 2, determining client's goals, the pros and cons of fitness testing
Chapter 15, evaluating resistance training exercises

Table 19. Specificity Chart

Relative Loading	Outcome	% 1 RM	Rep Range	# of Sets	Rest Between Sets
Light	Muscular Endurance	< 70	12-20	1-3	20-30 seconds
Moderate	Hypertrophy and Strength	70-80	8-12	1-6	30-120 seconds
Heavy	Maximum Strength and Power	80-100	1-8	1-5+	2-5 minutes

Adapted from Baechle et al. 1992

Note: Generally, assume a heavier load as soon as you are able to complete the required number of reps listed in the Specificity Chart.

Continuum of Training Programs

Figure 6. Training Program Continuum

Cardio Fitness	Muscle Endurance	Muscle Strength	Maximal Muscle Power

There is a wide continuum of training programs that range from what I call the "far left" of cardiorespiratory training to the "far right" of maximal muscular strength and power. There is a *huge* gap in terms of similarity, that exists between cardio fitness and muscular endurance (Fig. 6).

Cardiorespiratory fitness gains result in a physiologic adaptation that is very different from those adaptations seen in the muscular strength and endurance component. The overload and activities that are required to stimulate change in these components of fitness are very distinct. Optimal cardiorespiratory, and muscular strength and endurance, conditioning cannot be developed simultaneously.

Figure 7. Muscular Endurance, Strength and Power Continuum

Muscle Endurance	Muscle Strength	Maximal Muscle Power

This continuum (Fig. 7) represents the difference between muscle endurance, strength and power. The number of reps, sets and loads used in a resistance-training protocol will largely determine which of these areas will be developed predominantly by your client. Refer to Table 19, Specificity Chart.

Bioenergenics and Its Implication for Recovery

Bioenergenics refers to the sources of energy for muscular contraction in a biological system, such as your client's body. High-intensity resistance training relies primarily on the ATP-CP and lactic acid energy systems. Both the ATP-CP and lactic acid energy systems are replenished using the long-term aerobic energy system. Table 7, Important Energy System Characteristics, reviews the intensity and duration of effort that influences the predominance of one energy system over the other. This has important implications for muscular strength and endurance conditioning.

Table 7. Important Energy System Characteristics

	Immediate Energy/ ATP-CP System	Short-term Energy/ Lactic Acid or Glycolytic System	Long-term Energy or Oxidative System
	Anaerobic System	Anaerobic System	Aerobic System
Fuel or Substrate	• Creatin Phosphate • Stored ATP	• Blood Glucose • Glycogen	• Fatty Acids • Blood Glucose • Glycogen
Intensity	• Very, very hard • 9-10 Borg scale	• Very hard • 7 Borg scale	• Moderate to somewhat hard • 3-4 Borg scale
% VO2 =	• > 95% max	• 85-95% max	• < 85% max
Time to Fatigue	• Very short duration • 1-10 seconds	• Short duration • 60-180 seconds	• Longer duration • > 3 minutes
Limits to ATP Production	• Limited muscle stores of CP and ATP	• Lactic acid accumulation • Rapid fatigue	• Depletion of muscle glycogen and glucose • Insufficient oxygen delivery/utilization

At any given time, all 3 energy systems are functioning simultaneously. The percentage of contribution from each system is determined primarily by the intensity and duration of the activity. "Activity" may be viewed as a continuum from rest to maximal effort.

Once ATP has liberated energy from its bonds and been broken down to ADP, aerobic sources help reform ADP back to ATP, regardless of what energy system is most active for a particular intensity of exercise. ATP that is stored or reformed by oxidative processes is used to reform C and P back to CP. ATP and CP and their recoupled bonds represent limited amounts of stored energy in the body. The complete rebuilding of these energy sources that are depleted through the predominance of the ATP-CP system and short bursts of maximal effort takes about 2-5 minutes, depends on the aerobic energy system and oxygen during recovery or periods of lesser activity and probably occurs most efficiently during complete rest.

Oxygen debt is a reflection of oxygen taken in above what is normally taken in at rest (this includes oxygen deficit). Maximal or one RM lifts are examples of exercise that increase oxygen debt. The portion of oxygen debt that the ATP-CP system is responsible for is called alactacid and occurs during a set performed at maximal effort in about 10-seconds or less. **Alactacid** means energy production "without producing lactic acid." But even though no lactic acid is produced in this system, it is still limited in its ability to produce energy because of minimal supplies of stored ATP-CP. Therefore, sufficient time and oxygen are required to replenish the alactacid portion of oxygen debt through oxidative (aerobic) processes. In other words, reforming ATP and CP.

The half-life of the alactacid portion of oxygen debt occurs within the following time frame:

- Within 20 seconds, 50% of the depleted ATP and CP is replenished.
- Within 40 seconds, 75% of the depleted ATP and CP is replenished.
- Within 60 seconds, 87% of the depleted ATP and CP is replenished.
- Within 3-5 minutes, the majority of intramuscular stores of ATP and CP are replenished.

The complete recovery of the ATP-CP energy system has significant implications for skill, speed, form and safety that must occur during short, maximal, all-out work efforts.

> **Key Point**
>
> That is why, for example, power lifters and Olympic lifters take up to 5 minutes to recover from all-out maximal lifts, or one RMs. For these athletes to correctly execute the next effort, it is necessary for the ATP-CP energy system to fully recover.

The lactic acid system contributes the **lactacid,** or lactic acid-producing portion of oxygen debt. As maximal or strenuous efforts go beyond about 10-seconds, the short-term lactic acid system starts to contribute substantially to energy production to sustain high-level, predominantly anaerobic effort (failure or muscle fatigue in about 30-90 seconds).

The accumulated lactic acid in the muscle and blood is metabolized (oxidized) in the presence of oxygen in the muscle and liver. Excess oxygen that is taken in during recovery (there is an excess because workload has been decreased or eliminated) is used to pay back or re-create depleted stores of ATP-CP and to oxidize (reduce to a usable source) lactic acid. This usually occurs during recovery or lessened work efforts and helps reduce oxygen debt (Chapter 5, Fig.1).

Expediting Lactic Acid Clearance

The half-life of the lactacid portion of oxygen debt is considerably longer than the alactacid portion. It takes significantly more time to *completely* clear or metabolize significant accumulations of lactate from repeated maximal anaerobic effort when compared to replenishment of stored ATP-CP.

However, in sets of exercise to exhaustion, it would not be practical to rest between sets for the necessary duration to completely clear lactate from the body. Can you imagine your clients waiting 25 minutes to an hour between sets of resistance training exercise? Let's look at the time it does take and that relationship to exercise.

The half-life of the lactacid portion of oxygen debt is:

- Within 25 minutes, 50% of accumulated lactic acid is metabolized.
- Within 75 minutes, 95% of accumulated lactic acid is metabolized.
- Some experts believe that within 30-45 minutes, the *majority* of lactic acid is
cleared or oxidized.

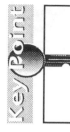

> The body and its musculature can sustain quality activity without a complete recovery to pre-exercise blood levels of lactate.

Here are facts you can use to help your client clear lactic acid.

• Light activity facilitates lactic acid removal.

• Lactic acid can be metabolized in the presence of oxygen (oxidized) to produce ATP (energy), and then be used as energy to recouple ADP + P; and C + P. The Cori cycle also provides a means for removing lactic acid formed in the muscle through a gluconeogenic process that results in more blood glucose and muscle glycogen.

• Rest periods that use light activity to facilitate lactic acid removal must be of at least 2 minutes to be of significant value, if *significant* lactate is accumulated and recovery from accumulated lactate levels is required or important to subsequent performance. In many cases, anywhere from 20-seconds to 2-minutes may be sufficient. Simply ask your client if they feel ready for another "hard" set. And, consider using active rest.

The lactic acid system is important in terms of significant energy contribution during "hard" workouts where sets to failure are performed in one to 3 minutes. Unless muscular endurance and increased tolerance to high levels of lactate is a goal, I recommend that your clients attain muscular fatigue in about 30-90 seconds. This is time efficient and will probably enhance most of your clients health, fitness, and muscular strength and endurance goals.

Quick Index:
Chapter 4, details on interactions between energy systems

Recovery Periods for Resistance Training

Recovery Between Workouts. Recovery between workouts is based on the intensity of the workout and the individual "recovery ability" of your client. Generally, about 48 hours is appropriate between workouts that are intense, or of an overload to which the body is not accustomed. Remember, resistance training should result in a positive building process (anabolic), versus a negative or breakdown (catabolic) process. Adequate recovery is essential to avoid overtraining and strength plateaus, and for progressive improvements in muscular strength and endurance.

Intensity is relative to—and dependent on—your client's current fitness level. An absolute weight that is lifted may reflect a light loading for one of your clients, whereas for another client it may represent a heavy or even maximal loading.

For example, a deconditioned client who performs a traditional push-up may find he can perform only 4 repetitions. For this individual, this equates to a heavy 4 RM load or greater than 80% of one RM. One of your more fit clients may be able to perform 50-100 push-ups. This is, relatively, a very light load, and represents much less than 50% of one RM.

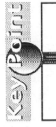

> The deconditioned client needs a significant recovery between workouts, at least 48 hours. And, any client working against a progressive overload to which they are not accustomed, requires a similar recovery.

The fit client probably can perform push-up reps every day of the week. Recovery is not required because a new and unfamiliar workload has not been introduced to the body. Note that by performing 100 push ups, the fit client is not creating gains in strength or cardiorespiratory fitness. If the goal is increased muscular strength, his time could be used more effectively by progressively overloading and fatiguing the body's musculature in 8-20 repetitions.

Recovery Between Sets. Recovery must allow for sufficient restoration of the ATP- PC and lactic acid energy systems. Adequate recovery results in the ability of your clients to prepare for and be able to give another quality effort or set of training.

The Specificity Chart (Table 19) shows a recommended amount of rest between sets for light, moderate and heavy loading by resistance. You will notice that the longest recovery period is 5 minutes. Shorter recovery times increase relative intensity. Your choice of recovery duration will depend on the answers to these questions:

• Is recovery duration relative to your client's program goals?

• Is recovery duration relative to your client's fitness level?

• What are you trying to optimize? Is it strength, endurance, hypertrophy and/or exercise compliance and health-related returns?

Now, this question must be answered. Why is it *not* necessary to recover longer than the recommended 20-seconds to 2-minutes for sets of exhaustive work (8-20 reps to fatigue in about 30-90 seconds), where major contributions of both the ATP-CP and lactic acid systems are prevalent?

First, the question of recovery has been answered regarding the depletion of ATP-CP sources, for example, with one RM lifts and heavy relative loading. About 2-5 minutes are required for complete recovery in lifts that require maximal effort in about 10-seconds or less. During relatively light or moderate loading (8-20 repetitions and less than 80% of one RM) there are no *maximal* contributions from either anaerobic energy system (ATP-CP and lactic acid systems). Therefore, *complete* exhaustion of the ATP-CP system does not occur, nor do significant accumulations of lactate occur via use of the lactic acid system.

Short rests of 20-30 seconds for light loads are usually adequate for recovery and allow another quality set of training by your client. Even moderate loading (about 8-12 repetitions and 30-90 seconds) does not require extreme contribution from either the ATP-CP or lactic acid systems. About 30-120 seconds of rest between sets is sufficient.

Active recovery is a great option to consider using with your clients if sport-specific goals are not the focus and accomplishing the most amount of work possible in a limited time span is the focus. Here's an example: Have your client perform a chest exercise followed by an abdominal exercise, followed by a lower-body exercise. Then repeat another set of exercise for the chest. Even though the client has been active, this will allow sufficient recovery of the chest musculature. Your client will be ready for another quality chest set, and this results in productive use of time.

Always let your clients who are looking for health returns and enjoyment in their exercise routine determine if more time is necessary. In instances where your clients need more recovery, consider using active recovery and sequence your exercises as suggested above, and/or include a stretch or 2 after the set is completed.

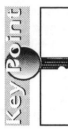

Energy-system recovery information has important implications, for example, to power lifters and Olympic lifters, as well as average clients. Optimal recovery of the energy systems is essential to performance and safety, and should be directed to your client's training goals and level of intensity to which he is currently prepared.

Quick Index:

Applying an Understanding of Motor Units

To better anticipate how to apply intensity toward achieving your client's goal(s), let's review what we learned about motor units in Chapter 7. A single **motor unit** is defined as a motor nerve and all the muscle fibers it stimulates or innervates. Motor units are composed of either all slow-twitch (ST) or all fast-twitch (FT) fibers. However, muscles are composed of *both* ST and FT motor units. The "all or none" principle applies to *single* motor units. If a load is strong enough to stimulate the motor nerve, the motor unit and all of the fibers it innervates will produce force (contract). Motor units have different thresholds at which a stimulus will cause them to fire. This has implications for strength gains. But innervation of single motor unit *does not* mean stimulation of the entire muscle.

In designing effective resistance-training programs, it is important to distinguish between the whole muscle(s) and numerous motor units within a *single muscle*. Also, proper intensity, related to motor-unit metabolic and physical characteristics, needs to be identified so the threshold of both the ST and FT motor units can be challenged. This results in more motor-unit involvement, which means more muscle mass is being engaged. This will help optimize results for individual clients.

Table 20. ST and FT Fibers

Motor units are classified into categories depending on:
- Their speed of contraction.
- The amount of force they generate.
- How easily the fibers are fatigued or how resistant the fibers are to fatigue.

Type I: ST	Low Tension Production	Fatigue Resistant
Type IIa: FT	Moderate Force Production	Fatigue Resistant
Type IIb: FT	High Force Production	Quick Fatigue

ST — Type I
- High aerobic enzyme activity
- High mitochondria concentration
- High myoglobin concentration
- High capillary density
- High levels of stored intramuscular triglycerides and LPL
- Difficult to fatigue
- Long sets (i.e., 20 reps/ >) exemplify the predominance of their (ST) use

FT — Type IIa and IIb
- High anaerobic enzyme activity
- High levels of intramuscular ATP/PC
- High glycolytic enzyme activity
- Suited for high force, maximal efforts
- Suited to activities of short duration
- Susceptible to fatigue
- 1 RM and short sets, such as 2-12 RM to fatigue, exemplify FT predominance
- Contain about 12% more protein, which if stimulated, enhance hypertrophy

The neuro-physiological principle of motor-unit recruitment order, ensures that slow-twitch (ST) motor units are predominantly recruited to perform low-intensity, long-duration activities. FT motor units (especially FT IIb) are predominantly recruited when high-intensity (anaerobic) activity is performed. FT motor units are held in reserve until the ST motor units can no longer perform the particular muscular contraction (Fleck and Kraemer, 1987; McArdle et al. 1991; Wilmore and Costill, 1994). This order of recruitment, based on firing thresholds of the ST and FT motor units, reflects a ramp-like recruitment effect (Fig. 3, Chapter 7).

In order to recruit FT fibers and attain an *optimal* training effect, the exercise must be intense: loads that are 70% or greater of one RM will most likely activate this motor unit. This equates to fatiguing the musculature in about 12 reps or fewer.

This is the theoretical foundation on which the ACSM guidelines (1990) of 8-12 reps (progress to this from a base of 12-20 reps) to muscle fatigue, are at least partially founded. This is intense, anaerobic work and is usually completed in 30-90 seconds. Of course, this time bench mark is not precise and may vary considerably, but is a good recommendation.

Correct intensity has huge implications for involving greater amounts of muscle mass, which can influence increases in resting metabolic rate and gains in strength through both hypertrophy and nervous system adaptations. Light loads involve only ST fibers, whereas heavy loads will involve *all* 3 fiber types. If light to moderate muscular force is used, only about 50% of your client's muscle mass will be challenged (an average person's motor unit ratio is about 50% ST to 50% FT).

What happens when a client always uses the same light weight and performs numerous repetitions? Since the activity is not of an intense nature, ST fibers will be recruited to perform the work. If the intensity of exercise remains low, the threshold necessary to activate FT motor units will not be exceeded and they will remain inactive and untrained. Continued use of high-repetition overload is not only ineffective, but essentially a waste of time for most clients, and could lead to overuse injuries because of the repetitive nature of high rep/low load overloads.

Having said that, in relation to program design *nothing* is written in stone. It is best *not* to view the whole topic of program design as an issue of "right" and "wrong," or "always," but more importantly, to understand the boundaries you should operate from to maintain a scientifically valid approach. You have many options from which to choose to maximize your clients' training results and individual program needs.

This discussion leads to several important points that need to be highlighted.

• Both ST and FT Fibers can hypertrophy.

• "Selective" or "preferential" hypertrophy is not limited to FT fibers, but based on FT fibers' physical and biochemical (metabolic) characteristics, they are likely to be more of a major contributing factor to gains in strength and hypertrophy. This especially seems true when combined with the fact that many individuals do not train intensely enough to elicit significant response from FT motor units.

> Key Point
>
> The practical application pearl of wisdom is to recognize the importance of using variety in your overall approach to program design.

• Use various repetition schemes within an approximate range of one RM to 20 RM. This will ensure a diversity of motor-unit recruitment patterns and optimize both ST and FT motor-unit recruitment.

• Periodize for a stimulating and well-rounded approach. Periodization attempts to provide maximum stimulation while simultaneously providing for recovery. It prevents detraining or overtraining.

• For athletes and individuals participating in activities that require a significant combination of speed and strength, trained FT fibers will create more power than trained ST fibers. In fact, low-intensity training may not even prepare your client for daily emergencies such as slipping, then righting himself to prevent a fall or strain.

Quick Index:

Speed of Movement
For the average person, gains in strength are best accomplished by moving the weight slowly (about 4-5 seconds per repetition), through a full range of motion and accomplishing FT recruitment by using an appropriately intense overload. Following are 7 reasons to control speed of movement (Westcott, 1991):

1. Consistent application of force.

2. More total muscle tension produced.

3. More total muscle force produced.

4. More muscle fiber activation (both ST and FT)

5. Greater muscle-power potential through high-intensity force development using controlled speed of movement and appropriately intense overload.

6. Less tissue trauma.

7. Greater momentum increases injury potential and reduces training effect on target muscle groups.

Exceptions to the above may be appropriate in sport-specific applications and when the risks are understood by your client.

Five Program Design Scenarios

How do you mix reps, sets and loads? Following are outlines for 5 program design scenarios ranging from health and fitness to competitive athletics. These sketches are designed to further clarify the multitude of approaches available to you to meet the diverse needs of your clients. Don't evaluate these approaches in terms of absolute correctness, but in relation to the appropriateness of the training approach when compared to the training goal and your client.

Health and Fitness Gains
Most of your clients' health and fitness goals can be optimized by using **active recovery**. The use of active recovery between sets allows for more productive use of limited time. For example, a stretching exercise or exercising another body part can serve to facilitate recovery from a previous strength exercise without requiring total inactivity.

Following the ACSM guidelines can also encourage effective use of time. By working out twice per week, with 10 exercises that target all of the major muscle groups, where 8-12 reps are completed to fatigue, and at least one set per exercise is performed, excellent gains in strength and muscular endurance can be realized. (Remember to progress from performing 12-20 repetitions before attempting 8-12 reps.) And regardless of your client's age, it is easy to excite him toward engaging in resistance training because the health benefits associated with resistance training occur at any age.

Quick Index:

Chapter 10, planning for health versus fitness

Plateaus and Program Variety

Plateaus and overtraining often result from the indefinite use of one training program approach. The following ideas can help minimize the possibilities of a situation where your client's training is going nowhere.

• Initially, change the exercise sequence or change the exercise while leaving the relative intensity, or reps, sets and load the same.

• Manipulate frequency, intensity (load) and volume (reps and sets) both up and down within the 8- to 20-repetition framework if no sport-specific application is needed. Both higher-rep and lower-rep schemes contribute to muscle hypertrophy and additional results.

• Increase the number of sets for the targeted muscle group.

• Sequence the exercises so there is very little recovery between sets targeting the same muscle group. This will allow for a different motor-unit recruitment pattern—and thus new stimulation.

For very fit and highly motivated clients, use one of the following techniques. These are **high-intensity training techniques**, so be sure your client is interested in them before you begin. They require a high degree of physical effort and are associated with physical discomfort:

Breakdown or Pyramid Training. Upon reaching momentary muscle failure, each exercise is performed with slightly less or more weight than the one preceding it.

Assisted Training or "Forced Reps." The trainer assists the client in completing a number of reps he could not have completed on his own. Typically, the spotter lifts 10-15% of the weight load to assist the client in completing the reps.

Negative Training. Negative training allows for 30% more force production than concentric contraction. Typically, negative training is accomplished by adding manual resistance on the lowering phase of any lift, by adjusting the weight lifted and lowered when using a selectorized plate machine, or by assisting your client through a concentric phase with an amount of weight he could not lift on his own, and then allowing him to lower the weight during the eccentric phase.

Negative training is used with a highly trained individual who is plateaued. Delayed-onset muscle soreness is highly associated with this type of training, so it should not be used with deconditioned clients.

Super Slow Training. Super slow training is often referred to as **10-second training**. It is usually comprised of a 10-second concentric lifting phase, followed by a 5-second lowering phase for each repetition. Failure is often attained in 4-6 reps. There are variations with regard to the number of seconds assigned to each lifting phase. There is no "miracle" number of seconds that will produce the "best" results. Record your results and experiment.

Super Set and Compound Training. Super setting usually refers to working agonist and antagonist muscle groups in succession. Compound training, as the name implies, generally consists of working the same muscle group back to back—two sets of consecutive exercises target the same muscle group, but not necessarily with the same exercise.

High-intensity training may be the edge you need to move advanced clients off strength plateaus. High-volume work is not realistic in limited time schedules, and while effective with elite body builders, can lead to overuse injury and burnout in many of your clients. Quality reigns over quantity. In fact, many competitive lifters are experimenting with decreasing volume of overload and increasing intensity of effort.

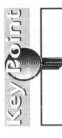

> It seems that the best stimulus for increased gains in strength is to make the muscle work harder, not longer.

Periodization encompasses some or all of these techniques. Periodized programs typically cycle volume (sets and reps) and intensity (load or resistance) over specific time periods. The time periods usually last 3-4 weeks (microcycle), and there are usually 4 phases to the year-long periodization program. This allows for progression relative to the program goals and assigned training loads.

Quick Index:

Functional Training

The number of reps, sets and load is probably least defined when training your client for gains in functional strength. **Functional strength** development is related to how your client normally engages in activity during a typical day. Though any given day's activity may require a maximal exertion, probably the most important "usable" strength is muscular endurance in key postural muscles. Postural muscles are important for maintaining correct spinal alignment most hours of the day. However, functional training can also involve other major muscle groups. Additionally, significant gains in *both* muscular strength and endurance help prevent injuries.

Resistance training can use both open-chain and closed-chain exercises. **Open chain exercise** (OCE) can be defined as isolated movement. An example of OCE is a seated leg extension. **Closed chain exercise** (CCE) can be defined as an integrated and coordinated response by the body to perform a movement safely and correctly. CCE is demonstrated by performing a squat, lunge or balancing movement on one leg.

CCE activity closely parallels the way your client moves in performing daily tasks, such as picking up a child or righting himself after a loss of balance. Functional training requires an integration of balance and intrinsic muscular stability while exerting muscular force. An excellent tool to train stability and balance that carries over functionally is a large, round, air-filled stability ball.

Body Building

The training goal for body builders centers around balanced muscular size, symmetry and definition. A variety of exercises is used in the training routine because it is *believed* that this promotes optimal gains in size and symmetry. Generally, a moderate intensity (8-12 reps to fatigue) is used. This allows for the completion of high volume, which is determined by load times reps times sets.

A load of 8-12 reps to fatigue seems logical, as the goal of body building is not superior maximal strength. Hypertrophy seems to be developed best within this repetition framework. Research suggests training should emphasize increases in resistance, not just volume (reps and sets) for maximal hypertrophy gains. Additionally, the order of exercises for a specific body part (i.e., biceps) is more important than which body part (i.e., chest/back) precedes the other.

Multiple or giant sets are used for volume overload and may contain 3-6 sets, although they can go as high as 10-15 sets per exercise. Short rest periods are a distinctive feature of body building. A 30- to 90-second rest *seems* to promote muscular definition, vascularity and a high metabolic intensity which may help in lowering body fat.

Body builders generally follow a full-body routine that targets all of the major muscle groups. Split routines, which work different body parts on an alternate schedule of days, allow for 2 workouts per week for most muscle groups. Generally, a split routine schedule requires 4-6 workouts per week. Some research suggests that 3 full-body workouts per week may be sufficient to stimulate optimal adaptive responses. This is important information to consider because more frequent, all-out training increases the potential for overuse symptoms and poor adaptive responses to the work load.

Professional/Competitive Athlete

Plyometrics and skill practice attempt to preserve movement speed with a load reflective of that required by the sport. Are sport-specific strength training movements better than developing base strength using a traditional approach? Regardless of what any of us *think*, the ultimate factor that dictates the athlete's training approach will be improved training results.

Science has not been able to answer definitively which type of training is better for performance. Experiment using a combination of both approaches. Individual response and results will dictate the approach you follow.

When Is the Right Time to Change a Strength Program?

The first question to ask when considering a change in a resistance-training program is, "Why?" Is it you, the trainer, who needs a change? Or is it the client?

A program that is plateaued in terms of resistance (intensity) that can be lifted or number of reps and sets that can be completed may or may not be a problem. If the client is pleased with his body image and strength, such a program can be termed "maintenance." Maintenance is a positive state of training, meaning you are keeping your client's fitness at an optimal level.

Valid reasons for changing a resistance-training program include client boredom, lack of motivation, lack of results, desire for change in muscle strength, hypertrophy or muscle endurance, or a need to change the training environment (type of equipment being used, location etc.). Variety encourages optimal training. It helps alleviate injury and unproductive training.

Before any changes are made to overload, your client should have a base of muscular strength and endurance. Establish this **strength foundation** by training your clients for at least 4-6 weeks. Establish strength and muscular endurance by using ACSM (1990) recommendations of resistance training 2 times per week, with 8-10 well-chosen resistance training exercises (balanced muscular fitness), using one to 2 sets of 12-20 repetitions executed to the point of muscle fatigue.

Using Cross Training. If your client simply needs variety, try cross training *without* initially changing the intensity. An easy first step is to change the sequence of exercises that the client is already doing to create variety and a new overload. Because of this change, it is theorized that the fatigue pattern of the involved motor units will be changed, causing them to adapt to the new stimulus.

The next step is to replace all the exercises, or those you think necessary, in the foundation routine with new ones. Look at the joint action(s) and muscle group(s) being utilized and choose the replacement exercise accordingly. Take care to replace each exercise with one that targets the same muscle group(s) to preserve balance.

For example, a bench press can be "replaced" by push-ups, dumbbell presses, or incline and decline presses, dumbbell or elastic resistance chest flyes (uses horizontal adduction only) because all these copy elbow extension and horizontal adduction at the shoulder. Machine pull-over movements can be replaced by movements that replicate shoulder extension, such as dumbbell or elastic resistance pullovers, one arm or double arm "low" rows, or straight-arm pull-backs with dumbbells or elastic resistance.

Any changes in movement patterns (new exercises or slight body position changes), even if you are targeting the same muscle group(s) and utilizing similar joint actions, will require a different motor-unit recruitment pattern (Fleck and Kraemer, 1987). This recruitment of muscle fibers (motor units) in a different order can act as a stimulus (overload) to create further strength gains. Cross training *within* the muscular strength and endurance component can positively affect compliance, motivation and interest, as well as stimulate the body toward additional strength gains. For optimal muscular development, variety is the name of the game.

Quick Index:

Changing Intensity for the Well-Trained Client

If your client has been training with you for more than 6 months (2-3 times per week, 10-20 exercises per session) and is looking for additional size and/or strength gains, look in depth at 2 factors: intensity and periodization. Periodization plans are discussed in Chapter 13, but here is how intensity is applied.

Remember that up to 80% of the gains in muscle strength can be attributed to motor learning. This involves the nervous system's ability to recruit muscle fibers not previously used, or to utilize them in a more efficient manner. That is why individuals (very common in women) who lift more weight and perform more repetitions can show strength gains as evidenced by the increased reps and weight they can lift, but may not necessarily show continued or significant increases in muscle size. Approximately 20-25% of the gains may be attributed to a physical change in the muscle (hypertrophy or size increase).

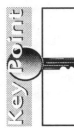

To increase strength and/or size, you must maintain intensity and train within anaerobic pathways. This means the client must *fatigue* the musculature within a time period of about 30-90 seconds.

Remember, the best stimulus for increased gains in strength is to make the muscle work harder, as opposed to longer. The typical person, when working at 75% of his one repetition maximum (one RM), will fatigue at about 10 repetitions, when performing each rep in 4-5 seconds. This level of intensity seems optimal from a safety standpoint and from a physiological standpoint, in terms of maximizing adaptations in the neuromuscular systems.

Utilize the high-intensity overload techniques mentioned previously under program design scenario 2, Plateaus and Program Variety. High-intensity training may be the edge you need to move your advanced clients off strength plateaus. Quality reigns over quantity. For the body's musculature to grow stronger and/or larger in size, favorable genetics are a necessity. However, by applying these principles, every person, regardless of genetics, can realize a huge degree of success.

Do High Repetitions Work?

Muscle endurance is defined as the ability to sustain repeated contractions without undue fatigue over a longer time period (for example about 12-25 reps). As your client becomes stronger his muscles become more enduring and he can perform more reps at a given resistance. As reps increase beyond 25, the movement starts to *resemble* the overload definition for cardiorespiratory conditioning (continuous, rhythmic movement).

However, *do not* interpret this statement to imply that significant cardiorespiratory conditioning takes place with high-repetition resistance training schemes. Actually, the load generally does not engage enough muscle mass to generate significant cardiorespiratory training effect.

For increases in strength, you have to present an intensity to the body's musculature to which it is unaccustomed on a regular and progressive basis. This type of intensity is necessary to stimulate the "cellular machinery" for muscle growth, or to stimulate motor learning for synchronous and additional motor unit recruitment. For the beginning to conditioned exerciser, that means 8-20 repetitions to muscular fatigue. The number works as well for older adults as it does for athletes, since it does not define an absolute weight. Instead, the amount of weight lifted reflects the current strength level of the individual.

High-repetition schemes are usually highly ineffective in promoting any kind of health and fitness gains. They do not produce significant gains in muscular strength and endurance over an extended period of time and have little to no effect on cardiorespiratory conditioning. Repetitions that are redundantly high can lead to overuse injuries, not to mention lack of results and frustration.

Changing Intensity for Strength Gains

• **Vary the number of reps** *either* up or down. Either method will stimulate an adaptation. Any kind of variety will help break plateaus and stimulate the body to adapt. Both higher-rep schemes (12-20), as well as lower-rep sets (8-12) contribute to muscle hypertrophy. Rest and/or lighter weights are often warranted because many participants do not allow for the recovery/building process. Train in a manner that you regularly do not!

• **Increase the number of sets** for the targeted muscle group.

• **Sequence** so there is very little recovery between sets targeting the same muscle group. This will allow for a different motor-unit recruitment pattern to occur, thus new stimulation.

• Utilize **high-intensity training** techniques and systems. Training examples include trisetting, pyramiding, compound training to the same muscle group (often called super setting), breakdown (breaking down the weight being lifted, not the muscle which you stimulate to build), super slow (10-15 seconds per repetition) and forced reps or assisted training.

• **Periodize** training using some or all of these techniques. A periodized program cycles volume (sets and reps) and intensity (load or resistance) over specific time periods. This type of organization encourages a process that maximizes adaptation and progression specific to program goals and intensities.

Case Study: Bridging Systems to Clients

Do you have a client focusing on elite or advanced strength? Are you dealing with an asymptomatic, average client or an older adult? There is much confusion surrounding the number of reps and sets and the amount of resistance, or load, one should use with varying populations. The confusion is related to physiological responses to loads (resistance) put on the musculature of the body. By looking at 2 case studies, one of an Olympic-style lifter and the other of an older adult (aged 63), I hope to clear up some of the confusion and seemingly contradictory recommendations.

Many proposed programs are based on anecdotal and empirical evidence. Often the results are linked to the specific system of reps, sets and loads that is popularized, when in fact, the reasons for the results have little to do with the actual regimen and its supposed "magical" features.

Case Study 1: Olympic Lifter

John is an Olympic lifter. Olympic lifting is a competitive sport that involves 2 technical and explosive lifting movements known as the "clean and jerk," and the "snatch." John maintains high levels of muscle strength, joint flexibility and neuromuscular coordination. He has had years of specialized training.

His goals are based on the demands of the sport: to accomplish maximal strength development and one RM lifts. You'll see how this is represented in Table 21, which shows a typical protocol for Olympic lifters.

Table 21. Workout Protocol for an Olympic Lifter

Load (resistance)	1-6 RM	For maximum strength development
Sets	Multiple sets: 3-6	For each exercise
Repetitions	1-10 per set, to fatigue	For strength and power development
Rest / Recovery	2-5 minutes	Between each set for full energy system recovery
Frequency	1-3 sessions per day and 4-6 days per week	

Examples of exercises that John uses include: clean and jerk lifts, snatch lifts, bench presses, squat variations, good morning lift, jerks from the rack, military presses, shoulder shrugs, back hyperextensions, abdominal and leg curls.

Since the requirements of the sport dictate the training regimen, most of John's training is centered around preparing for the required lifts. Some of these exercises are high risk, but they are what the sport demands. When John's goal is increasing strength, he does 1-6 reps. When he is training for overall program goals and practicing technique, he does 1-10 reps.

Case Study 2: Older Adult Exerciser

Janet is 63 years old and participates in a regular walking program. She has just begun a muscular strength-and-endurance conditioning program. She was motivated by reports that resistance training can positively affect osteoporosis, increase metabolism and calorie burning, influence posture and help her maintain her physical independence. Janet's program resembles the one shown in Table 22.

Table 22. Exercise Protocol for an Older Adult		
Load (resistance)	12-20 RM to muscular fatigue	Introduction to training
Load (resistance)	8-12 RM to muscular fatigue	After 6-8 weeks of training
Sets	Initially 1 per exercise	Introduction to training
Sets	1-2 per exercise after progressive buildup	After 4-6 weeks of training
Number of exercises	8-10	To challenge all major muscle groups
Repetitions	8-20 range per set	Number of reps depends on the load: See "load" above
Recovery	20-seconds to 2-minutes between sets	Using "active" recovery to minimize downtime
Frequency	2 times per week	For excellent gains in strength and muscular endurance

Exercise examples for Janet include: pressing movements (dumbbell presses, cable presses), pulling movements (dumbbell rows, rowing machine), overhead presses, lat pull-downs, leg extensions, leg curls, balance training for leg abductors/adductors, leg presses, squats, lunges, abdominal and back exercises.

Traditionally, clients like Janet are encouraged to perform 3 sets. I feel that performing one to 2 sets with the appropriate overload is more time efficient and will get her the results she is looking for. Although exercising 3 days per week might be better (although not significantly), exercising twice per week may be an advantage for client compliance and interest.

Analyzing the Case Studies

Notice that I have not mentioned *how much weight* either person should lift. The load is determined by an appropriate resistance that fatigues the muscle within the stated repetition goal range. The key to strength development is high-intensity effort. Resistance (load) should be sufficient to fatigue the target muscle group within about 30-90 seconds after the exercise is begun.

Rather than comparing apples (John) to oranges (Janet), let's compare oranges to oranges. Janet's friend Joe, who is also 63, has joined in the same fitness pursuit as Janet. Since their goals are similar, their exercise protocols will be the same. But this does not mean they will lift an identical amount of weight. For example, after Joe has trained for 8 weeks, both may fatigue at 10 RM. However, Janet may use a 12-pound weight for a given lift, while Joe—who joined the program later and has not been training as long—may use an 8-pound weight to reach muscle fatigue at 10 RM.

When would you change John's or Janet's program? For an Olympic lifter who wants to be competitive, there is really no flexibility. The demands of the sport determine how John will train. Periodization will create the only variation.

Janet's program, on the other hand, can be as varied as her needs and wants. Her results are based on personal goals, not on sports performance. Even if she is physiologically ready to increase the weight load, only her interest in doing so will give you the go-ahead to change her program. When the client is ready for a change, you use your knowledge to execute the change and determine its appropriateness.

Make the Most of the Systems

It is imperative to determine the goal of the individual or program before you ever start training. The Specificity Chart will always help you sort out the seemingly contradictory statements regarding resistance training reps, sets and loads and what they can or can not provide. Most systems, regardless of their format, have been proved to be effective (Fleck and Kraemer, 1987). Any stimulus to which a client is not accustomed to will cause his body to adapt to the new overload. This produces a training effect.

Fortunately, regardless of how we train ourselves or others, we sometimes still get results. Whether the method meets your client's needs and safety concerns is another story. Do not join the ranks of many trainers who create programs that are too hard for their clients. Even if you do not injure them, you surely will defeat them.

It is likely that no 2 people will respond in the same manner to a given training program. Make sure you keep accurate lifting records (reps, sets, resistance, order of exercise and periodization planning program) so that you can determine the combinations that best stimulate your client's mind and body. Your records, client feedback, appropriate testing and body fat and circumference measurements will help determine the program's effectiveness. Resistance training program design is a process that demands constant evaluation, manipulation and change!

The Bridge

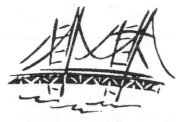

No training system is better than another. The most important factor to consider is whether the system is appropriate to your client's goals. Intensity is relative to the individual, so err on the side of conservatism. You must know your client's physical limits and his perception of what is too much. To effectively plan intensity, volume and frequency: (1) Design systems with specific goals in mind; (2) Fit all systems designed into the Specificity Chart; (3) Encourage consistent, regular and varied efforts; (4) Allow for the recovery/building process; and (5) Keep accurate records.

References and Recommended Reading

Also, refer to the complete reference listing at the end of this book.

Baechle, Thomas, editor (1994). **Essentials of Strength Training and Conditioning—NSCA.** *Human Kinetic Publishers, Champaign, IL. (800) 747-4457*

Baechle, Thomas, and Groves, Barney (1992). **Weight Training - Steps to Success.** *Human Kinetics Publishers, Champaign, IL.*

Basmajian, John, and DeLuca, Carlo (1979). **Muscles Alive - Their Functions Revealed By Electromyography.** *4th edition, Williams and Wilkins, Baltimore, MD. (800) 638-0672*

Brooks, Douglas, editor (1995). **Resist-A-Ball™ (stability ball) Programming Guide For Fitness Professionals.** *Moves International (619) 934-0312*

Brooks, Douglas, and Copeland-Brooks, Candice (1993). **Uncovering the Myths of Abdominal Exercise,** *IDEA Today, April, pp. 42-49.*

Cailliet, Rene (1988). **Low Back Pain Syndrome,** *4th edition. F.A. Davis Co., Philadelphia, PA.*

Ellison, Deborah (1993). **Advanced Exercise Design for Lower Body.** *2nd edition, Movement That Matters, Vista, CA.*

Fleck, Steven, and Kraemer, William (1987). **Designing Resistance Training Programs.** *Human Kinetics Publishers, Champaign, IL.*

Francis, Peter et al. (1994). **The effectiveness of elastic resistance in strength overload.** *Pilot study, San Diego State University.*

Kendall, Florence, et al. (1993). **Muscles - Testing and Function.** *4th edition. Williams and Wilkins, Baltimore, MD. (800) 638-0672*

Komi, P.V., editor (1992). **Strength and Power in Sport,** *Distributed by Human Kinetics Publishers, Champaign, IL. (800) 747-4457*

Kraemer, William, and Fleck, Steven (1993). **Strength Training for Young Athletes.** *Human Kinetics Publishers, Champaign, IL.*

Purvis, Tom (1994). **Trainer's Video Lecture and Hands-On Series.** *Focus On Fitness: Oklahoma City, Oklahoma. (405) 755-3082*

Siff, Mel et al. (1993). *Super Training-Special Strength Training For Sporting Excellence.* Published by: The School of Mechanical Engineering, University of the Witwatersrand, South Africa.

Stone, Michael, and O'Bryant, Harold (1987). *Weight Training - A Scientific Approach.* Burgess International Group, Minneapolis, MN.

Thompson, Clem (1989). *Manual of Structural Kinesiology.* 11th edition, Times/Mirror/Mosby, St. Louis, MO. (314) 872-8370

Townsend, Hal et al. (1991) Electromyographic analysis of the glenohumeral muscles during a baseball rehabilitation program. *The American Journal of Sports Medicine*, Vol. 19, No. 3.

Westcott, Wayne (1991). *Strength Fitness.* 3rd edition, Wm. C. Brown Publishers, Dubuque, IA. (319) 588-1451

Wilmore, Jack, and David Costill (1994). *Physiology of Sport and Exercise.* Human Kinetics Publishers, Champaign, IL.

CHAPTER 15

EVALUATING RESISTANCE TRAINING EXERCISES

In the weight room you can always observe a number of interesting, sometimes "amazing," strength exercises. Consumer fitness magazines are laced with strength-training exercise variations. You can select from an enormous variety of exercises and equipment, and you can hear all types of conflicting advice. With such an array of choices, how do you know which is the "best" resistance-training exercise?

Rarely is the *type* of resistance-training equipment a limiting factor in creating strength training results. Whether you are using sophisticated and costly machinery, free-weights, water as a resistance medium or elastic resistance, the *process* for developing resistance-training exercises stays the same. The necessary skill you must possess as a trainer is an ability to evaluate each exercise and fit it to each client's unique combination of abilities, interests and health circumstances. You can do that by following the 10-step **Any Exercise Drill**. The "Drill" is a systematic method I developed to make fitting exercise to your client fast and accurate. You can use it to make the "best" resistance exercise choices, *and* you can use the process to modify or create new exercises that meet current biomechanical standards of safety and effectiveness.

The "best" resistance exercise for each client maximizes effectiveness and client compliance because it is safe and uses proper biomechanics and muscle function. When you maintain quality control over exercise selection, you are never at the mercy of the latest, untested exercise variation.

Even traditional exercises that have been performed for years in the gym should be put to the test of the Any Exercise Drill. Why? Many times their value and mechanics have never been analyzed or questioned. When put to the test, many of these seemingly effective—or at worst harmless—exercises are either ineffective or high risk for the average client or competitive athlete. This holds true especially when the goals of clients are not in line with the training method or exercise. Training procedures, exercise selection and exercise creation must go hand in hand with individual exercise goals.

Any Exercise Drill—10 Steps to Effective Resistance-Training Exercises

This drill, which consists of 10 key questions, will help you evaluate the effectiveness of a *given* resistance-training exercise. The drill also helps you weigh exercise effectiveness against safety concerns. And, it can be used as a creative process for developing *new* resistance exercises.

1. What is the goal?

The goal of the exercise usually relates to a particular body part, muscle or groups of muscles. For example, if your goal is to target the chest, it is important to identify a number of effective exercises for this body part using different body positions and equipment.

2. What is (are) the joint action(s)?

There are a finite number of *intended* joint actions in the body. Joint actions are largely determined by anatomical structure of the joint and muscle-attachment points. Having mastery and understanding of the key joint actions that are related to gross motor movement is important to see through the *seemingly* infinite number of movements available to the body. An excellent resource to learn joint actions is *The Manual of Structural Kinesiology* by Clem Thompson (Times Mirror/Mosby, publisher).

3. What muscle(s) is (are) being used to create movement at the joint(s)?

Once the joint action(s) has been identified and the motion(s) that you need to replicate has been defined, you can identify the muscle(s) involved in the movement. As is true for joint actions, it is imperative that you have a solid understanding of the function of muscles that contribute to the large, or gross, motor movements of the body. Understanding muscle function is most easily accomplished by visualizing attachment points of key muscles. Muscles contract along the lines of their fiber direction. By "seeing" attachment points and knowing joint actions, it's easy to understand what movements can and should occur at the joints. An excellent resource to visualize muscle-attachment points is *The Manual of Structural Kinesiology* by Clem Thompson.

4. What is the proper path of motion?

Specific joint action(s) and muscles that contribute to a proper path of motion must be identified in relation to any anatomical considerations, muscle attachments (fiber direction), body position, the type of equipment being used and the goal of the exercise. For example, if the goal of a lateral shoulder raise is to challenge shoulder abduction and the middle deltoid, versus the anterior deltoid, a specific body position and path of motion of the arms must be maintained. Remember, mechanics are mechanics! Do not alter or compromise correct movement because of limitations imposed by external factors such as machine design.

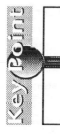

> Neither the type of equipment nor the position of the body during an exercise should alter correct mechanics.

5. What is the proper range of motion (ROM) at the joint?

Range of motion at the joint can be estimated by learning the average, or so-called "normal," range of motion at each joint of the body. This information is provided in various textbooks. For example, the commonly cited ROM for knee flexion is 135 degrees. However, each of your clients has special and different circumstance related to ROM. Though textbook ROM characterization may provide a good estimate of general movement capabilities at each joint, the best starting point with your clients is to determine their active range of motion.

6. What is the active range of motion (AROM) at the joint?

Flexibility, or range of motion about a joint or joints, is generally limited by the strength of the agonist muscle(s) at the joint, lack of flexibility in the antagonistic muscles (specifically the muscle fascia) and natural or other anatomical limitations. Although there are textbook descriptions of appropriate or average ROM for each joint, AROM is specific to your client's individual situation. To determine your client's AROM for any joint, have her perform the desired movement pattern with no resistance. Subsequently, the client should work the resistance-training exercise within this AROM.

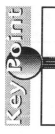

> Proper ROM at a joint or joints is probably most accurately identified and safely determined by your client's AROM.

7. Is the overload effective in terms of the amount of resistance?

Effective overload for the majority of your clients means working at or close to muscle fatigue, or to the point where the client is thinking, "This is about the last repetition I can do with good form." Muscle fatigue should be attained for most of your clients, in about 8-20 repetitions, or in about 30-90 seconds.

8. Is the direction of force or resistance in direct opposition (or as close as possible) to the movement pattern?

Is your client's body properly positioned in relation to the *type of equipment* being used and to the *direction of force* created by a particular piece of resistance-training equipment? For example, because of gravity, the direction of force created by free weights is always down or toward the floor. Selectorized plates and their forces are generally routed through a system of pulleys and cables, whereas elastic resistance generally affords resistance that is directly opposite and in line with its attachment point.

Direction of force as provided by free weights is, for example, the reason that a standing chest press using dumbbells is *not* effective. Regardless of equipment, always position the body so that the direction of force created by a particular piece of equipment is in direct opposition to the movement pattern.

9. Has the necessary stabilization occurred in the body prior to the movement, and has it been maintained during the movement?

The most important initial step in any strength-training exercise is stabilization. **Stabilization** generally refers to a position that is assumed before the exercise is started and maintained during the exercise, with no variance. (Notable exceptions to this general rule include trunk exercise, where it is essential to move in and out of neutral lumbar spine to work the proper range of motion, and some sport-specific resistance training movements.) Effective stabilization occurs when your client maintains the position from which she started until the exercise is completed. An effective cue is, "Where you start is where you stay."

Maintaining and/or returning to a neutral lumbar and cervical posture is critical for effective, safe and functional movement. Stabilization may also occur in other areas of the body, such as the upper back (scapular stabilization), shoulders, hips and knees.

10. Do the risks of the exercise outweigh its potential effectiveness? What about orthopedic concerns?

An exercise may be effective in challenging a particular body part(s) or group of muscles and in creating excellent functional strength gains. However, the risks may outweigh any potential benefits of some exercises when you consider known orthopedic concerns, such as sustained, unsupported forward flexion, loaded and hyperflexed knees, shoulder impingement and speed of movement.

Quick Index:

Chapter 2, understanding client's goal
Chapter 8, explanation of ROM in relation to joint structures
Chapter 14, using overload in resistance training

Any Exercise Drill

1. What is the goal?

2. What is (are) the joint action(s)?

3. What muscle(s) is (are) being used to create movement at the joint(s)?

4. What is the proper path of motion?

5. What is the proper range of motion (ROM) at the joint?

6. What is the active range of motion (AROM) at the joint?

7. Is the overload effective in terms of the amount of resistance?

8. Is the direction of force or resistance in direct opposition (or as close as possible) to the movement pattern?

9. Has the necessary stabilization occurred in the body prior to the movement and has it been maintained during the movement?

10. Do the risks of the exercise outweigh its potential effectiveness? What about orthopedic concerns?

Applying the Drill

Here's an example of how to use the Any Exercise Drill to evaluate an exercise.

Exercise: unsupported bent-over row

In this position the exerciser is standing on her feet and flexed 90 degrees at the hips. Neutral lumbar posture is not maintained (the spine is flexed). The weight being lifted is suspended from the arms. Now, let's look at how this exercise stacks up against the drill.

The **goal (1)** of this exercise could be to target the upper arm, back of the shoulder and the upper back musculature. The **major muscles (3)** involved in this movement are the biceps, posterior deltoid, latissimus dorsi, trapezius I and II, and the rhomboids. The **joint actions (2)** include elbow flexion, horizontal shoulder abduction or extension, and scapular adduction or retraction.

The body is in a position of 90 degrees flexion at the hip, with some lumbar spinal flexion as well. From this position, the **direction of force or resistance (8)**, due to the weights and gravity's effect, is in direct opposition to this movement.

So far, this exercise has passed most of the criteria set forth in the Any Exercise Drill. **Stabilization (9)**, **AROM (5, 6)**, **effective overload (7)** and **correct movement path (4)** still need to be investigated, but in theory, your client could execute these properly.

However, regardless of the many positives of this exercise, when you get to the question regarding **orthopedic concerns (10)**, the unsupported bent-over row fails. While it is very effective in overloading the musculature, the risk of injury and accumulative stress to the low-back region is high. This exercise places the body in a position of unsupported forward flexion, which requires the spine to be supported passively by the ligaments and fascia of the low-back region. The stress is multiplied by the addition of weights. The risk is particularly high if trunk flexion (rather than hip flexion and full knee extension) is allowed during its execution.

A combination of any of these factors can compromise the stabilizing effects that ligaments and fascia have on the vertebral joints. Furthermore, there is considerable stress to the discs between the lumbar vertebrae. While the effectiveness of the exercise is high in its ability to overload your client's musculature, any potential advantage is far outweighed by the high risk of potential injury or cumulative stress to the spine.

The Creative Way to Adapt Exercises

How can you redirect the good qualities of the unsupported bent-over row? Use the drill as a checklist to adapt exercises. Often, the same muscles and joint actions can be safely and effectively challenged by putting the body in a different position, and/or by using a different piece of exercise equipment.

For example, with the unsupported bent-over row, the client could simply lie face down on a flat bench with dumbbells in each hand, or perform a one-arm row with one knee and hand on a bench for support. The spine is safely supported and the movement path is effective. Alternatively, the client could be positioned in a standing or seated position. Cables or elastic resistance that are attached to a wall or a selectorized cable pulley system could provide resistance in opposition to the movement.

As long as you have a solid foundation in kinesiology and movement mechanics, using the Any Exercise Drill system will allow you to enjoy unlimited creative freedom in exercise selection and creation. If an exercise is not recommended or its relative risk is high, you can usually find a solution. That is your challenge.

Five Principles to Incorporate in All Resistance Exercises

These 5 principles evolve from the Any Exercise Drill system. During the execution or creation of an *excellent* resistance-training exercise, all of the drill's criteria should be fulfilled. In addition:

• Attempt to emphasize *movements that are natural* to the body. Joint action and muscle function, as related to anatomical considerations, muscle fiber direction and attachment points, will provide the "clues" to natural movement.

• Increase the joints' *active range of motion (AROM)* if not contraindicated by injury or other medical limitation by working through a full and controlled plane(s) of movement.

• Maximize motor-unit recruitment and efficient muscle contraction by utilizing all joint actions appropriate to the movement, full AROM and proper overload (intensity).

• Create resistance that is, as closely as possible, in *direct opposition* to the path of movement.

• Decrease the likelihood of injury by taking into account known orthopedic principles and orthopedic concerns of the client.

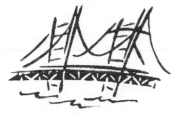

The Bridge

Every exercise must meet certain criteria for safety as well as effectiveness. Joint and muscle actions must be analyzed, along with movement path, line of resistance and active range of motion. Is there risk involved in the exercise? Using the Any Exercise Drill allows you to quickly and accurately analyze each exercise and determine if it is appropriate for your client.

References and Recommended Reading

Videos

Brooks, Douglas (1995). *The Best Strength Training Exercises: Upper Body.* Moves International: Mammoth Lakes, CA (619) 934-0312.

Brooks, Douglas (1995). *The Best Strength Training Exercises: Lower Body.* Moves International: Mammoth Lakes, CA (619) 934-0312.

Brooks, Douglas (1995). *The Best Strength Training Exercises: Trunk.* Moves International: Mammoth Lakes, CA (619) 934-0312.

Brooks, Douglas (1991). *One on One: Strength Training Workouts for Everyone.* Moves International: Mammoth Lakes, CA (619) 934-0312.

Purvis, Tom (1994). *Trainer's Video Lecture and Hands-On Series.* Oklahoma City, OK (405) 755-3082.

Articles

Brooks, Douglas (1995). *Planning Your Strength Program.* IDEA Today: San Diego, CA, September.

Brooks, Douglas (1995). *Shaping the Shoulder.* IDEA Today: San Diego, CA, October.

Brooks, Douglas (1995). *Training the Upper Back.* IDEA Today: San Diego, CA, November/December.

Brooks, Douglas (1996). *Sculpting the Chest.* IDEA Today: San Diego, CA, January.

Brooks, Douglas (1996). *Strengthening the Upper Arms.* IDEA Today: San Diego, CA, March.

CHAPTER 16

WORKING WITH MINIMAL EQUIPMENT

Many trainers feel helpless if they are presented with limited equipment options—especially if they are accustomed to being surrounded by a multitude of equipment choices. However, the effectiveness, or lack of effectiveness, of exercise is generally not determined by the amount, cost or type of training equipment. The basis of program design, *regardless* of equipment options, is in the physiology of the energy, cardiorespiratory and muscular systems and the methods used to manipulate them. Equipment options do not limit the specific joint action and body parts you can target, nor do they limit the effectiveness of your client's cardiorespiratory workouts.

Armed with the following approach, you will no longer be limited by the so-called "lack of equipment" syndrome. Even if you have a variety of equipment choices, it is easy to fall into the rut of numbly "going through a line of equipment." This chapter gives you an approach that puts the thought process, control and direction of the workout back into your hands.

> **Key Point**
>
> Your clients will be more excited about the changes they feel and see in their bodies than about any equipment you bring to them! Focus on effective training versus variety of equipment. You'll increase your value as a trainer in their eyes and overcome *seemingly* limited situations with practical and effective solutions.

For example, trainers who work in clients' homes generally have limited equipment choices. Yet clients may already have equipment that just needs to be dusted off. If you're bringing the equipment, search for equipment that can serve more than one function. For example, use a step platform for cardio conditioning or as a weight bench. Consider activities or training methods that do not require equipment. Outdoor training, cross training, walking, running and the use of "real" stairs are practical examples. And, remember that manual resistance (trainer resisted) and client body weight are valid and effective methods to overload major muscle groups for strength training. With all these options, workouts are certainly not limited.

The Essential Equipment

When purchasing equipment for an exercise environment, 5 important qualities come to mind:

1. diversity

2. variety

3. portability

4. space efficiency

5. cost

An example of these qualities is a bench that inclines, declines and lies flat. Elastic resistance is a prime example of a tool that can be used to challenge many different body movements and it can provide progressive overload. Both types of equipment can be easily transported, take up minimum space and are reasonably priced.

When training a client in his home, these qualities are especially important. At the beginning of a program, your client is probably not sure of his commitment to you and training in general. He wants an effective workout, but may not initially want to invest a significant dollar amount into equipment. You can alleviate these concerns by telling him that superb workouts are possible with little equipment, and that you possess all of the equipment needed to get his program started. After weeks of training, your client will probably be interested in expanding his home gym. Though not an absolute necessity, expanding the gym is usually a natural response to a positive relationship with you.

Equipment and Methods

Following is a list of equipment and methods that are inexpensive, portable and versatile. Several of these tools and methods are nice to use even in an atmosphere where there is a wide assortment of equipment. *None* of them compromises the workout. Even in situations where I have every equipment option, I often return to these choices because they are fun and effective variety for a client who is tired of the same workout.

Versatile *Equipment* Options:

1. Dumbbells

   a. The Power Block™ is equivalent to 28 pairs of dumbbells, ranging from 10 to 95 pounds. Power Block is available at many sporting good stores that carry resistance-training equipment.

   b. An alternative is several pairs of fixed dumbbells that are appropriate to your client's current strength level.

   c. Changeable (non-fixed) dumbbells are another good choice, but be aware of safety issues. Secure the quick-release locking collars before every exercise.

2. Elastic Resistance (tubing, bands, etc.)

   a. Provides variable resistance and many different strengths of tubing.

   b. Attached handles and bars make it easy to perform a variety of exercises.

c. Door attachments and wall-mounted units increase elastic resistance versatility. Lifeline and SPRI are 2 excellent companies that supply elastic resistance training systems.

3. Stability Ball

a. Provides major muscle group overload and flexibility training.

b. Especially effective for abdominal and back (or trunk) strengthening.

c. Can provide progressive resistance overload by adjusting body position.

d. Can be used as an exercise bench.

4. Manual Resistance (trainer resisted)

a. Trainer-assisted resistance is very effective and allows you to add overload and assist with range of motion, or correct technique.

b. T.O.U.C.H. Training™ does not apply resistance, but it enhances the client's mental image of the muscle being worked and facilitates contraction through reflexive pathways (Rothenberg and Rothenberg, 1995, Human Kinetics Publishers).

5. Client's Body Weight as Resistance

a. A variety of exercise positions, such as a push-up or heel raise, can utilize this technique.

6. Adjustable Step Platform

a. Can be used for cardio and strength training in combination with weight or tubing.

b. Doubles as a flat, incline or decline bench.

7. Adjustable Exercise Bench

a. Replaces the need for 2 benches because it is adjustable from flat to vertical.

b. Many exercises can be performed from standing or seated positions.

8. Manual Rowing Machine (non flywheel)

a. Can be used for cardio or strength training by changing resistance.

b. By changing seat position, works the arms, chest and upper back.

Versatile *Methods* Options:

1. Circuit Training

a. Can be modified to challenge strength and cardiorespiratory fitness, cardio only or strength only.

2. Interval Training

a. Can be used with any cardiorespiratory training.

3. Step Training (adjustable platform)

a. athletic approach (with or without music).

b. stylized approach (choreography and music).

4. Slide Training

   a. athletic approach (with or without music).

   b. stylized approach (choreography and music).

5. Walk or Run Training

   a. Can be performed outside or indoors on a treadmill.

   b. Can be combined with interval and circuit training.

6. Water Training

   a. Can train cardio, strength or flexibility.

7. Outdoor Cross Training

   a. Can use a variety of activities such as biking and hiking. The activity will depend somewhat on the type of outdoor environment you have access to and equipment availability.

Quick Index:

The Muscular Analysis Process

Replicating movement patterns with minimal equipment is easy when the Any Exercise Drill (Chapter 15) is used. The Any Exercise Drill identifies the goal, the body part you want to target, or the machine movement you want to replicate. Next, the joint actions and muscles involved in the movement are determined. Force—whether provided by elastic resistance, dumbbells, client's body weight or trainer resistance—is placed in direct opposition to the movement pattern by positioning the body correctly. Finally, risk versus effectiveness of the exercise is determined.

By becoming a "thinker," you can help your client accomplish his goals with minimal equipment. The first step is to determine the goal—the body part you want to isolate or the piece of equipment you want to replicate. Next, determine the joint actions and muscles involved that challenge this area of the body. Finally, observe what equipment is available to you. Many times you will find useful equipment in the client's home that long ago had been converted to a clothes rack or relegated to stored "junk" status. The examples in the "Goals, Equipment and Methods" chart will bring this methodology to life.

Table 23. Goals, Equipment and Methods

Piece of Equipment to Replicate or Body Part to Challenge	Major Joint Action(s)	Major Muscle(s) Involved	Equipment	Methods
Replicate "pec deck"; target chest	shoulder horizontal adduction; scapular retraction (stabilization)	anterior deltoid; pectoralis major; rhomboids; mid trapezius	flat bench; dumbbells	manual resistance; spotter assisted
Replicate barbell press; target chest	elbow extension; shoulder horizontal adduction; scapular retraction (stabilization)	triceps brachii; anterior deltoid; pectoralis major; rhomboids; mid trapezius	rowing machine; stability ball; elastic resistance	manual resistance; client's body weight; spotter assisted
Replicate high elbow row; back of shoulder; upper back	elbow flexion; shoulder horizontal abduction; scapular retraction (stabilization)	biceps brachii; posterior deltoid; latissimus; rhomboids; mid trapezius	rowing machine; elastic resistance	manual resistance; spotter assisted
Replicate leg curl; isolate back of leg	knee flexion	hamstring group	elastic resistance	manual resistance
Replicate reverse abdominal curl; emphasize fibers in lower abdominal region	trunk flexion or 9-degrees of posterior pelvic tilt	rectus abdominis; external obliques	adjustable step; flat or incline bench	manual resistance; client's body weight against gravity
Replicate hyper-extension machine; target low back	trunk extension	erector spinae group; quadratus lumborum	adjustable step; bench; stability ball	manual resistance; spotter assisted

Let's take a closer look at a couple of the examples in the chart.

Replicate the "pec deck." To satisfy this goal, I gave an example of a supine position, using dumbbells, on a flat bench. Of course, this is hardly novel. You know that a chest flye targets the chest. This is not the key point. What's important is to identify the muscles and (probably more importantly) joint actions, so you can recognize the flye is a substitute movement that effectively challenges this area of the body and mimics the joint action required by the "pec deck."

Replicate the barbell press. When using the stability ball (a large air-filled ball), your client could perform a push-up with his feet elevated on the ball. This copies the joint actions used during a barbell press. An added dimension to using this tool is the stability needed to maintain body position while keeping the ball centered under the feet. Thus, your client's muscles are being challenged as both movers (the push-up/barbell press action) and stabilizers (the trunk, hip and leg muscles) that keep the ball from moving excessively.

Using the rowing machine as a resistance training tool. For resistance training, the rowing machine must be of the traditional type where there are 2 rowing "arms" attached to the machine. Single-cable rowing simulators do not work well for this application. To work the posterior musculature of the upper body, your client sits in the rower, straps his feet into the machine as if to row a boat and then pulls the rowing "arms" toward himself. This replicates a seated "high-elbow" row or a high-elbow one-arm dumbbell row. Be sure to increase the resistance supplied by the rowing arms to challenge the strength level of the individual. Since the goal is strength development, don't perform high-repetition work typically done on this machine.

To isolate the opposing or anterior musculature of the upper body, as exemplified by a bench press or push-up movement, your client removes his feet from the straps, swivels around and slides the seat back to face in the opposite direction. He sits tall with an extended spine and pushes the rowing arms of the machine away from his body. The seat does not slide. You can support your client's spine from behind with the side of your leg. It's a good idea to place a folded towel between your leg and his back.

Understanding direction of force. There is a variety of methods, types of equipment and body positions that can target the muscle groups and joint actions in these examples. However, the direction of force must be in direct opposition to the movement.

If you stand up and perform shoulder horizontal adduction (chest flye exercise) with dumbbells, you are performing the correct joint action, but the exercise is ineffective. Because of the effects of gravity, the direction of force exerted by any dumbbell or free weight is toward the ground. This is not in opposition to the movement.

However, if you attach a piece of elastic resistance behind your client at shoulder height, take an end in each hand, have him walk out from the wall or attachment point, stabilize himself and perform the flye movement, this would be effective. Why? Because the line of resistance supplied by the cable is in direct opposition to the movement. You could effectively resist this same movement with the dumbbells by placing your client in a supine position.

Once the joint actions that effectively isolate specific body segments are known, the world of effective options is yours. Just be sure the resistance tool you choose can provide resistance that is opposite to the movement being performed.

The Bridge

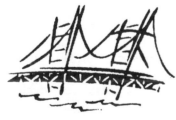

It's essential not to let equipment availability determine what cardiovascular or resistance training exercises you choose to use, and what body parts you can challenge. Lack of equipment does not limit your effectiveness, and a successful program is not determined by the amount, cost or type of equipment available. Armed with a little creativity and a good understanding of physiology, anatomy and biomechanics, you can create programs that are interesting, exciting and will give your clients great results.

References and Recommended Reading

Lifeline and SPRI (elastic resistance-training systems) and Resist-A-Ball (stability ball) Programming are listed in the resources section at the back of this book.

CHAPTER 17

FLEXIBILITY TRAINING

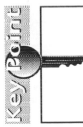Flexibility training is probably one of the most overlooked, poorly executed, poorly understood and undervalued components of physical fitness and overall personal health. Yet achieving and maintaining flexibility is an important factor in reaching optimal physical potential. Flexibility is most simply defined as range of motion (ROM) available to a joint or joints. However, the joint's *normal* ROM is not always healthy, or adequate, for individual movement pattern needs.

Functional flexibility (Siff, 1992) or **functional range of motion (FROM)** is a relatively new concept that is gaining momentum. According to Siff, with this philosophy the goal of stretching changes from simply increasing range of motion (ROM) to improving the flexibility necessary for a specific activity, sport, or daily chore—without compromising joint stability. This could also be termed "usable" flexibility and represents the concept of FROM.

Aren't most clients looking to gain "usable" flexibility with minimal risk, discomfort and time commitment? Extreme ranges of motion and contorted stretch postures are high risk for the majority of the population. But static, active, passive and proprioceptive neuromuscular facilitation (PNF) stretching will all yield favorable results when performed correctly. Stretching can be a very enjoyable, relaxing part of your client's workout.

> **Key Point**
>
> Maintaining functional movement capability is important to every person.

Physiological and Biomechanical Basics

There is a multitude of circumstances that can add to or detract from the success of a flexibility training program. It has been well established that increases in *intramuscular temperature*, through warm-up, decrease viscosity or a tissue's resistance to stretch (Sapega, 1981). According to Kravitz and Kosich (1993), there does not appear to be a *body build* that consistently represents "good flexibility."

Several authors report that females tend to be more flexible, in general, than males (Alter, 1988; Holland, 1968, reported by Kravitz and Kosich, 1993). Though conclusive evidence is lacking in regard to *gender* differences, a female's tendency to be more flexible in the pelvic region than most males may be related to the female's role in childbearing. Beyond these issues, it seems that a regular commitment to exercise is the most influential variable that can affect flexibility gains or losses.

The degree of movement is specific to each joint. Being "flexible" in one joint does not influence flexibility in another joint. Gains in flexibility are limited largely by 4 factors: (1) The elastic limits of the ligaments and tendons crossing the joint, (2) the elasticity of the muscle fibers themselves and muscle fascia that "encases" single muscle fibers, groups of muscle fibers and the entire muscle, (3) the bone and joint structure, and (4) the skin.

The greatest improvement in flexibility seems to be related to the ability of a stretching program to target the muscle's fascial sheath (which seems to be the most modifiable factor with regard to limitations to gains in ROM). When the fascia is warm, it is "stretchable." When it is cold, it is "brittle and breakable." Ligaments and tendons have a high resistance to stretch. Muscle fascia has a low resistance to stretch.

The (1) type of force, (2) mechanics of the stretch and exercise position, (3) duration of the stretch, (4) intensity of the stretch, and (5) temperature of the muscle during the stretch determine if elongation of tissue is permanent or temporary, and whether the stretch is helpful or harmful. If the muscles are stretched too fast, muscle spindles initiate a stretch reflex, which causes the affected muscle group to reflexively shorten and protect it from being overstretched. The resultant increase in muscular tension inhibits the stretching process. If the stretch is performed slowly and controlled, the stretch reflex may be avoided or be of low intensity.

Quick Index:

Chapter 8, details on the neurophysiology of muscles and stretching

Types and Relative Risks of Stretching

There are 5 types of stretching techniques available:

1. Static Stretching. Static stretching is defined as a controlled stretch, held at the point of mild tension. This places the muscle in a lengthened position, and the stretch is sustained for about 10-60 seconds.

2. Dynamic or Ballistic Stretching. Dynamic or ballistic stretching uses bouncing, jerking or abrupt movements to gain momentum to facilitate overstretching.

3. Active Stretching. Active stretching is voluntary, unassisted movement that requires strength and muscular contraction of the agonist muscle or prime mover. For example, in a supine position the hip flexors can contract actively to draw the leg forward, resulting in hip flexion. The agonist is unassisted by external (passive) forces. The purpose of the stretch is to actively stretch the hip extensors (gluteus maximus and hamstrings) by using only the muscular effort and strength provided by the agonist hip flexors.

4. Passive Stretching. Passive stretching occurs when movements are accomplished through the use of an outside (external) force such as that provided by a partner, exerting pull on your own body part with another limb, gravity or momentum.

5. Proprioceptive Neuromuscular Facilitation (PNF). PNF stretching works by first putting the targeted muscle on a stretch that is fairly intense. The intensity of the stretch is at, or approaches, the elastic limit of the muscle fascia. Then, a maximal force is generated in the muscle that is "on stretch." This procedure can activate a sensory organ called the Golgi tendon organ, which causes the muscle to relax. A muscle that is relaxed or free of tension will more easily allow the muscle fascia to be stretched.

The types of stretching can further be categorized as to their relative risk based on muscular force and tension. These categories are in Table 24, Relative Risk of Types of Stretching.

Table 24. Relative Risk of Types of Stretching

Active	Low force	Low tension	Low risk
Controlled Passive	Low force	Low tension	Low risk
Passive	Higher *potential* force, tension and risk		
Static	Low force	Controlled tension	Low risk
Ballistic	High force	High tension	High risk
PNF (high skill)	High force	High tension	High risk

Which Stretching Method or Methods Work Best?

Scientists generally think that the major limiting factor affecting flexibility, that can be changed, is muscle fascia (Johns and Wright, 1962). Almost half of the resistance to ROM is related to muscle fascia. This is a factor that can be modified without negatively affecting joint stability and creating an increased risk for injury.

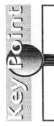

When deciding what technique or combination of techniques to use, look to science first, then balance this factual information with each client's individual makeup.

Static stretching, in its various forms, gains the most support in terms of safety and effectiveness. The amount of tissue lengthening that remains after the stretching force is removed is greatest when using low-force, long-duration, static stretches. This could encompass active-static, passive-static, PNF followed by an active and/or passive stretch into a static hold, or some combination thereof. Static stretching offers a low incidence of injury potential. If your client's goal is to attain "functional flexibility," this can easily and effectively be attained with static stretching.

Active stretching, while in theory sound and currently promoted to some extent, can be tedious and demanding for the average client. Many clients lack the requisite agonist strength and mental concentration to bring the limb through an effective and *increased* ROM. Many clients prefer **passive stretching** because they seem to be able to "relax" into the stretch, or a combination of active and passive stretching.

Ballistic stretching involves the use of momentum to gain an advantage in "overstretching" an area of the body. Ballistic stretching has a tendency to encourage *recoverable* fascial tissue elongation (no change in available ROM) and *non-recoverable* muscle or ligament elongation, or in other words, injury. Arguments *against* ballistic stretching, based on negative short-term and long-term adaptations, include:

• Increased muscle soreness.

• Lack of tissue adaptation. Tissue adaptation is time dependent. Ballistic stretching does not allow for a lengthened position of the fascia to be sustained.

• Initiates the stretch reflex and increases muscular tension.

• Decreased neurological adaptations, especially the muscle spindle and its time-dependent threshold. If the goal is to reset the muscle spindle to a higher level, ballistic stretching will not facilitate this adaptation.

Though there is sufficient reasoning to justify this type of stretching for performance preparation in elite athletic participation, the risk versus effectiveness should be carefully examined. For example, a professional tennis player needs sufficient dynamic flexibility in the shoulder to slam a tennis serve 120 mph. However, a recreational exerciser may need only sufficient dynamic flexibility to play softball on the weekends. Normal ROM attained through static stretching may be sufficient to meet the "dynamic" needs of the recreational exerciser, whereas dynamic flexibility training may be required to meet the demands imposed on the body of a professional tennis player.

Many professionals associate ballistic stretching with *dynamic* stretching. Is it the same? The answer is both yes and no. Ballistic stretching, which has fallen mostly out of favor, is only one technique of many that could be grouped under the heading of dynamic stretching.

Dynamic stretching can be performed actively, passively or as a combination of both. Regardless, momentum is used to gain an edge for increasing ROM. Whether it can be done safely is dependent upon the speed and range of motion at which the stretch is being executed, and the individual performing the maneuver. Murphy (1991) suggests that for this type of stretching (1) the ROM should be normal, and (2) it should take about 4-5 seconds to complete the full, intended range of motion at any given joint. In other words, the dynamic ROM should be *controlled.*

This type of dynamic stretching can be used to prepare an athlete for an aggressive event or for sport-specific activity. Professional gymnasts, divers and dancers use dynamic stretching extensively. There is no specific scientific literature that conclusively suggests dynamic stretching is more effective than other methods in producing flexibility gains, and certainly, there is a higher risk for injury when compared to static stretching.

Though it is often quoted that **PNF stretching** in its various forms yields far greater results than standard static stretching, experts in the field, including Etnyre et al. (1987) and Hutton (1992) disagree with this popular notion. When you read that one method is the "best," you need to ask, "for whom and for what?" If attaining "functional flexibility" is the goal, PNF stretching and its associated risks might be inappropriate. Functional flexibility can be attained easily and effectively with static stretching.

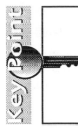

> Many of the gains in any fitness component are often related to a client's effort, focus, concentration and consistency in the effort, as well as the appropriateness of the approach to the individual, rather than any "one best way."

Quick Index:

This chapter, special section on PNF

How to Develop Flexibility

A variety of stretching methods improves flexibility. The goal of each client, current fitness level, individual limitations to ROM, the type of activity the client regularly participates in and risk versus effectiveness must carefully be considered.

A **flexibility warm-up** and **cool-down** can be defined as stretching that is participated in before or after an activity to improve performance, reduce the risk of injury or enhance recovery. The goal is *not* to increase ROM, but to prepare your client's body for upcoming activity or to facilitate recovery from activity.

Flexibility training is defined as a planned, deliberate, progressive and regular program of stretching that causes permanent (plastic) elongation of soft tissues without causing, or contributing to, injury. Flexibility training's focus is to aggressively pursue increases in ROM available at the joint, or joints, being stretched.

An excellent approach is to use a *combination* of active, controlled passive and static stretching technique. Using this approach, an active contraction is initiated with agonist muscles. This begins the stretch process and defines an individual's **active range of motion (AROM)**. Once the AROM is determined, the trainer has a better idea of a participant's elastic limit and associated constraints to safe movement. This step may, or may not, be followed by an application of an outside or passive force that is used to enhance movement through a greater ROM. And finally, a static and sustained stretch is held.

Following are basic guidelines for safe and effective flexibility improvement with most clients:

• Stretch all of the major muscle groups of the body for balance and bodily symmetry, because flexibility is specific to each joint. But, concentrate on the areas of the body that generally lack adequate flexibility. These include the chest, anterior shoulder, hip flexors, hamstrings and the gastrocnemius/soleus muscle groups of the lower leg.

• Perform static stretching after a thorough warm-up of at least 3-5 minutes. This increases body and muscle temperature, and the likelihood that good gains in range of motion will be attained. (Note: Duration and intensity of stretch may have the greatest impact on flexibility gains.)

• Sustain stretches for about 10-60 seconds. Hold each stretch at the point of mild tension or "tightness." This represents the load or exercise intensity. Stretch to the point where movement or ROM is limited at the joint. Stretching to an intensity that could be described as "comfortably uncomfortable" is okay if the stretch can be sustained. Do not stretch to the point of pain.

• The recommended frequency for stretching is a *minimum* of 3 times per week, though stretching may be performed daily.

• Perform 1-4 set(s) of a stretch or stretches per muscle group each time you stretch.

• Stretches should be performed after the muscle is relaxed, in a slow and controlled manner. Progress gradually to greater ranges of motion. When "coming out" of a stretch, release slowly.

• Use subtle variations for given positions to stretch muscles in a variety of ways. The muscles of the body generally have various fiber direction alignments and orientations. By varying stretches, these structural arrangements within a given muscle, or muscles, will more likely be challenged. This may lead to overall greater flexibility improvement.

• Focus on proper stretching position and biomechanics that do not put your client at risk because of extreme or contorted postures. Sullivan et al. (1992) reported that the effect of pelvic position (anterior versus posterior tilt) was more important than the stretching *method* utilized for gains in flexibility.

Key Point

It is important to position your clients in biomechanically correct postures to facilitate stretching gains and limit any increased risk for injury.

• Design programming and assessment that measure improvement in flexibility. Assess and evaluate weaknesses and improvement in flexibility or areas of postural concern on an ongoing basis. For an excellent reference, see Francis and Francis (1988).

• Participate in a stretching program on a regular basis. Possibly the most important factor in stretching, after identifying and using correct stretching methods, is consistency and patience.

These guidelines are, of course, not black and white. Recent research (Taylor et al. 1990) suggests that 4 sets of 15-20 seconds per stretch might result in *optimal* flexibility gains. However, the guidelines written above can encompass a wide range of personal goals and available time commitments, while still ensuring excellent flexibility gains.

Using a combination of stretching techniques will probably be most effective with your clients. You can attempt to challenge your clients to become "involved" in the stretch even if you are not utilizing a PNF technique. A good way to do so is to ask your client to contract the muscle(s) opposite those being stretched. This invokes the nervous system reflex called **reciprocal innervation**, and causes the antagonist muscle(s) on the opposite side to relax. This is also a good lead into an active stretch, and will trigger this relaxation reflex. In general motor movement, reciprocal innervation is important because it allows coordinated motor movement to occur. During stretching, it is a reflex mechanism that can be taken advantage of to create a relaxed muscle that is being targeted for flexibility gains. Potentially, invoking reciprocal innervation will allow for more-effective stretching to take place.

Quick Index:

When to Stretch

When is the best time to fit stretching into your client's program? The answer, of course, is when it is most enjoyed and *accepted* by your client. Some clients don't like to take time for stretching that lasts more than a minute. If this is your client's personality, "sneak" stretches in between resistance-training exercises as "active recovery." Other clients will look forward to the quiet "time-out," relaxation and stress reduction that an extended series of stretches provides. Work with your client's preferences so that you can maintain and improve upon this important component of fitness.

The optimal time to stretch depends upon the (1) goal of the client, (2) degree of warm-up that has taken place, and (3) type of activity. A well-rounded approach to maintaining or increasing FROM will utilize a variety of stretching techniques.

Graduated, low-level, rhythmic warm-up movement is essential prior to stretching. The warm-up activity should move through an easy range of motion, never going beyond a point perceived as excessive strain. The movements should be kept fluid, rhythmic and controlled.

Duration of a warm-up depends on the activity being participated in, and the client. However, for general activity, a minimum of 3-5 minutes is recommended to increase your client's core temperature sufficiently to reduce viscosity or resistance to stretch in the muscle. High-intensity activity, where accentuated or extreme ROM is necessary, may require 5-15 minutes of warm-up, as well as an extended stretching period.

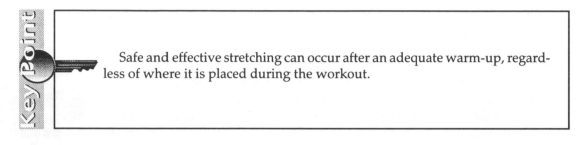

Safe and effective stretching can occur after an adequate warm-up, regardless of where it is placed during the workout.

If stretches are performed during the warm-up preceding cardiorespiratory activity, the stretches should not last more than about 10 seconds and should be interspersed throughout the warm-up (Kravitz and Kosich, 1993). In this case, the goal of the warm-up is to allow for a redistribution of blood to the working muscles (McArdle et al. 1991). Holds longer than 10 seconds may inhibit an effective blood shift or shunt to working muscles.

To increase ROM, it may be best to perform stretching after cardiorespiratory training because the soft tissues will be very warm and more likely to respond to flexibility training.

Stretch During Strength Training. While it is a good idea to perform resistance training exercise through an active and full ROM, this type of training *does not* replace flexibility training. Remember, active stretching which occurs during resistance training can be limited by the strength of the agonist and/or lack of flexibility in the antagonist, which resists the agonist's movement.

Sport-Specific Stretching. If going out for a leisurely or steady-rate run, it may not be necessary—and in fact, may cause more harm—to stretch prior to the run. If your client starts at a slow pace, and gradually increases the pace, there is little risk for injury. No extreme ranges of motion or ballistic movement must be prepared for in this case.

Competitive sports are a different situation. An elite cross country team might engage in a 10- or 15-minute run to warm the soft tissues of their bodies. If the team is going to train with intervals, which demand all-out efforts and extreme ROM relative to steady-rate training, stretching is a prudent choice before interval conditioning. After initially stretching, the team may go for an additional jog of 2-3 miles, intersperse speed play during the jog, perform the interval workout, cool down with a jog and engage in stretching or flexibility training again, post-workout. This approach is time intensive, yet very effective and appropriate for an athlete's commitment.

When *Not* to Stretch

Some situations when it may not be best for your clients to stretch include:

- Within the first 24-72 hours of muscular or tendinous trauma.
- Following muscle strains and ligament sprains.
- When joints or muscles are infected or inflamed.
- Stretching tissues or areas of the body associated with an area of recent fracture.
- "Working through" or "stretching out" when discomfort is felt.
- When sharp pains are felt in the joint or muscle.
- If osteoporosis is present or suspected.

Consult with the appropriate medical professional. Rest and ice may be the simple solution in many of the instances cited. However, expert and accurate professional opinion is necessary before proceeding.

The Bridge

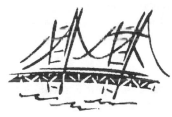

Combining active, passive and static combinations of stretching, with or without stimulating the GTO response (Chapter 8), may lead to the best improvements in flexibility. Furthermore, when results are coupled with manageable and enjoyable effort, and efficient use of time, the outcome is often the highest degree of compliance, which is possibly the most important factor thus far mentioned in getting results. Review the science and your client's individual needs and physical status before deciding which type of stretching to use. A combination will probably give the best results.

SPECIAL SECTION
PNF Stretching

Have you ever wondered what proprioceptive neuromuscular facilitation (PNF) stretching really is? Of course, we have all heard of it. PNF is an aggressive stretching technique designed to facilitate an increased ROM at the joint(s). Three questions often asked regarding PNF stretching are:

1. Does PNF stretching belong in a training program?
2. If so, where and when does PNF stretching fit into a training program?
3. Is PNF more effective than static stretching?

Quick Index:

Chapter 8, details on the neurophysiology of PNF stretching

Stretching Procedures

Although there are numerous techniques, PNF stretching typically involves some variation on these 3 methods:

1. contract-relax (CR), followed by passive stretch

2. contract-relax followed by agonist contraction (CRAC)

3. contract-relax followed by agonist contraction, followed by a passive stretch (CRAC-P)

By definition, agonist contraction occurring in the second and third methods tells you that these methods utilize active stretching. All 3 PNF techniques are trying to invoke or create neurological responses to facilitate the stretching process.

In the first method, **CR, passive stretch**, the target muscle is "put on stretch." For the average client, the degree or intensity of stretch is at the point of mild tension. This amount of intensity approximates approaching a client's muscle fascial elastic limit. Next, the client will be asked to produce a maximal contraction in the muscle being stretched. During this process it is important to increase the magnitude of the contraction over time, as opposed to an all-out, immediate, 100% effort. A muscle on full stretch that is asked to produce a maximal contraction is very vulnerable to injury. Rather than "turning on" the contraction as "all or none," which is analogous to turning a light switch on and off, think of this step as something more like slowly intensifying the contraction to a point of maximum. Dr. Robert Stephens (1992) likens this to using a dimmer switch to intensify the light of a bulb to maximum brightness or intensity.

For example, to stretch the hamstring muscle your client lies in a supine position and the hamstring is "put on stretch." Next, she isometrically contracts her hamstring for 3-10 seconds against an "immovable" force. Generally, use your body and have your client attempt to aggressively, yet in a controlled manner, "push you away." I prefer to use about 8 seconds to gradually peak the contraction to maximal. The intensity must be "turned on" slowly to lessen the likelihood of injury. This maximum contraction is then followed by a passive (outside force) force/stretch application. The client relaxes, and you move her leg forward to flex the hip and stretch the hamstrings.

The **CRAC, agonist contraction** technique is similar, but after the maximal contraction an active stretch technique is applied. Using the preceding example, the hamstring is stretched and brought to a maximal contraction in 8 seconds. Next, the quadriceps contracts actively to extend the knee, thus straightening the leg, and the hip flexors actively flex the hip, creating an active stretch on the hamstrings. The stretch force is applied actively by contracting these agonist muscles. No outside (passive) force is applied.

In the **CRAC-P, agonist contraction, passive stretch**, all of the steps used for CRAC remain the same. The only difference between the 2 is the addition of "P," or an outside passive force, to complete the stretch. The passive stretch is increased to a point of *maintainable* intensity ("comfortably uncomfortable") and is generally held for 10-60 seconds.

Research Is Controversial

In Robert Hutton's (1992) excellent review on the neuromuscular basis of stretching, he notes that a great deal of attention has been placed on the use of PNF stretching techniques on the *assumption* that they are the "most" effective methods for increasing ROM. However, other reports have shown no significant differences between ROM achieved by PNF techniques and static stretching procedures. Part of this disparity is associated with study design. Historically, the results have been rather mixed, but the CRAC-P procedure has often been shown to produce the greatest "absolute" gains in ROM over other PNF procedures, static stretch or ballistic stretch, although the results emphasized are sometimes not statistically significant.

Hutton (1992) continues by saying it is generally assumed that a maximum contraction prior to stretch, as is done in the PNF procedure, promotes muscle relaxation through mechanisms previously discussed. Contrary to the general assumptions, recent findings suggest that, overall, PNF procedures produce greater electromyographic (EMG) activity in muscle. Thus, current PNF procedures seem to produce *more tension* in the muscle, not less. Hutton concludes that constraints within the muscle component in determining ROM have long been *underestimated* and the role of connective tissue as the major resistance to stretch is possibly *overestimated*.

It is obvious that the exact mechanisms for flexibility gains are not known. Certain procedures are associated with gains, although the exact science is not understood. Based on soft-tissue characteristics (muscle fascia, its taffy-like characteristics and the effect of temperature increases on fascial tissue) and the body of stretch research that exists, the above techniques can be used with a reasonable sense of security in their safety and efficacy. Current research (Osternig, 1990; Hutton 1992; Moore and Hutton, 1989) may soon influence a change in how PNF stretching is administered, or at least provide a better understanding of how PNF stretching works.

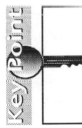

While PNF stretching will remain open to controversy, there are few scientists who would argue against the superb results that the combinations of active-static, passive-static or active-passive-static stretching give the majority of your clients.

When to Use PNF Stretching

I recommend using PNF techniques with participants who are fairly fit, have good body awareness, physical control and a base level of strength. (Of course, this recommendation may not be applicable in a medically supervised setting.) Additionally, your client should have a desire to experience this more physically and mentally involved, and intense type of training. Ask the following questions when considering its use:

1. What are the stretching goals and needs of my client? Are the goals related to sport performance, extreme range of motion or simply functional flexibility?

2. What is the conditioning level of my client?

3. What is her sense of body awareness (proprioceptive) and skill level in performing bodily movements?

4. What is the motivation level of my client?

5. Are my skill and knowledge adequate to administer this technique in a timely, safe and effective manner?

PNF stretches can be used with a variety of clients, including deconditioned participants, patients in rehabilitation under trained and expert care, and competitive athletes. Having said that, it is important to emphasize that most clients can attain their flexibility goals with static stretching. It may not be necessary to stimulate the GTO with a maximal contraction (PNF) or a highly intense and sustained static stretch. The exception to this statement might be a specific rehabilitation situation. In this case, a trained professional, such as a licensed physical therapist, will have the necessary expertise to work with this patient's needs.

Safely teaching PNF stretches requires a clear understanding of neurophysiology, an accurate sense of the limits of a client's body, and constant verbal and nonverbal communication *during* the stretch. Remember, clients can achieve very acceptable flexibility gains with static stretches, which generally are more comfortable and less likely to cause an injury.

Correct PNF teaching technique is best learned from an experienced practitioner of this art. One way to gain this experience is to work with a physical therapist or sports medicine doctor in your professional network. She can help you determine when PNF is appropriate for a client and show you how to perform the stretches properly. Come prepared with a good fundamental knowledge of physiology so you can speak the same language. Hands-on PNF teaching methods can also be experienced at workshops, where practicing with other attendees is encouraged. Most presenters are receptive to specific application questions following the presentation.

References and Recommended Reading

Located at the end of Chapter 8, Neurophysiology of Flexibility

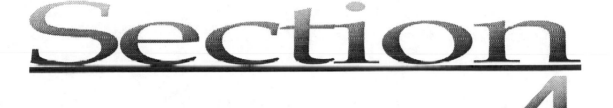

Section 4

Building More Bridges

"Those who think they have not time for exercise will sooner or later have to find time for illness."

Edward Stanley

"One of the biggest reasons people cannot mobilize themselves is that they try to accomplish great things. Most worthwhile achievements are the result of many little things done in a single direction."

Nido Quebin

CHAPTER 18

CAN YOU WORK WITH SPECIAL-NEED CLIENTS?

Sooner or later, you will have the opportunity to work with a special-need and/or high-risk client. That can be good news because it expands your market potential for prospective clients and increases your positive impact on the lives of others.

Today's personal trainers have many opportunities for education and certification, which may better qualify them to individualize workouts. Because of this development, trainers have become more credible and attractive for referral by licensed and allied health professionals. Many members of the medical profession now recognize a qualified personal trainer as an important adjunct to their patients' treatment and ongoing health programs (Couzens, *The Physician and Sportsmedicine*, 1992).

Special-need populations and high-risk conditions that you may encounter include:

- cardiac rehabilitation
- obesity
- neurological and chronic degenerative diseases
- diabetes
- asthma
- youth
- older adult and aging population
- women requiring perinatal care (before, during and after pregnancy)

When you first encounter a special need client, you will have to answer the question, "Do I have the abilities and desire to work with this person?" The keys to working with special-need clientele are:

1. Receive guidance or an exercise prescription from a qualified professional, such as a physician, osteopathic doctor, physical therapist, chiropractor or registered dietitian.

2. Work within the scope of your training. What is within your scope of practice? If you completely understand the necessary precautions or modifications recommended for a client by his health-care provider, and you feel you can adhere to them, then that client is probably

within your scope of practice. If you do not understand a training principle, are unfamiliar with the condition or are not confident about the training regimen, then you should refer the client elsewhere.

I have received a large number of medical and high-risk referrals over the years. I think this has occurred for 3 reasons. First, many trainers simply prefer not to work with high-need clients and this creates a huge market for trainers who can. Second, my credentials, desire, interest and ability to investigate special-need situations give me the necessary background and confidence to work with these clients. In turn, my security and enthusiasm toward the situation promotes confidence in the referring professional, family member, friend and/or potential client. And third, I unfailingly follow the licensed professional's directions.

If I have any concern about the accuracy of the prescription or safety to the client/patient, I discuss it with the referring professional. The discussion remains private and the client/patient may, or may not, have knowledge of the contact. This approach preserves the integrity and credibility of all parties involved. Because I prepare before the contact, have a working knowledge of the high-need situation and come from a position of creating what is best for the client/patient, most referring parties positively embrace my concern and input. In fact, this has often placed me, in the eyes of the doctor, as an integral part of his patient's and my new client's health team.

How to Identify a High-Need Client

Regardless of actual, reported or perceived health status, *all* of your clients need to go through a screening process. This involves a written health-history questionnaire plus dialogue with the client and his health-care provider. Your health-history form should contain items that require responses that would indicate a need for special attention, such as a heart condition, high blood pressure, diabetes, pregnancy, medications or obesity.

Though it seems logical that you would discover a higher risk situation when you speak with a client, I find this is not always the case. Many clients erroneously report their current health status. They may not have an accurate grasp of their current situation, or they may have dealt with a condition for so long they no longer consider it significant enough to mention. A client undergoing cardiac rehabilitation may be in denial and blithely say, "I can do anything." A diabetic person may be so accustomed to insulin injections that he forgets to mention them. And clients who have controlled their asthma for years with medication may not feel it is important to discuss. Sometimes I don't identify a special need until I read the health history, talk with their health-care professional or dialogue extensively with the client.

When something is out of the ordinary, I identify it as a "red flag." Red flags generally need some kind of attention or follow-up that is beyond your expertise. It could also signify an area where you simply need more information to create the best, and safest, program for your client.

Quick Index:

Chapter 2, sample health-history questionnaires

Can I Work With This Person?

Most of the time, the answer to this question is "yes!" It is remarkable how closely an obese client's program may parallel that of a cardiac patient, a postpartum mom or a diabetic. Though any special-need program has significant modifications that make it unique, specific and safe, educated professionals who "speak the language" can easily follow most changes. After all, these modifications deal with frequency, intensity, duration and mode—the same elements that are juggled for any exercise session.

For a cardiac rehab client, the physician may say that the person is "out of immediate danger," but his heart rate should never go above 135 unless the doctor prescribes a new training prescription based on your client's progression. For a type II diabetic, the instruction may be to monitor blood-glucose level (easily done with a glucose testing strip or kit) and keep candy or fruit juice around in case of hypoglycemia. For a client with multiple sclerosis, the health care provider may warn you about heat buildup or intolerance that could exacerbate existing symptoms and recommend intermittent exercise or water workouts.

Whenever possible, develop an ongoing line of communication with the health-care professional to help monitor changes in the client's needs. If you combine this dialogue, your education, common sense and the client's practical experience and apply it to the situation, you should be able to contribute effectively to a higher-risk person's health program.

> If you have the slightest doubt about your ability to meet the client's needs safely and effectively, it shows greater intelligence and a higher level of sophistication to refer the client to another trainer who is qualified.

Expand Your Area of Professional Capability

Realize that you are *not* the expert in most high-risk situations. None of us can know everything about all specialty areas, but you can "grow into" them. Where do you get information on special conditions?

Self-study and Continuing Education. I have found that "life's events" tend to introduce us to high-risk or special-need situations rather magically. Since I have 2 young sons, over the years I have become extremely interested in pregnancy and exercise, as well as youth fitness. Through my personal training business I have been introduced to diabetics, asthmatics, obese and cardiac patients.

Whenever I encounter a special need, I seek information related to it with limitless enthusiasm and an open mind. Over several years I have become well versed and comfortable with the topics just mentioned. Obviously, I have grown into and expanded my area of professional capability over time.

When I work with clients who have perinatal concerns, I often get a comment that is quite revealing. Many of my female clients have commented along the lines, "It's amazing how much you know and are comfortable talking about the anatomy of a pregnant female body. You really seem to empathize with the joys, discomfort and physical changes that have occurred during my pregnancy." I believe it is refreshing, a confidence-builder and encouraging to the client and her obstetrician to know they have found an allied professional who "knows her situation." This is another instance of doing your homework. (And, it helps having a family of my own!)

Build a library. To ensure that you have current and relevant information regarding specialty areas, create a filing system that contains articles, pamphlets and other information. I begin with broad topic areas like asthma, diabetes, cardiac rehabilitation, aging, physically challenged and pregnancy, and then subdivide them into more specialized categories within each topic, as the files grow. Oftentimes, I don't even read the articles as I file them, but I anticipate needing them one day in the future. That way, when the situation arises, I have current information at my fingertips.

The Client. You will learn some of your most valuable and practical information from your client. This person undoubtedly has become an expert concerning his own situation. For example, a diabetic knows when to take an insulin injection and can probably educate you about any warning signals pertaining to hypoglycemia.

Health-Care Professional. Most physicians, chiropractors, physical therapists and other health-care professionals who treat your clients expect you to have a baseline understanding of their patients' situation. In fact, many might ask you how *you* would go about planning a program of exercise with their patients.

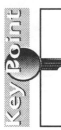

Be thorough! The efficacy of your programming and client's safety is, ultimately, still *your* responsibility.

Some clients and their doctors simply want a trainer who knows exercise principles and can follow their exact guidelines and modifications. Even in this situation, I think it is preferable to be well versed in the condition. If you have any questions or concerns with the prescribed approach, it is important to discuss them privately and in a professional manner with the doctor. Your knowledge creates confidence and excitement in the person with whom you will be working, as well as your client's health team.

Tips for Working With Health-Care Providers

When you first contact an attending health-care professional, it is important to establish credibility and professionalism. If you do this successfully and handle your special-need clients well, this professional could become an incredible source of clients to you in the future.

Because time is usually of the essence, a quick phone call is quite appropriate. Do not be intimidated when you call. Remember, you have the blessing and clout of a client who has given you permission to contact his specialist. Prepare your questions and concerns ahead of time so that you can cover crucial information quickly. Careful preparation facilitates minimum time investment by both parties, and maximizes the benefit to your client. It will gain you the physician's respect and encourage a productive relationship. Be thorough during this initial phone call. That way, you will cut out the need for frequent and often irritating calls to the specialist. Do not wear out your welcome.

Even though the physician is the expert and diagnostician, you need to be able to "speak the same language" and demonstrate an awareness of potential adjustments to your client's exercise and diet program. You may have to "dig" a bit for the information. Let's say your client has a history of high blood pressure. A physician might comment, "Oh, there's nothing to be currently concerned with—he can really do anything." Nonetheless, you may still want to ask for confirmation of a plan to strength train with high reps and low weight. It may remind the physician to mention another fact; for example, the client is taking a beta blocker to manage blood pressure and control heart rate.

If there is any problem gaining access to the specialist, enlist the help of your client. This works well because it is in the client's interest that you obtain the information you need, and in the doctor's interest to keep the patient/doctor relationship positive and intact. If you have difficulty reaching a health-care provider, never indicate that this person was "wrong" or "uncooperative." Focus only on your goal of obtaining the most pertinent information regarding your client's condition, so that you can better serve your client.

Follow your phone call with a letter of introduction and a resume or "presentation packet" to detail your credentials. Most professionals look for documentation of updated, formal university degrees and/or current industry certifications.

If appropriate, or if requested by your client or specialist, send the specialist occasional updates of progress. Regardless, document these changes and updates in your files.

Like almost every service business today, personal training has entered into a specialization phase. For you, as a personal trainer, this means that the more special-need clients that you can work with, such as cardiac rehabilitation patients, diabetics, asthmatics, the obese, the elderly, children/youth and the pregnant client, the more marketable you will be. Versatility and depth will be the hallmark of successful training businesses today and into the future.

The Bridge

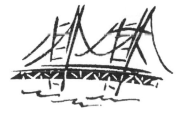

You can train clients with special needs if you have the appropriate training and knowledge, and if you unequivocally follow the licensed health-care professional's instructions. Educate yourself by researching each condition as you encounter it and speaking with the health-care provider. Proper care of a client with special needs can lead to regular referrals and a highly rewarding feeling of personal accomplishment.

References and Recommended Reading

American Council on Exercise (ACE) (1991). **Personal Trainer Manual.** *Published by ACE, San Diego, CA.*

American College of Sports Medicine (ACSM) (1991). **Guidelines for Exercise Testing and Prescription.** *4th edition, Lea and Febiger, Philadelphia, PA.*

Evans, William, and Rosenberg, Irwin (1991). **Biomarkers.** *Simon and Schuster, New York, NY.*

Gordon, Neil (1993). **Diabetes: Your Complete Exercise Guide.** *Human Kinetics Publishers, Champaign, IL.*

Gordon, Neil (1993). **Breathing Disorders: Your Complete Exercise Guide.** *Human Kinetics Publishers, Champaign, IL.*

Gordon, Neil (1993). **Arthritis: Your Complete Exercise Guide.** *Human Kinetics Publishers, Champaign, IL.*

Ornish, Dean et al. (1990). Can Lifestyle Changes Reverse Coronary Heart Disease?" **The Lancet,** *336, pps. 129-133.*

Sherman, Carl (1994). Reversing Heart Disease: Are Lifestyle Changes Enough? **The Physician And Sportsmedicine,** *Vol. 22, No. 1, January, pps. 91-94.*

Spirduso, Waneen (1995). **Physical Dimensions of Aging.** *Human Kinetics Publishers, Champaign, IL.*

Wichmann, Susan, and Martin, D.R. (1992). Heart Disease: Not For Men Only. **The Physician And Sports Medicine,** *Vol. 20, No. 8, August, pps. 138-48.*

A "presentation packet" is detailed in Going Solo... The Art of Personal Training, *by Douglas Brooks, 1990, Moves International (619) 934-0312.*

CHAPTER 19

GUIDING CLIENTS TOWARD HEALTHY EATING HABITS

Clients are constantly asking questions. Does the latest nutritional aid work? What about that new weight-loss system advertised on television? What's the food pyramid? How can I count fat grams? How much should I eat? These questions are fueled by inaccurate and sensationalized reporting by the media. For instance, recent headlines have suggested "pasta makes you fat," and "a low-fat diet may be harmful to your health." Of course, my clients want my opinion on the latest "controversy." And, as you and I know, there really is no controversy, only confusion, contradiction and inaccurate media messages.

A personal trainer is not a substitute for a registered dietitian (R.D.) or other licensed and/or degreed nutrition expert. However, as a personal trainer you will be asked many nutritional questions by your clients and you should be able to give them accurate, general nutritional guidelines.

Though your main concern may be healthy eating habits, your clients may be coming to you for an answer to the million-dollar question, "What's the best way to lose weight and keep it off?" Of course, the answer is a sensible and realistic approach that incorporates exercise and a low-fat approach to eating. That message alone may be an ongoing challenge to communicate. But you have an even more important message to send. Your client needs to realize that losing weight in the pursuit of *perfection* will end in failure. The "perfect body" does not exist, although a personal body image that your client *can* be comfortable with, surely does. Perfection is only an illusion that the *mind* grasps for in futility—and never reaches. Set your clients up for success and don't play the weight-loss yo-yo game! Communicating this message is as much a part of each client's overall health picture as interpreting blood cholesterol levels, recognizing risk factors for heart disease and working out.

The Weight Loss Game

All of your clients know that poor eating habits can lead to poor health. High cholesterol, high LDLs (the "bad" cholesterol), heart disease, diabetes, poor self-image and low energy are a few of the potential outcomes for your clients who may not be getting enough exercise, and/or consuming too many calories, cholesterol and fat from poor food selections. Yet, we are fatter than ever as a society, and one out of 3 American adults is overweight (*Nutrition Action Health Letter*, May 1995).

Our culture promotes a sedentary way of life with little physical activity, indulgent eating and the hope for a quick fix for our overweight problems that does not require much thought or personal time investment. Does that last point sound too good to be true? Of course it is, and the billions of dollars that are spent each year for weight-loss schemes and nutritional supplements reflects this futile approach. Michael Jacobson, Ph.D., (*Nutrition Action Health Letter*, May 1995) suggests that the cure for our obesity problem lies in creating a network of bike paths and jogging trails, cities and neighborhoods that are designed for walking and biking, schools that encourage and develop a lifelong love of physical activity, restaurants that disclose calories on their menus and activities that are fun and do-able, so that kids and adults will turn off the television, get out of the easy chair and "into the streets."

I believe what Dr. Jacobson is talking about is a societal behavior and attitude change. It is time to ask our clients for a personal investment and commitment of time and attention with regard to healthy eating habits. It is appropriate that you lead by example, and in turn, ask your clients to influence their family and friends by strong example.

At the forefront of that quick-fix mentality is the word "diet." To me, a diet is usually associated with severe calorie restriction, deprivation or some other extreme, unscientific approach. There is the *Why Women Need Chocolate* diet, the *Zone Favorable High-Fat* diet, *Carbohydrate Addict's* diet, the *Fit for Life* diet, the *Eat Smart, Think Smart* diet, *Eat 'till You Puke and Still Lose Weight* diet, and dozens more. According to Kelly Brownell, director of the Center for Eating and Weight Disorders at Yale University, all of these diets have equally compelling testimonials from "pseudo experts" who think, or want you to believe, that they have something new.

But, not all diets are bad. You and your clients have been hearing for years about a "low-fat diet." The premise is that by cutting down the fat in your diet and replacing it with healthier choices, you can easily and automatically cut calories. Quite a few researchers believe that it doesn't matter *what* you eat as long as you cut total calories. Fat has over twice the calories per gram as carbohydrate or protein, so you can eat the same or larger *amount* of food with food selections that limit fat intake, and still take in fewer calories.

When you answer client questions by offering sensible eating guidelines, ideas for low-fat eating should be intermingled with every suggestion. That is the basis of a healthy diet.

Help Clients Learn How to Eat Healthfully

Empower Your Clients. Confidence, support and a realistic approach are the key ingredients to healthy eating habits and weight control. Many of the empowerment tools discussed in this chapter, such as label reading and the food pyramid, will strengthen your client's ability to eat healthfully and lose weight. Additionally, stress the theme of moderation. Reinforce there is no need to be obsessed with weight control, which is ultimately counterproductive. Keep the focus on health. Help your clients learn to know and like themselves better, and be easier on themselves. Encourage them to be more compassionate and patient with *their* progress and effort.

Phase in Behavior Change. Your clients don't have to immediately—or for that matter ever—go from fat to thin. Their health can be greatly impacted with small changes. Total cholesterol, LDL cholesterol and triglycerides significantly drop—and HDL cholesterol significantly rises—every time your client drops 5 pounds. In one study, 60% of people with high blood pressure were able to discontinue their blood pressure medication after losing 10 pounds. And, over-weight diabetics who lost at least 15 pounds over a year lowered their blood sugar levels by 15%, without medication. Those who lost 30 pounds reduced their blood sugar by more than 40% *even though they remained overweight* (reported in *Nutrition Action Health Letter*, May 1995).

Transition to Healthy Food Choices. Evolving to healthier eating is very rewarding. How-ever, remind your clients that tastes are learned. Although some experts would argue that it's easier to make a complete change to a more wholesome diet—vegetables, grains, fruits and legumes diet—I believe a moderate approach will work well with most of your clients. For example, replace high-fat dairy products with low-fat options before proceeding to nonfat sources. Another progression might be to eat meat less often and purchase cuts that are lowest in fat rather than completely eliminating it from the diet.

Increase Formal Exercise and/or Activity Habits. The best kept secret regarding weight loss is regular activity, of any kind. Your clients are lucky to have you to guide them while they identify activities they can enjoy for a lifetime. Also, research indicates that people who exercise regularly usually start eating more healthfully.

Encourage Healthful Eating Habits. Your clients should, for example, drink copious amounts of fluids and eat lots of fruits, vegetables, legumes and grains—instead of fat-free cakes and cookies loaded with "fake fat" and sugar. Reduce the intake of refined carbohydrates, that in-clude white flour, white sugar and white rice to name a few, by choosing whole-grain products and natural sweeteners such as fruits, juices and syrup. Reduce red meat, poultry and fish. Limit hydrogenated oils or trans fat (be sure to read labels). They raise blood cholesterol as much as saturated fat (*Nutrition Action Healthletter*, September 1996). Gradually reduce both butter and margarine in their diet. Switch to nonfat or low-fat versions of prepared foods and dairy products.

Teach Accurate Calorie Needs. Though your clients should not be obsessed with an inflex-ible approach to calorie counting, they need to have some sense of portion control and total daily caloric intake. Both the food pyramid and reading labels can help your client get a feel for her daily caloric intake, without going overboard toward a rigid calorie-counting regimen. Also, your clients will quickly learn that not all single servings are the same. For example, an 8-ounce serving of nonfat milk carries with it about 90 calories, whereas an 8-ounce serving of whole milk contains about 150 calories.

Encourage Clients to Consume Calories Evenly Throughout the Day. When the typical diet is analyzed, most of the daily caloric intake is consumed at night. Today's social patterns en-courage a light or skipped breakfast, quick lunch and late dinner, with over-consumption at this evening meal. Calories may be best consumed throughout the day to optimize alertness, energy and the caloric needs required for basic metabolic maintenance and daily physical activity. Continually eating or grazing throughout the day may not be the best idea, but 3-5 solid meals and low-fat nutritional snacks, such as fruit, may work best.

How to Help With Weight Loss

Do Not Reduce Daily Caloric Intakes by More Than About 20%. Severe calorie restriction can not be maintained. And severe restriction ultimately leads to weight-loss maintenance failure in a majority of cases, commonly referred to as yo-yo dieting and weight cycling. Small reductions, done consistently over an extended period of time are tolerable and can lead to safe and permanent weight loss. On the other hand, don't interpret this message as one that discourages obese clients from attempting to lose weight because of concerns about the hazards of weight cycling. The National Institutes of Health (1994) say, "Obese individuals should not allow concerns about the hazards of weight cycling to deter them from efforts to control their body weight."

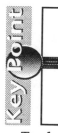

This is strong support for continued attempts at weight loss, even if the weight is regained. Even small amounts of weight loss can positively impact health.

Teach Correct Food Portion Size by Using a Food Scale. I often use a food scale with my clients to drive home the important issue of portion control. It is not a shock to me that a majority of my clients vastly *underestimate* the amount of food they eat. (Do realize that for some of your clients who border on under-eating, too small portions can also jeopardize their health and weight management goals.) For example, many of my clients thought an acceptable serving from the fish, poultry or meat group was anything set in front of them. Obviously, a 16-ounce steak is over 5 times the recommended 3-ounce serving! I have asked clients to pour 3-4 ounces of cereal (3-4 servings) in a bowl, and to their amazement the scale reveals anywhere from 6-8 ounces.

By using the food scale with your clients, they can quickly learn to accurately judge serving sizes. The visual image of, for example, what an ounce of cereal actually *looks* like is a very powerful teaching tool. This approach has helped many of my clients who have struggled, not so much with poor food choices, but with simply consuming too much food. My clients jokingly refer to this syndrome as, "Too much of a good thing."

Reverse Small Weight Gains Immediately. Any of your clients who struggle with losing weight know that the difficult aspect is not initially losing weight, but keeping it off. The key to keeping weight off for a group of 160 men and women who have successfully kept off an average of 63 pounds for 3 years is to immediately reverse gains of 3-5 pounds [Fletcher, Anne

(1994) *Thin for Life: 10 Keys to Success From People Who Have Lost Weight and Kept It Off*, Chapters Publishing: Shelbourne, VT, as reported in *Nutrition Action Health Letter*, May 1996].

Offer Suggestions for Changes in Daily Habits. Here's a list of suggestions you can give clients:

• Read food labels consistently and carefully. Make sure the serving size listed on the label is in line with the food pyramid recommendations. (The food pyramid and label reading is discussed later in this chapter.)

• Order all toppings and salad dressings on the side. This allows you to control the amount you use. Ask for light, low or nonfat options. If low-fat options are not available, dressings and toppings can be mixed with vinegar and lemon juice, too.

• Reduce the use of cooking oils and oil-based salad dressings. Using Dijon mustard and nonfat plain yogurt is a great substitute for an oil-based salad dressing.

• Limit your intake of baked goods that are high in fat. Cookie, pie and doughnut calories are often at least 50% fat.

• Replace mayonnaise or butter on your sandwiches with mustard. Eat bread plain.

• Instead of using margarine, butter or regular sour cream on your baked potato, use non-fat yogurt or nonfat sour cream.

• Instead of frying food, bake, boil or poach.

• Sauté food in a low-fat broth or small amount of olive oil. Avoid using solid fats.

• Use low or nonfat yogurt and cottage cheese, and either skim (nonfat) or 1% fat milk.

• Purchase lean cuts of meat and trim any visible fat.

• Buy chicken and turkey without the skin or remove the skin before eating.

• Buy ground beef only if it is labeled as 96% fat-free. Don't be fooled by "extra-lean ground beef."

• For dessert, try sorbet, sherbet, nonfat or low-fat frozen yogurt and fresh fruit.

• Add water or seltzer to dilute juices and cut calories. Recognize that juices are a food and can add significant calories to your total daily intake.

• When eating out, in general, order vegetarian, seafood or poultry dishes instead of beef or pork. Order side dishes that are filling yet low in fat, such as rice. Don't forget that alcoholic beverages count about the same as fat calories. In movie theaters request air-popped popcorn.

Personal Reality Check—Let's Get Honest! Randy Eichner calls self-delusion the "most popular indoor sport" (*Sports Medicine Digest*, December 1993). What he's getting at is that most of us overestimate how much we exercise and underestimate how much we eat. While weight maintenance and weight loss are very complex, part of the reason that some obese people can't lose weight, according to Dr. Eichner, is because of self-delusion. He refers to a sophisticated study in the *New England Journal of Medicine* (1992; 327:1893-8) that reports in the failed diet group, subjects ate 1,000 calories more than they recorded in their diaries and burned 250 fewer calories than their exercise records indicated. Interestingly, this same pattern is seen in young, old, fat or slim people. Four out of 5 people believe that they eat less and exercise more than they actually do (Eichner, 1993). Regardless of your goal, results depend on what you do, not what you *believe* you are doing.

How to Read the New Food Labels

Though the new food labels are not as useful and easy to understand as they could be, they still can help your clients assess the food they are buying. The new labels can help your clients be more aware of fat intake, quickly see food portion or serving size and identify what kinds of nutrients are present in the serving. Following is a description of the elements of a label.

The New Food Label

Serving size (#1). While this may seem mundane, serving size helps with realistic estimates of total caloric intake and keeping track of the number of servings of a particular food group. A food scale is an effective teaching tool to learn serving size. Actually seeing a serving size on a scale will help your client understand and observe, for example, what a one-ounce serving looks like. This will help your client accurately estimate appropriate portion or serving sizes.

The **percent daily value (#2)** column tells you how much of the day's worth of fat, cholesterol, sodium, carbohydrates, dietary fiber and sugars the food provides. If a food contains 20% or more of the daily value, whether fat or carbohydrate, it could be considered "high" in that nutrient. "Low" is probably no more than 5%.

Saturated fat (#3). This particular percentage of the daily value is important to

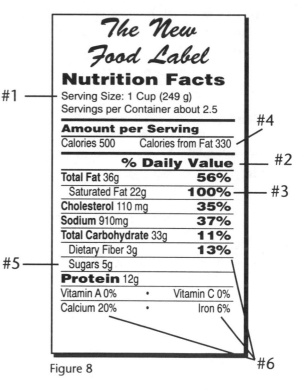

Figure 8

note because this nutrient probably causes the most damage to your client's health. (Unfortunately, trans fat or hydrogenated oil, which is just as damaging, is not reported.)

Calories from fat (#4) help your client quickly see how much fat is in each serving of this particular food. In this example, 330 calories of each 500-calorie serving is from fat. If you divide 330 by 550, you can calculate that 60% of each serving is fat! Many experts recommend a daily fat intake of no more than 20% of total daily calories. This does not mean that you shouldn't eat this food, because it's only *part* of your total daily calories, but it must be balanced with the overall daily intake.

The FDA has not set a daily value for **sugar (#5)** because health experts have not yet set a limit on how much should be eaten on a daily basis. Furthermore, this number is not very accurate because it does not contain all types of sugars. Limit intake of simple sugars whenever possible.

The **percent daily values (#6)** are based on a daily intake of 2,000 calories. This is very interesting because it allows you to compare the **percentage** daily value for healthier nutrients (vitamins A and C, minerals calcium and iron, and dietary fiber) against fat, sodium and cholesterol.

The information on food labels can be used to improve food selection and overall health. The typical diet is high in sodium, cholesterol, saturated fat and total calories. It is well documented that this type of diet greatly increases the risk of heart disease, stroke, diabetes and some cancers. An aggressive recommendation (for optimal health) is to keep fat intake below 20% of daily total caloric intake. Based on a 2,000-calorie diet, that's about 40-50 grams of fat per day. I have found that many of my clients find it easier to focus solely on fat gram intake versus the myriad of other diet variables. Daily sodium intake should be kept below 2,000 mg.

Quick Index:
Chapter 3, blood lipid profiles and saturated fat
Chapter 20, for intake of vitamins and minerals

How to Use the Food Pyramid

Did you know there is more than one food pyramid model to choose from? The 2 that I am going to discuss can help you teach your clients to moderate their eating and choose better foods. Both are similar and practical to implement in your client's busy life.

The USDA (United States Department of Agriculture) finally replaced its "Basic 4" chart first introduced in the 1950s. The USDA's new nutritional educational tool is the food pyramid. It has been received with mixed reviews by nutrition experts, but certainly is a helpful improvement when compared to earlier models. One weakness of the USDA pyramid is that it does not make a distinction among foods within groups. For example, extremely healthful legumes are in the same high-protein category as bacon.

Another approach that builds on the "power of the pyramid" is the Center for Science in the Public Interest (CSPI) healthy-eating pyramid. CSPI, the publisher of *Nutrition Action Health Letter*, uses a 3-D design that allows for 3 times the detail of other pyramids. It classifies foods into groups and tells you what foods within the group are best eaten "anytime," "sometimes" or "seldom." For example, a potato and fruit fit into the "anytime" category whereas french fries and avocado are placed in the "sometimes" category. This is a strong message that suggests how food is prepared (french fries) can greatly determine how healthy it may or may not be for your client. And, although foods may technically be lumped in the same healthy food groups, some (i.e., avocado) may not actually be that good for you. The CSPI pyramid emphasizes plant-based protein sources, for example nuts and legumes, over animal-based products. This is exemplified by positioning beans in a higher priority group with vegetables and fruits.

Both the USDA and CSPI models specify number of servings in each food group and offer examples of serving sizes.

One of the most important aspects of the pyramid is its focus on food portions. This shows a shift away from concerns of undernourishment and a growing awareness that the real risk is dietary excess, especially concerning too much simple sugar and fat.

When using the pyramids, the practical solution is to focus on the pyramids' similarities rather than their differences. The pyramids tell you: eat more whole grain products, fruits and vegetables, and avoid fats and excessive sweets. Both also emphasize portion control and dietary variety.

The USDA Food Pyramid

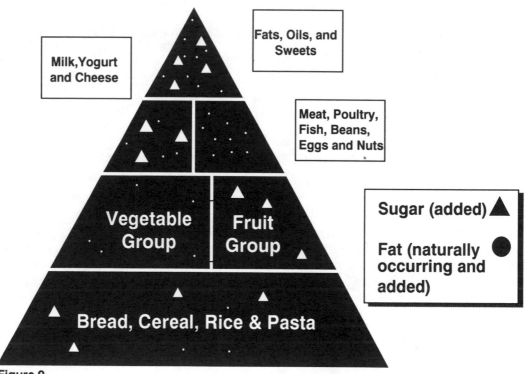

Figure 9

The best place to start, for healthy eating, is at the base of the food pyramid.

Bread, cereal, rice and pasta food group, 6-11 servings per day. Examples of one serving include one slice of bread, one-ounce of breakfast cereal, one-half cup of cooked pasta, rice or cereal and 4 crackers.

Vegetable group, 3-5 servings a day and fruit group, 2-4 servings. Serving size examples include one-half cup of raw or cooked broccoli or other vegetables, one cup of leafy raw vegetables, three-quarters of a cup of vegetable juice, one piece of medium-sized fruit such as an apple, banana or orange, one-half cup of chopped, cooked or canned fruit, one cup of strawberries or grapes, 6-ounces of fruit juice and one-quarter cup of dried fruit.

Milk, yogurt and cheese group, 2-3 servings a day and meat, poultry, fish, beans, eggs and nuts food group, 2-3 servings a day. Choose nonfat or low-fat servings. Serving sizes include one cup or 8-ounces of milk, one cup of yogurt, 1 cup of cottage cheese, one and one-half to 2-

ounces of cheese, 3-ounces of fish, meat or poultry, 2 tablespoons of nuts, one egg and one-half cup of beans.

Lastly, the USDA Food Pyramid tells you to use fats, oils and sweets sparingly. There are no recommended number of daily servings for these categories.

Share the Big Picture of Health and Well-Being With Your Clients

Some of your clients may set themselves up for failure by trying to be perfect, all of the time. Many times they may approach health-related issues, such as food choices, with an all-or-none attitude. For example, they may feel they have to follow the food pyramid, low-fat and eating portion recommendations 100% of the time—to perfection—or they "may as well toss in the towel."

Whether it's exercise or eating habits, it's the *perfect* setup for personal failure. Eating should not be approached from the fringe of extreme choices. Let your clients know that perfection is *not* normal. Many distractions, in the form of travel, job and family may come up on a daily basis. That's why you need a flexible approach that encourages consistency, not perfection.

In *Get Real: A Personal Guide to Real-Life Weight Management*, (IDEA Press, 1995, San Diego, CA) Dr. Daniel Kosich discusses what he calls "the 80/20 rule." Follow an eating and exercise plan 80% of the time, and don't worry if you slip 20% of the time. The 80/20 rule reminds me of my antiquated 90/10 principle. That is, 90% of the time I used to make the "right" and healthy choices, and 10% of the time I wouldn't.

Over the years I have realized that my clients, as well as I, need to bend the 90/10 principle more if an approach to healthier eating is going to work in a real-life, practical sense. With the addition of 2 young sons, my personal 90/10 principle has eroded to 80/20 or 70/30 on occasion. Funny how a family can impact your eating habits. However, you can still eat healthfully by eating "right" *most* of the time. Both of my children, my wife, my clients and your clients need some operating room to enjoy eating and to be successful!

The Bridge

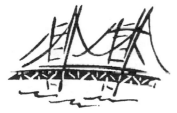

When clients ask you questions about eating, you should be able to give them reasonable guidelines and dispel myths. You should refer specific diet concerns that are beyond your expertise. However, by teaching clients about the new food pyramid and how to read labels, you can help them move toward sensible eating and weight control goals. Offer suggestions for low-fat eating, and constantly reinforce a reasonable, non-obsessive approach to nutrition.

CHAPTER 20

RATIONALE FOR RESPONSIBLE NUTRITIONAL SUPPLEMENTATION

With Kendra Gibson, R.D.

The purpose of this rationale is to provide evidence and documentation supporting the safety and potential benefits of nutritional supplementation. Responsible nutritional supplementation is in conflict with a standard nutritional approach that usually ends with the cliché recommendation that "adequate nutrition can be obtained through your diet." While science has not been able to prove all the benefits attributed to a generous intake of nutrients, sufficient evidence supports the use of dietary supplements.

For example, Michael Jacobson, Ph.D., executive director of Center for Science in the Public Interest, in May 1992 stated, "I believe there is now sufficient evidence to warrant people taking supplements, some at many times the USRDA, *on top of an excellent diet*. But, don't count (only) on pills to reverse the effects of a quiche-and-candy diet."

Why do standard nutritional guidelines often ignore or recommend against supplementation? Marmot (1986) observed that opposing views on public health issues arise "as much from ideological or political belief as from scientific judgment." It is hard to influence tradition, even in light of convincing scientific evidence. In the area of nutritional supplementation, this certainly holds true. Marmot concludes that "the argument that we should wait for certainty is an argument for never taking action—we shall never be certain."

Top scientists and health experts have taken the lead in proclaiming the necessity for responsible supplementation. Proponents include: Kenneth Cooper, M.D., president and founder of the Cooper Aerobics Center in Dallas, Texas; John Erdmand, Ph.D., director of the division of nutritional sciences at the University of Illinois; Simin Meydani, D.V.M., Ph.D., chief of the nutritional immunology laboratory at the Human Nutrition Research Center on Aging at Tufts University in Massachusetts; William Castelli, M.D., director of the Framingham Heart Study, Framingham, Massachusetts; Jeffrey Blumberg, Ph.D., professor of nutrition at Tufts University; Walter Willett, M.D., professor of epidemiology and nutrition at Harvard School of Public Health, Boston; Matthew P. Longnecker, M.D., assistant professor of epidemiology, UCLA School of Public Health, Los Angeles; and Bruce Ames, Ph.D., director of the National Institute of Environmental Health Sciences Center at the University of California at Berkeley.

In light of the current scientific evidence, the appropriate use of nutritional supplements can and probably should be included in a balanced approach to *optimize* personal fitness and health. This means that personal trainers should become knowledgeable and enlightened so that an appropriate stance with regard to nutritional supplementation can be confidently assumed.

The consumer is confused by the often-quoted opinion of many professionals in the fitness industry that nutritional supplementation is a complete waste of time and money. I am afraid a credibility gap has been created between what the average consumer believes and what scientific literature supports versus the position of many health professionals who may have never studied nutrition or may not have updated themselves with regard to new research.

If you do not guide and counsel your clients, they will try to figure out the nutritional equation for themselves. The Food and Drug Administration estimates that 40% of the United States public uses nutritional supplements. If you choose not to help them and quote cliché, your clients will probably not listen to this rhetoric, and will take it upon themselves to create optimal nutritional intake. You would be more powerful working as a team!

Fitness professionals have a responsibility to promote public health through improved nutrition. There are many population groups (including asymptomatic, apparently healthy people) that may need supplements. Other groups that need special attention include women of child-bearing age, women who are pregnant or breast feeding, people who are inactive or who do not eat very much, as well as people who are older and taking medications that may interfere with nutrient absorption. Furthermore, recent evidence suggests that if a high-level intake of protective antioxidants is to be achieved, food intake alone can not satisfy this goal.

Rather than recommending against supplement use because of the remote chance that the public may go overboard in its enthusiasm—if some is good, more is better—it seems preferable to inform the public clearly about the range of safe intake of supplements and about the levels of nutrient intake which have been shown to be protective. Nutritional supplements can and should be an integral part of both a healthy diet and a healthy lifestyle.

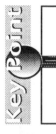

It is professionally *irresponsible* to ignore your role in providing guidance to your clientele in the area of nutritional supplementation. It is this important role of honest and ethical guidance that you, the fitness professional, must take.

Evaluating Products and Needs

For busy personal trainers, the task of assimilating nutritional information is not easy. Most trainers do not have the time or expertise to interpret the rapidly changing literature. Currently, at best, guidelines are confusing, contradictory and vague. The following analysis of vitamins and minerals resulted from an evaluation I did on one multi-vitamin and mineral supplement. I couldn't find a single source that clearly presented the information that I needed, and my clients were requesting information about supplementation that they had read about or watched on television. Out of desperation, I did a literature review.

I spent many hours focusing on toxicity levels, and analyzed recommendations that were in excess of the recommended daily or dietary allowances (RDA). From this research I was able to formulate responsible recommendations for my clients for proper amounts of minerals and vitamins.

I hope this research begins to help you sort through the maze of information. My clients' interest stimulated me to become involved and informed, so that I could assist them with intelligent and safe choices. I encourage you to let nutritional experts know that we need their help in formulating responsible nutritional recommendations! Fitness professionals need a source of reliable information that is easy to access and regularly updated.

Generally, vitamin and mineral supplements act as nutritional insurance for clients. Some of your clients do not choose the right foods or do not consume enough calories from their daily diet. Vitamin and mineral supplements can work as a nutritional catalyst by enhancing the energy and recovery processes in the body. Furthermore, many scientific studies indicate that supplements may provide a degree of nutritional insurance against the ravages of free radicals.

Free radicals cause oxidative damage within the body that results in injured, altered and killed cells. Environmental hazards such as pollutants, smoke, automobile fumes and the everyday oxidative (energy) processes in the body can lead to oxidative damage. Research has also directly implicated free radicals in the development of cancer, heart disease (atherosclerosis), emphysema, rheumatoid arthritis, Parkinson's disease and the aging process.

Supplements are often formulated with a protective antioxidant system. This may include vitamin C, vitamin E, and beta carotene for potentially neutralizing free radicals. The USDA Research Center on Aging and the National Cancer Institute have reported evidence indicating these 3 vitamins may help reduce risks of developing diseases such as cataracts, cancer and heart disease. Many products contain "energy activators" that theoretically facilitate energy production in the body.

How to Take Supplements

As a nutritional supplement, vitamin caplets (or some other form, such as liquid) should probably be taken to complement the active part of any client's day, which often means taking them with the morning meal. Food consumption with supplementation generally increases the absorption of the nutrients because there are other "factors and nutrients" within food that enhance this process. Plenty of fluids should be taken at meal time and throughout the day. Most important, however, is to encourage a time that allows your client to be compliant with their supplementation.

Many supplements are formulated to enhance the sleep cycle. That is why some supplements involve taking tablets in both the morning (vitamins) and evening (minerals). One set enhances daily activities, while the other enhances the recuperative effects of the body during sleep. Sleep is known to be essential to recovery and well-being. Sleep and proper nutrition are very important because of their positive effect on the body's building processes related to bone and lean-tissue development, and cellular formation. The mineral design or formulation is often what helps to rebuild or maintain the skeletal system.

Most nutritional experts who advocate nutritional supplementation for *optimal health* state that it is very difficult to derive sufficient nutritional needs from a one-per-day tablet. Simply, there is not enough physical space in one tablet to allow for the necessary amounts of nutrients to facilitate preventive and optimal nutrition.

A month's supply of most supplements includes a 30-day (or greater) supply of caplets at a cost between 20 cents and one dollar or more per day. To some degree, the old saying "you get what you pay for" holds true. However, more is not always better in terms of cost. Justify what you are paying for by making sure the nutrients complement your client's nutritional needs.

Formulation

The margin of safety (toxicity level) for most vitamins and minerals is substantial when responsible manufacturing practices and product formulation are maintained. The formulation of any products you recommend should be in line with state-of-the-art manufacturing guidelines and current dosage parameters for safe administration of vitamins and minerals. One sign of responsible manufacturing is a company's policy of voluntarily adapting the standards of the Council for Responsible Nutrition (CRN) and the U.S. Pharmacopoeia. CRN recently issued guidelines for correcting potential safety problems surrounding vitamin A, vitamin B-6 (pyridoxine), niacin, chromium and iron intakes. These adjustments to product formulation based on new, accumulated and ever-changing research must be implemented, regardless of cost, by responsible manufacturers.

Many vitamin and mineral supplements are processed with nutrients that manufacturers claim may make the ingredients more "cell friendly" or more likely to be used by the body. **Bio-potentiation** and **chelation** are examples of manufacturing processes that are used to *theoretically* increase the cell's ability to use a particular vitamin or mineral. The formulation of "bio-friendly" nutrients is claimed by manufacturers to be an important reason why certain (their) products have been associated with such "outstanding personal results." Peer-reviewed research is mixed on this claim.

Possibly more important, in terms of cellular absorption and use, is a fast disintegration and dissolution of the product once it enters the stomach. Nutrients that dissolve in the stomach in less than 30 minutes are more likely to be absorbed by the body (U.S. Pharmacopoeia standards). Place tablets in a weak solution of vinegar water to test. They should dissolve in about 30 minutes.

"**Cold processing**" is an example of a manufacturing method that may preserve the integrity of the nutrients, especially botanicals. Heat, sonic or over drying techniques may negatively affect nutrient quality.

Look for products that contain no soy, egg, yeast, sugar, wheat, gluten, artificial coloring or preservatives.

Multi-Vitamin and Mineral Nutritional Analysis

The following is a breakdown of the ingredients in one brand of a multi-vitamin and mineral supplement. The user is instructed to take 3 of the multi-vitamin caplets with a morning meal and 3 of the mineral caplets with an evening meal.

Beta Carotene (pro vitamin A). Each 3 multi-vitamin caplets contain 10,000 IU, which is 200% of the RDA. Over 20 human studies have described the beneficial effect of beta carotene in lowering the risk of lung cancer and cancers of the mouth, throat, stomach, bladder and rectum.

Several carotene pigments (i.e., beta carotene) found in food can be converted to vitamin A.

They are referred to as pro vitamin A. Recommended amounts for antioxidant protection range from 10,000-25,000 IU per day (*Berkeley Wellness Letter*, July 1994). When analyzing products, note that your client's normal diet and other products will provide additional sources of beta carotene.

Currently, 12 additional studies are in progress to evaluate the effectiveness of beta carotene supplements in the range of 15,000-25,000 IU. Theoretically your client could consume this amount of beta carotene through dietary food intake, but it would be difficult to do so consistently. In fact, research indicates that for most individuals, proper nutrition attained solely through diet is all but impossible.

Conversion of vitamin A is regulated so that excess vitamin A is not absorbed from carotene sources (Mahan, 1992). Because of this, carotenoids are not known to be toxic, even when ingested in very large amounts for extended periods of time. To benefit from antioxidant protection, the recommended range of intake is from 10,000-25,000 IU per day.

Vitamin A (palmitate). Each 3 multi-vitamin caplets of this product contain 5,000 IU, which is 100% of the RDA. Visual changes, skin dryness and increased infections are associated with vitamin A deficiencies (Haas, 1992).

Retinol is another name for *pre*formed vitamin A, so named because of its importance for vision. Several carotene pigments found in food can be converted to vitamin A in the body and are called *pro* vitamin A. Beta carotene is the most available and yields the highest amount of A. About 10,000-15,000 IU of beta carotene will probably yield about 5,000 IU of vitamin A in the body (Haas, 1992), though other research indicates far less vitamin A would be formed (*Committee on Dietary Allowances*, 1989, reported by Dickinson, 1991). The bioavailability of carotenoids (i.e., beta carotene) is uncertain because of variable absorption and conversion to vitamin A. Conversion of vitamin A is regulated in the body so that excess vitamin A is not absorbed from carotene sources (Mahan, 1992).

Dickinson (1991) and the Council for Responsible Nutrition, after extensive reviews, report an adequate safety margin for vitamin A (from retinol) at doses up to at least 10,000 IU. Prenatal supplements for vitamin A products should be limited to 5-8,000 IU from retinol. Any recommendations for special populations should be done in consultation with the person's heath-care professional.

Vitamin C (esterified or buffered). Each 3 multi-vitamin caplets contain 1,000 mg, which is 1,667% of the RDA. Though vitamin C will not prevent colds (*Nutrition Action Health Letter-CSPI*, November 1994), there is significant data that indicates a reduction in the severity of symptoms and duration of colds. Most intervention trials use about 1,000 mg or less. It's too early to tell regarding vitamin C's effect on raising good cholesterol, preventing LDL oxidation, lowering blood pressure, preventing cataracts, protecting against cancer and strengthening the immune system.

For an antioxidant effect, 250-500 mg of vitamin C is recommended (*Berkeley Wellness Letter*, July 1994). Daily intakes of 100-1,000 mg of vitamin C can deactivate free radicals within the blood stream, rendering them ineffective in contributing to cell damage.

Some research indicates that 500 mg per day can cause oxidant activity and interfere with the body's use of other nutrients, such as excessive absorption of iron and interference with copper absorption. However, the Select Committee on GRAS (Generally Recognized As Safe), 1979, stated that the findings of various studies that focused on concerns including oxalate excretion, renal tract stones, effects on the utilization of copper, iron and other metals, need for vitamin B-12, blood coagulation and reproductive performance *indicate that the tolerance to excessive amounts of absorbic acid (vitamin C) and its sodium salt is high.*

The Council for Responsible Nutrition (1990) reports an adequate safety margin for vitamin C in doses as high as 1,000 mg per day in adults. Some people may experience diarrhea when taking levels of 1,000 mg or even lower. People taking anticoagulant drugs should tell their doctors they are taking vitamin C. People with hemochromatosis, who can easily absorb toxic levels of iron (vitamin C improves absorption), should discuss vitamin C intake with their physicians. Taking C doesn't appear to promote kidney stones in people who aren't prone to getting them.

For most people (*CSPI*, November 1994), tissue saturation of vitamin C is reached with about 250-500 mg per day, according to Balz Frei of Boston University. However, since the body eliminates C in about 12 hours, taking an additional dose of about 500 mg after this time period will keep blood levels high throughout the day (*Berkeley Wellness Letter*, February 1995).

Vitamin C appears to be safe, even at doses of several thousand milligrams per day. The most common reaction is diarrhea, which occurs in 10% of study volunteers when they take anywhere from 500-2,000 mg at a time. If diarrhea is a problem, take smaller doses spread out over the course of the day.

B-Complex Vitamins. The essential nature of vitamin B in the diet was first observed in 1897, as it related to the prevention of beriberi. In 1911, scientists described this as an essential food factor they designated as vitamin B. Ten vitamin B factors have now been identified, thus their grouping under the term B-complex. The B-complex umbrella is based upon their similar source of distribution (i.e., food groups) and their functional interrelationships. An inadequate intake of one of the B vitamins may impair the utilization of other B vitamins.

Vitamin B-1 (thiamine mononitrate). Each 3 multi-vitamin caplets contain 25 mg, which is 1,667% of the RDA. Thiamine has essential roles in energy transformation (glycolysis) and membrane and nerve conduction. Although thiamine is needed for the metabolism of fats, proteins and nucleic acids, it is most strongly linked with carbohydrate metabolism. Thiamine needs may increase with physical activity.

There is no known toxicity level for thiamine (Mahan, 1992).

Vitamin B-2 (riboflavin). Each 3 multi-vitamin caplets contain 15 mg or 882% of the RDA. Riboflavin functions primarily as a component of two coenzymes (FAD and FMN) that are essential components of energy production via the respiratory chain. Some research indicates that riboflavin requirements increase with increased activity (Van der Beek et al. 1988). Requirements increase during pregnancy and lactation to meet the needs of increased tissue synthesis and to replace the riboflavin secreted in milk.

There is no known toxicity level for riboflavin (Mahan, 1992). The absorption of riboflavin is increased by the presence of food in the gastrointestinal tract, thus the importance of ingesting the nutrient with food (Mahan, 1992).

Niacin (niacinamide and nicotinic acid). Each 3 multi-vitamin caplets contain 50 mg of niacinamide, which is 250% of the RDA. Niacin is the generic term for nicotinamide (niacinamide) and nicotinic acid. Niacinamide is the preferred form of niacin, since it does not have the side effects seen with nicotinic acid. Niacin functions as a component of coenzymes (NAD and NADP) that are present in cells.

Niacinamide has no observed toxicity up to a range of 3,000-9,000 mg daily, whereas doses of *nicotinic acid* above 50 mg have produced flushing and itching of skin, as well as other symptoms. Liver damage has been reported in a few subjects taking 3,000 mg of nicotinic acid or 9,000 mg of niacinamide (Dickinson, 1991). The OTC (Over The Counter) Review Panel (1979) concludes that *nicotinic acid* produces side effects beginning with single 50-mg oral doses daily, whereas no untoward effects accompany intakes of *niacinamide* until 3,000-9,000 mg doses are reached.

The Council for Responsible Nutrition (reported by Dickinson, 1991) reports that research demonstrates the safety of niacin (in the form of niacinamide) at doses up to several hundred milligrams per day in adults. Little storage occurs in the body and any excess is eliminated through the urine.

Niacin (in the form of nicotinic acid) may cause side effects in some subjects at doses above 50 mg. Niacin (nicotinic acid) in pharmacologic doses of 3,000 mg per day or more lowers serum cholesterol in some people (Mahan, 1992). Niacin at these levels is considered a drug and should be administered by a physician who can monitor its effects with blood tests (*Berkeley Wellness Letter,* September 1994). Side effects include facial flushing as a result of vascular dilation and histamine release. The histamine release could be injurious to people with asthma or peptic ulcer disease.

CRN recommends cautionary labeling on niacin products in excess of 100 mg and advises consumers not to take more than 500 mg of niacin per day except under supervision of a physician. CRN also recommends the discontinued marketing of sustained-release niacin products pending development of a fuller understanding of their effects.

Vitamin B-6 (pyridoxine-HCL, pyridoxal and pyridoxamine). Each 3 multi-vitamin caplets contain 25 mg of vitamin B-6, which is 1,250% of the RDA. Derivatives of pyridoxine or vitamin B-6 are coenzymes that function primarily in transamination and other reactions related to protein metabolism. Another derivative is important for the formation of the precursor of heme in hemoglobin. Vitamin B-6 is essential for the metabolism of tryptophan and for the conversion of tryptophan to niacin. Research indicates that when the intake of folacin, B-6 and B-12 is low, the risk of heart disease increases and is associated with high homocysteine levels. These vitamins help convert homocysteine into amino acids the body can use. This may limit high levels of homocysteine in the blood and prevent atherosclerosis and blood-vessel damage (*Berkeley Wellness Letter,* March 1995).

CRN concludes, based on its review of research and various committee reports, that the safety of pyridoxine (vitamin B-6) in doses up to at least 200 mg is demonstrated. Massive doses (2,000-6,000 mg) have caused neuropathy or nerve damage.

Folate (folic acid or folacin). Each 3 multi-vitamin caplets contain 400 mcg of folic acid, which is 100% of the RDA. High folic acid intakes may prevent at least 2 types of cancer, colorectal cancer and cervical cancer (*Berkeley Wellness Report,* 1994), as well as neural tube defects during pregnancy.

Folacin is now recognized as a critical factor in preventing neural tube defects (*Berkeley Wellness Report,* 1994). This includes spina bifida (a defect in which the spinal cord is improperly encased in bone) and anencephaly (a fatal defect in which a major part of the brain never develops). However, it works only if taken 30 days before and 30 days after conception. A woman shouldn't wait until she knows she is pregnant to begin consuming high levels of folacin. The defects occur in the first 2 weeks of pregnancy, long before most women know conception has taken place (*Berkeley Wellness Report,* 1994). The evidence of folic acid for reducing the risk of neural-tube defects is so strong that the Food and Drug Administration (FDA) now allows the labels of folic acid containing supplement or foods to describe or "claim the health benefits" of folacin on birth defects (*CSPI*, December 1993).

Consuming more than 800 mcg of folacin daily is not advised. Many people get about 200 mcg from diet, though only about 50% may be absorbed. The RDA for pregnant women is 400 mcg. CRN concludes that the safety of folic acid is easily demonstrated by various reports and research. Because of the potential for masking the symptoms of B-12 deficiency, food-additive regulations limit the use of folate in nutritional supplements and other foods to 100 mcg for infants, 300 mcg for children, 400 mcg for adults and 800 mcg for pregnant women (Dickinson, 1991).

Vitamin B-12 (cobalamin concentrate). Each 3 multi-vitamin caplets contain 50 mcg of Vitamin B-12, which is 833% of the RDA. Vitamin B-12 is effective in the treatment of pernicious anemia. Pernicious anemia occurs when the stomach fails to secrete intrinsic factor, which is needed to absorb B-12. Vitamin B-12 is essential for normal red blood cell development, maintenance of nerve tissue and the formation of myelin. It is essential for normal function in the metabolism of all cells, especially for those of the gastrointestinal tract, bone marrow and nerve tissue.

It appears that vitamins B-12, B-6 and folic acid may play a complex but possibly key role in averting heart attacks. Research indicates that when the intake of folacin, B-6, and B-12 is low, the risk of heart disease increases and is associated with high homocysteine levels. These vitamins help convert homocysteine into amino acids the body can use. This may limit high levels of homocysteine in the blood and prevent atherosclerosis and blood vessel damage (*Berkeley Wellness Letter*, March 1995).

Though the body's store of this vitamin is substantial (Magan, 1992), B-12 deficiency is extremely common in apparently healthy older people, though it's not clear why (*American Journal of Clinical Nutrition*, 60: 2, 1994). Most of these individuals don't have pernicious anemia. It may be that the elderly population doesn't secrete enough acid and pepsin to liberate B-12 from food. Regardless of the cause, B-12 deficiency is dangerous, as it can irreversibly damage the nervous system. Part of the problem could be corrected by supplements.

No toxic effects are known for vitamin B-12 (Mahan, 1992). CRN corroborates this with a conclusion that no toxic effects of oral vitamin B-12 have been demonstrated in humans.

Pantothenic Acid (d-Cal pantothenate). Each 3 multi-vitamin caplets contain 50 mg of pantothenic acid, which is 500% of the RDA. Pantothenic acid's primary role is in cellular metabolism. Through coenzyme A, it is involved in the release of energy from carbohydrates and in the degradation and metabolism of fatty acids. It is involved in the synthesis of cholesterol, phospholipids, steroid hormones and porphyrin for hemoglobin.

No serious toxic effects of this substance are known. Some studies indicate that daily doses of 10-20 *grams* can result in occasional diarrhea and water retention (Dickinson, 1991).

Biotin. Each 3 multi-vitamin caplets contain 300 mcg of biotin, which is 100% of the RDA. Since biotin is the most expensive of the B vitamins, many supplements do not contain 100% of the RDA. Biotin is important in the synthesis of fat and glycogen (gluconeogenesis), oxidation of fat, amino acid metabolism and maintenance of nervous tissue. Biotin functions via biotin-dependent enzymes (Mahan, 1992). Biotin is closely related metabolically to folic acid, pantothenic acid and vitamin B-12.

There are known toxic effects from biotin (Mahan, 1992).

Vitamin E Complex. Each 3 multi-vitamin caplets contain 200 IU, which is 667% of the RDA. Adequate vitamin E supports cellular integrity, provides anti-aging protection, may be helpful in arthritic treatment and may lower the risk of heart disease. The Harvard Medical Group recently reported that vitamin E at levels greater than 100 IU could possibly lower the risk of cardiovascular disease by 40%. Vitamin E has been cited as a factor in reducing cancer, specifically cancers of the colon, rectum, esophagus and stomach. Vitamin E has been shown to reduce the risk of cataracts and boost the immune system.

This particular vitamin E complex is composed of d-Alpha Tocopheryl Acid Succinate and mixed Tocopherols Beta, Gamma and Delta. Vitamin E in its natural form of d-Alpha is the only vitamin that research contends is absorbed better than a synthetic derivative. Its inclusion in this formulation would serve to maximize absorption and utilization.

Antioxidant recommendation is 200-800 IU of vitamin E (*Berkeley Wellness Letter*, July 1994), whereas The National Academy of Sciences recommends 100-400 IU per day. The long-term effects of vitamin E supplementation are unknown. Compared with other fat-soluble vitamins, vitamin E is relatively nontoxic when taken by mouth (Dickinson, 1991). Doses over 400 IU per day have been shown to accelerate "rectinitis pigmentosa," a condition that can potentially lead to blindness in individuals who are *predisposed* to this risk via genetic inheritance. The Council for Responsible Nutrition report demonstrates the safety of vitamin E intake in adults at several hundred IU per day (Dickinson, 1991).

Branched-Chain Amino Acids. The amino acids **valine, isoleucine and leucine** are characterized as branched-chain amino acids. They are indispensable, or essential amino acids, because the body synthesis of these is inadequate to meet metabolic demands. Each 3 multi-vitamin caplets contain 50 mg of valine, isoleucine and leucine. No nutritional requirements have been established. Amino acids are organic compounds that function as the building blocks of protein. They are important in tissue synthesis and other special metabolic functions.

Data derived from studies of lysine, leucine, valine and threonine have suggested that requirements for these essential amino acids may be 2-3 times higher than those previously established (Young and Bier, 1987, as reported in Mahan, 1992).

With regard to other amino acids, there is no established USRDA for these nutrients. Estimates of amino acid requirements are available. Depending on the amino acid and individual requirements, adults require a certain number of milligrams per kilogram of body weight per day (Mahan, 1992). Amino acids methionine, cysteine and taurine may play key roles as antioxidants.

Phyto Nutrients/Food Factors. Phytochemicals are simply chemicals found in plants. They may explain why proper nutrition may help prevent cancer (*CSPI*, April 1994). Many substances in plants are now being investigated for potential anti-cancer as well as heart-protection effects. These compounds include flavonoids, carotenoids, isothiocyanates, cruciferous vegetables and indoles (*Berkeley Wellness Report-Nutrition, 1995*).

Each 3 multi-vitamin caplets contain 50 mg of green barley, chlorella, spirulina and lemon bioflavonoid complex.

Chromium. Each 3 multi-vitamin caplets contain 100 mcg of chromium in the form of a Kreb's cycle chelate (bio-friendly). This is similar to chromium picolinate, which is supposedly more easily absorbed than generic chromium. It has not been established how much chromium an individual needs to be healthy, so there is no established RDA, although chromium has been identified as an essential trace mineral. Chromium is important for *normal* carbohydrate and fat metabolism in the body, and in the proper functioning of insulin.

The estimated safe and adequate *daily* dietary intake (ESADDI) for chromium is 50-200 mcg per day for persons 7 years of age and older (Mahan, 1992 and National Academy of Sciences). It's hard to say how much chromium is in a given food because amounts vary, and some chromium is not bioavailable (easily absorbed) to the body. Though it is not clear whether chromium supplementation will induce weight loss, build lean muscle mass or reduce cholesterol—and current research seems to indicate that it won't—many experts believe it can not hurt anybody and might help prevent diabetes (*Berkeley Wellness Letter*, October 1994).

Since definitive studies are ongoing to determine chromium's absolute effectiveness in weight loss and lean body mass gain, and toxicity studies are not yet available, it is a prudent step to consult with a qualified expert if 200 mcg of chromium per day is exceeded.

Ginkgo Biloba. Each 3 caplets contain 50 mg of the herb ginkgo biloba. There are no nutritional requirements established. Ginkgo biloba is a popular ornamental tree grown world wide. Ginkgo biloba provides remarkable pharmacological action on the circulatory and nervous systems, according to Ross Pelton, R.Ph., Ph.D. in *Mind Food and Smart Pills*. Some of its attributes may include: acting as a vasodilator, preventing free-radical damage, protecting nervous tissue from damage, assisting the brain's metabolizing of glucose, improving nerve transmission and repairing lesions in cell membranes that have been damaged by free radicals. Since ginkgo biloba offers so many potential applications for keeping people healthy, it is not surprising that this herb is one of the most popular under scientific investigation (Hendler, 1990).

Calcium (Ca). Each 3 multi-mineral caplets contain 500 mg of the mineral calcium, which is 50% of the RDA. Calcium is an important nutrient and most Americans do not consume enough (*Berkeley Wellness Report-Nutrition,* 1994). In addition to its major function of building bones and teeth, calcium maintains bone strength and density, and regulates heartbeat, muscle contraction, nerve function and blood clotting. Calcium is an essential mineral in preventing or delaying the onset of osteoporosis, the age-related loss of bone mass and density that can lead to fragile bones, disability and sometimes death. Recent research suggests that calcium may have a role in preventing hypertension and cancer. Its importance in building and maintaining bone mass is undisputed (*Berkeley Wellness Report-Nutrition*, 1994).

Calcium is absorbed mainly in the part of the duodenum where an acid environment prevails. Absorption is greatly reduced in the lower part of the intestinal tract, where the contents become alkaline. Usually, only 20-30% of ingested calcium and sometimes as little as 10% is absorbed (Mahan, 1992). Normally, most of the ingested calcium (65-70%) is excreted in the feces and urine (Mahan, 1992). Vitamin D increases calcium absorption. The hydrochloric acid secreted in the stomach favors calcium absorption by lowering the pH (moving it toward an acidic versus alkaline environment) in the proximal duodenum. Moderate amounts of fat decrease transit time through the digestive tract, allowing more time for mineral absorption. Certain amino acids favorably influence pH in the intestinal tract. Taking calcium with a meal improves absorption (Heaney et al. 1989, Meal Effects on Calcium Absorption, *American Journal of Clinical Nutrition*, 49: 372).

Based on accumulated evidence, it seems prudent to increase the intake of calcium and vitamin D in most postmenopausal women. Calcium should be increased to at least 1,000 and preferably 1,500 mg per day, and vitamin D to 400-800 IU daily without waiting for further information (reported in *Berkeley Wellness Letter-Nutrition*, 1994). A good approach is to get at least 750 mg of calcium from one's diet, and to add a 1,000 mg supplement.

These conclusions were confirmed at the 1987 and 1990 conferences on "Research Advances in Osteoporosis," sponsored by the National Osteoporosis Foundation, the National Institutes of Health and the American Society for Bone and Mineral Research. The body builds bone mass during childhood and young adult years, thus peak bone mass isn't reached until age 25 or later. Adequate calcium is critical in these formative years, as well as in adult years. In a statement released at the 1990 conference, it was recommended that teenagers should get about 1,200 mg of calcium per day; postmenopausal women should get 1,000 mg a day if they are on hormone replacement therapy, and 1,500 mg if they are not. Other adults should get 800 mg of calcium per day. Obviously, if diet alone can not achieve this, the use of a supplement is warranted.

A calcium-rich diet may provide for a *lower* risk of kidney *stones (New England Journal of Medicine*, 1993). One explanation may be that many kidney stones are made of oxalate, and the calcium in foods may bind the oxalate before it can form or be deposited in an existing stone. Despite calcium's apparent safety, there is no reason to consume more than 1,500 mg per day (*CSPI, Nutrition Action Health Letter*, June 1994).

Reports reviewed by CRN demonstrate the safety of calcium in the dosage ranges currently being recommended for prevention of bone loss (Dickinson, 1991).

Magnesium (Mg). Each 3 multi-mineral caplets contain 250 mg of the mineral magnesium, which is 63% of the RDA. Magnesium occurs abundantly in food and is involved in a wide variety of biochemical and physiologic processes. These include muscle contraction and nerve excitability. It is a normal constituent of bone. Magnesium (along with calcium, vitamin D and boron) is important in building bone (*Berkeley Wellness Report-Nutrition*, 1994).

Magnesium and calcium, with similar functions, work somewhat in opposition to one another. Excess magnesium (thus a reason for 63% of the RDA and allowance for diet to provide additional mg) inhibits bone calcification. Many of the factors that govern calcium absorption from the upper intestine also influence bioavailability of magnesium (vitamin D has no effect on magnesium absorption). As dietary calcium is decreased, magnesium absorption is increased, thus the need for specific intakes of these nutrients within the stated guidelines.

CRN's review of literature demonstrates the safety of magnesium in doses of several hundred mg.

Iron (Fe). Each 3 multi-mineral caplets contain 9 mg of the mineral iron, which is 90% of the RDA for men.

Iron appears to be involved in the function of the immune system (Mahan, 1992). When iron intake is low or absorption is poor, the immune system is affected, placing it at higher risk for developing colds and infections. A person deficient in iron may feel sluggish or recover slowly after exercise. These symptoms can occur even when there are no signs of anemia, which is the final stage of iron deficiency.

Iron has a role in respiratory transport of oxygen and carbon dioxide. Hemoglobin is present in red blood cells. The iron-containing protein heme combines with oxygen in the lungs and with carbon dioxide. Myoglobin is also a heme protein and serves as an oxygen reservoir within the muscle. Oxidative production of ATP within the mitochondria involves many iron-containing enzymes, both heme and nonheme. The role of iron in cognitive performance has shown to make a difference in scholastic performance, sensorimotor competence, attention, learning and memory (Mahan, 1992).

The RDA for men is 10 mg, and for women age 25-50, the RDA is 15 mg. Nine mg of iron provided in this product equals 60% of the RDA for women. Unfortunately, even a well-balanced diet supplies only 6 mg of iron for every 1,000 calories (Elizabeth Somers, M.A., R.D., *The Essential Guide to Vitamins and Minerals and Nutrition for Women*, 1993 and Mahan, 1992). A menstruating, moderately active woman should consume at least 18 mg of iron daily (Somers, 1993).

The Food and Nutrition Board has recommended a daily intake of 10 mg of iron for men and postmenopausal women. An intake of 15 mg is recommended for women during child-bearing years to replace losses during menstruation and to provide for iron stores sufficient to support a pregnancy (Mahan, 1992). During pregnancy, the mother requires 30 mg per day of iron (twice her non-pregnant RDA of 15 mg per day), both to accommodate her increased blood volume and to have iron available for the fetus. Thus, pregnant women should receive 30 mg of supplemental elemental iron each day (*Sports Medicine Digest*, June 1990 and Mahan, 1992). Lactating mothers should receive 15 mg of iron per day (Mahan, 1992).

Iron deficiency can be aggravated by a poorly balanced diet containing insufficient iron, protein, folate and vitamins B-12, B-6 and C. Vitamin C (ascorbic acid) greatly enhances iron absorption. Attention also needs to be paid to the balance of iron, zinc and copper. By combining iron supplementation with iron-rich foods, such as black beans, oatmeal, whole-wheat bread, raisins, spinach and strawberries, it is reasonable to conclude that daily iron requirements can be met.

An additional supplement of elemental iron is usually required during pregnancy. Consult with the person's obstetrician/gynecologist concerning manipulations necessary for calcium (recommended 1200 mg), folic acid (at least 400 mcg but not more than 800 mcg), iron (30 mg of supplemental elemental iron) and any other nutritional concerns of the perinatal client.

Zinc (Zn). Each 3 multi-mineral caplets contain 15 mg of the mineral zinc, which is 100% of the RDA for men (the RDA for women is 12 mg). Zinc, in proper amounts, supports the immune system, helps with wound healing and is an essential component of many enzymes related to synthesis or degradation of carbohydrates, lipids and proteins. Zinc is also involved with one of the key antioxidant enzymes (superoxide dismutase).

CRN reports that research demonstrates the safety of zinc in doses several times the RDA. Mild diarrhea or nausea may be an indication the dose is excessive. Taking zinc with meals may alleviate such minor side effects. Attention needs to be paid to the balance of zinc, copper and iron. Levels of zinc greater than 15 mg may inhibit calcium absorption and affect the immune system if copper intake is low. Megadoses (10 times the RDA) can reduce levels of HDL and may impair blood cell formation and compromise immunity (*Berkeley Wellness Letter*, December 1994).

Excess oral ingestion of zinc to the point of toxicity (100-300 mg per day) is rare. Supplementation in excess of the RDA will interfere with copper absorption unless a balance is maintained (Mahan, 1992).

Copper (Cu). Each 3 multi-mineral caplets contain 2 mg of the mineral copper, which is within the range of the 1.5-3 mg per day (Mahan, 1992) recommended as an estimated safe and adequate daily dietary intake (ESADDI). Copper aids in the healing processes, red blood cell formation and is an essential component of many enzymes, including those essential to antioxidants functioning effectively and mitochondrial energy production. Copper is involved with one of the key antioxidant enzymes (superoxide dismutase).

CRN concludes that research demonstrates the safety of copper at intakes up to 5-10 mg per day, for adults. The Food and Drug Administration permits the inclusion of copper in nutritional supplements at doses within the "safe and adequate" range established by the Food and Nutrition Board.

Manganese (Mn). Each 3 multi-mineral caplets contain 25 mg of the mineral manganese. Manganese has been determined to be an essential nutrient, but actual requirements have not been established. It should not be confused with magnesium.

Manganese supports reproduction and growth, the formation of connective and bony tissues, carbohydrate and lipid metabolism and is involved in key free-radical-fighting enzymes (Mahan, 1992). Manganese is involved with one of the key antioxidant enzymes (superoxide dismutase). Along with calcium and magnesium, manganese may play an important role in preventing osteoporosis and may help diabetics who do not respond to insulin injections (*Environmental Nutrition*, November 1994). And while these findings are still preliminary, a manganese deficiency has never been diagnosed in humans. However, it's still a good idea to eat foods rich in manganese. These include whole grain breads, cereals and other plant foods.

Note that the recommended safe intake (National Academy of Sciences) is 5 mg per day. An ESADDI for manganese for adults and children 11 years and older ranges from 2-5 mg per day (Mahan, 1992). This product contains 25 mg of manganese, which is well in excess of these recommendations. Does that make this product a bad selection? Probably not. Manganese is one of the least toxic minerals. There is no known natural toxicity from manganese in food or from taking *reasonable* amounts in the form of supplements (Haas, 1992). Haas believes that manganese from supplements should be limited to about 10-15 mg per day, if taken regularly. Most supplements contain an average of 4 mg. He does note that 50 mg has been taken daily in some research studies without negative side effects. Though there seems to be little toxicity risk regarding this level of intake, you have to wonder why the manufacturer missed the "mark" on this particular nutrient, with regard to guidelines for recommended intake.

Selenium (L-Selenomethionine). Each 3 multi-mineral caplets contain 50 mcg of the mineral selenium. Selenium has been determined to be an essential nutrient, but actual requirements have not been established. Selenium is recognized as a free-radical fighter and supports the immune system. Selenium is involved with the enzyme glutathione peroxidase and this enzyme helps prevent the formation of hydroxyl radicals.

Recommended safe intake is 50 mcg per day (National Academy of Sciences). In 1989 the RDA for selenium was set for the first time. The recommended intake for males over 18 is 70 mcg, 55 mcg for females over 18, 65 mcg for pregnant women and 75 mcg for lactating women. It should be noted that indicators of selenium toxicity and the level of dietary intake at which toxicity occurs are not known (Mahan, 1992). Reports reviewed by CRN demonstrate the safety of selenium at doses well above the recommended dietary levels (Dickinson, 1991).

Molybdenum (Mb). Each 3 multi-mineral caplets contain 100 mcg of the mineral molybdenum. An interrelationship among molybdenum, copper and sulfate absorption has been demonstrated (Mahan, 1992). Molybdenum is a component of several enzyme systems whose function is the formation of uric acid and the shifting of iron into transport transferrin when more iron is required. Dosage recommendations range from 150-500 mcg (Stare, et al. *Living Nutrition*, 1981). The daily requirement of molybdenum is not known; however, the 1989 ESADDI is 75-250 mcg per day for adolescents and adults (Mahan, 1992).

Vanadium (V). Each 3 multi-mineral caplets contain 50 mcg of the mineral vanadium. Vanadium *in vitro* inhibits various transfer enzymes, but it is unclear whether it performs a regulatory function under normal physiologic conditions (Mahan, 1992). Vanadium is now known to be an essential nutrient but no RDA or ESADDI have been established (Mahan, 1992), nor a toxicity level identified.

Potassium (K). Each 3 multi-mineral caplets contain 99 mg of the mineral potassium. Potassium is a major cation (positive ion) in intracellular fluid. Along with sodium (Na), it is involved in the maintenance of normal water balance and acid base balance (Mahan, 1992). It is usually added to electrolyte-replacement drinks. Potassium also promotes cellular growth, and its level in muscle is related to muscle mass and glycogen storage. Therefore, if muscle is being formed, an adequate supply of potassium is essential (Mahan, 1992).

The minimum requirement for adults is 1,600-2,000 mg per day (Mahan, 1992), but higher levels may be recommended because of potassium's possible protective effect against hypertension (Food and Nutrition Board, 1989 and National Research Council, 1989). A potassium deficiency from an inadequate intake is not likely in healthy individuals, because potassium is widely distributed in foods.

Lipogenic Complex. Each 3 multi-mineral caplets contain 50 mg of **betaine HCL, choline** and **myo-inositol.** Choline is an essential component of animal tissues and is classified as having vitamin-like activity. Choline functions as a component of larger molecules (i.e., lecithin) that serve as structural components of cell membranes, as pulmonary surfactant and as a neurotransmitter (Magan, 1992). Choline is a precursor of acetylcholine (neuro-transmitter) and is often classed with the B-complex vitamins.

Daily requirements are not known, and no toxic effects have been observed. The average diet has been estimated to contain 400-900 mg per day of choline (Mahan, 1992). This amount is apparently adequate for health but should not be equated with dietary requirement.

Myo-inositol occurs abundantly in the average diet, usually as inositol phospholipids. It is estimated that a mixed North American diet provides the adult with 300-1,000 mg per day (Mahan, 1992). Myo-inositol is one of 9 isomers of inositol that has metabolic importance. Its physiologic role is related to the function of phospholipids in cell membranes. Inositol mediates cellular responses to stimuli, nerve transmissions and regulates enzyme activity. Inositol metabolism is partially affected by dietary choline content (Mahan, 1992).

Vitamin D-2 (ergocalciferol). Each 3 multi-mineral caplets contain 400 IU of vitamin D, which is 100% of the RDA. Vitamin D deficiency is manifested as rickets (malformation of bones) in children and osteomalacia (softening of the bones) in adults. Lack of the vitamin in adults may also contribute to the development of osteoporosis (Mahan, 1992).

Vitamin D is as essential as calcium for bone strength. Vitamin D plays a vital role in the body's absorption of calcium and phosphorus, and thus promotes the growth of strong bones. In older people, a vitamin D deficiency increases the severity of osteoporosis (loss of bone mass and weakening of bones) and the risk of osteomalacia, an adult form of rickets (*Berkeley Wellness Letter*, August 1994).

A group of recent studies suggests that adequate intake of vitamin D may reduce the risk of some cancers. Though the evidence is preliminary, since vitamin D works closely with calcium in the body and calcium seems to protect against certain cancers (notably colon cancer), this may explain why vitamin D may also be protective (*Berkeley Wellness Letter*, August 1994). Some researchers think the RDA for vitamin D should be raised to 800 IU because it works so closely with calcium in creating stronger bones (*Berkeley Wellness Report-Nutrition*, 1994).

CRN reports that research demonstrates the safety of vitamin D at daily intakes several times the RDA, which is 400 IU for men and women age 11-24, and 200 IU for men and women age 25 and over. The RDA for pregnant and lactating women is 400 IU.

Vitamin D toxicity develops over time. The toxic level has not been established for all ages, but toxicity should always be monitored when large doses of vitamin D (i.e., 1,000 IU or more) are given for an extended period (Mahan, 1992).

Iodine (kelp). Each 3 multi-mineral caplets contain 150 mcg of this mineral, which is 100% of the RDA. Iodine occurs in extremely variable amounts in food and drinking water. The only known function of iodine is its role as an integral part of thyroid hormones (Mahan, 1992). Lack of iodine intake is associated with the development of simple goiter, which is an enlargement of the thyroid gland.

In terms of toxicity, iodine has a wide margin of safety (Mahan, 1992). An intake of 150 mcg has been suggested as sufficient for all adults and adolescents. The RDA for pregnant women is 175 mcg and for lactating women, 200 mcg per day.

CRN's review of research indicates the safety of iodine at many times the recommended dietary levels. Food additive regulations limit the iodine content of nutritional supplements and fortified foods to 45 mcg for infants, 105 mcg for children, 225 mcg for adults and 300 mcg for pregnant or lactating women.

The Bridge

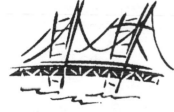

There is a continuing and expanding knowledge of the role of vitamins and minerals, and their contribution to overall health. (It is estimated that every few minutes thousands of "bits" of new information is generated regarding nutrition.) Since your clients will ask you questions about supplements they hear and read about, you are encouraged to acquire knowledge in this area. I believe that responsible supplementation is appropriate. Before you make any decisions, take the time to learn about the purpose of each vitamin and mineral and about toxicity levels.

The following references have been extremely helpful to me in forming my personal philosophy and recommendations regarding nutritional supplementation. Additionally, the scientific references have allowed me to confidently and accurately guide my clients to more efficient use of the money they were *already* spending on supplements. And most important, I believe I am helping them pursue another area of their total health and fitness program, safely and effectively. (One of my favorite references when I need information quickly is Haas, 1992.)

References and Recommended Reading

Council for Responsible Nutrition (1993). **Benefits of Nutritional Supplements.** Published by Council for Responsible Nutrition, (202) 872-1488

Council For Responsible Nutrition (1991). **The Safety of Vitamins and Minerals: A Summary of the Findings of Key Reviews.**

Bernardot, Dan, editor (1993). **Sports Nutrition—A Guide for the Professional Working With Active People.** The American Dietetic Association.

Dickinson, Annette, editor (1993). **Benefits of Nutritional Supplements.** Washington, D.C., The Council for Responsible Nutrition.

Dickinson, Annette, Editor (1991). **Safety of Vitamins and Minerals: A Summary of the Findings of Key Reviews.** Washington, D.C., The Council for Responsible Nutrition, June.

Haas, Elson (1992). **Staying Healthy with Nutrition.** Berkeley, CA: Celestial Art Publishing.

Hendler, Sheldon (1990). **The Doctors Vitamin and Mineral Encyclopedia.** New York: Simon and Schuster.

Jacobson, Michael, editor (1987). The Right Dose. **Nutrition Action Health Letter**, Washington, D.C., Center for Science in the Public Interest (CSPI).

Mahan, Kathleen, and Arlin, Marian (1992). **Krause's Food, Nutrition and Diet Therapy.** Philadelphia, PA: W. B. Saunders, 8th edition.

Margen, Sheldon, et al. editors (1994). Nutrition. **The University of California at Berkeley Wellness Reports.**

Marmot, M. G. (1986). Epidemiology and the Art of the Soluble. **Lancet:** i: 897-900.

Miller, S.A., and Stephenson, M.G. (1985). **Scientific and Public Health Rationale for the Dietary Guidelines for Americans.** Vol. 42:739-745.

Van der Beek et al. (1988). Thiamin, Riboflavin and Vitamin B-6, and C: Impact of Combined Restricted Intake on Functional Performance in Man. **American Journal of Clinical Nutrition**, 48: 601.

CHAPTER 21

THE TENTH STEP

Here's the vision: You have a waiting list of clients. Many former clients have successfully integrated exercise into their lives with your help—you know because they call to say hello and come back periodically for "refresher" courses. Other clients have stayed with you over the years and continue to refer clients to you. They like the ongoing motivation you offer, or have special needs that require your monitoring and expertise.

You have mastered Step 10—the reality factor. Lives change. Personal needs change. But a high-quality personal training business always has an abundance of clients, in my observation, because the trainer(s) leading the organization is able to customize programs to changing needs and has the "right" personality. In other words, she has an approach and style that is capable of meeting the diversity of an extensive client list.

Encouraging your clients' perception that they are successful may be the most important aspect of program design. Four important factors can ensure exercise adherence and a successful business.

1. **Time.** Keep beginning workouts around one hour, 2-3 times per week.

2. **Variety.** Use cross training when appropriate.

3. **Intrinsic Motivation.** Both you, and especially the clients, should know why they want to exercise (ask them!).

4. **Lifestyle Changes.** Your clients must like what they are doing to permanently incorporate new behavior into their lifelong habits.

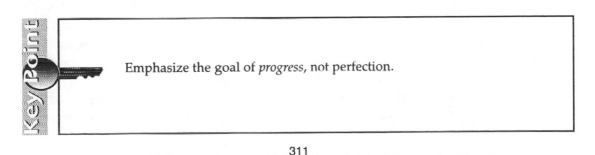

Emphasize the goal of *progress*, not perfection.

Successful program design means healthy, happy clients, as well as a thriving business. Most clients do not want to exercise "hard." Most individuals exercise to feel better and have more energy for daily living. As a trainer you need to step beyond your own biases and understand the preferences of your clients. Most of your clients would not plan their exercise programs like you plan your own. Consider this thought seriously and you are on your way to effective and safe program design that will keep your clients coming back for more!

I have worked with some personal training clients for as long as 9 years. Their "reality factor" or situations today, are similar to what you read about them in Chapter 1. Many still do not perform with perfect exercise technique. Some do not have all of the ideal components of a balanced fitness program comfortably inserted into their daily schedule. Others have never linked their moderate cardiorespiratory interval segments into a continual effort.

Though most of my clients are usually not perfect, their individual improvements are great. Their lives are better. My philosophy is to attempt to optimize my clients' involvement in fitness for a lifetime, with whatever techniques it takes. That means not becoming a robotic trainer who uses one recipe or program for every client. The measurement of your success is gauged by your actions, and in the eyes of your clients, by your service toward them.

> More often than not, an effective program and successful business offer a smorgasbord of options that is ever-changing with each client's individual fluctuations.

The 10 Steps

Are you using the 10 steps when planning programs? I feel these steps are extremely important. Here's a final review. You can achieve the 10th step only when you can knowledgeably apply the first nine.

Step 1: Information Gathering. The medical history/health questionnaire asks questions that elicit information you need to help identify medical concerns, and fitness testing is an *optional* motivational tool. The client interview that becomes an ongoing dialogue is a critical factor in long-term success.

Step 2: Balanced Physical Programming. Balanced physical programming walks a fine line between *listening* to what your client is telling you that she *wants*, and incorporating these interests into a program that also contains what she *needs* from a total wellness perspective. It's your challenge to plan for variety and effectiveness.

Step 3: Cardiorespiratory Conditioning. Not as straightforward as it might seem, a variety of cardiorespiratory activities (walking, running, biking, swimming) avoids an increased risk of overuse injury, maintains a high level of interest and keeps producing results.

Step 4: Muscular Strength and Endurance Conditioning. Most of your clients should engage in strength training, and you have an incredible array of options to change the program and influence results.

Step 5: Flexibility Training. An important part of the program, the development of functional or usable flexibility, entails challenging range of motion in a manner that closely mimics daily or functional movement.

Step 6: Active Rest. Your job is to incorporate active rest into the workout to optimize time availability and accommodate the fitness level of the individual. This is an excellent way to effectively use the finite time you have available.

Step 7: Cross Training. This is fun for you because it challenges your skills, and fun for your client because of the variety and results. Cross training is productive, time-efficient and motivates your clients to stick to their program.

Step 8: Special Needs for Healthy Populations. You can work with special populations when you recognize your boundaries of knowledge. "Special" includes issues such as safe weight maintenance or exercising safely through pregnancy.

Step 9: Success and Adherence. This is a key. Planning appropriate physical programs and encouraging the client's perception that she is successful is one—if not the most—important aspect of program design.

Step 10: The Reality Factor. This characterizes successful trainers. Optimize your client's involvement in fitness for a lifetime, with whatever techniques it takes.

Qualities for the Next Millennium

Essential qualities of successful trainers that will carry them (you!) into the next century include:

1. Formal education and/or nationally recognized industry certifications are important to help you establish credibility with licensed professionals, and an increasingly educated consumer.

2. Continuing education through home-study programs and by attendance at industry educational conferences. These are critical to your continued growth and crucial to providing accurate information to clients, as exercise science is always changing.

3. Depth and diversity in education will allow you to expand your client base, provide the best programming to your clients and help you keep interested and enthusiastic about your job.

4. An ability to identify the ever-changing needs of our population. This will allow you to become part of the cutting-edge group of professionals who are prepared to meet the constantly evolving and changing needs of society.

5. Interest in identifying and growing with fitness/health trends as they evolve so that you can be among the first to align with these new ideas and fill the need created by consumer interest, with appropriate service.

6. The capability of bringing your skills and training back to a personal level. If it isn't personal, your business isn't as special as it could be, and you're not taking advantage of a perfect learning environment—one on one.

7. Maintaining an ongoing dialogue with your clients and exhibiting people skills that communicate "I care about you." This is best shown by your attention to detail in regard to your clients' needs, your professional growth and behavior, and delivery of impeccable service.

You should have the ability to charm, cajole, educate, motivate and prod when necessary. You should not only convince and assist your clients to achieve their exercise goal(s), but also help them sustain their level of enthusiasm and commitment to health-related lifestyle changes and regular exercise.

The Bridge

The prized and intangible skill, that goes well beyond necessary technical competency, is your personality. Ultimately, the right combination of qualities leads to success for you and all of your clients—and keeps them coming back for more!

Appendix
Bibliography, References and Recommended Reading

Anderson, Owen (1993). *Running Research News* (general reference), Lansing, MI.

American Council on Exercise (ACE) (1991). *Personal Trainer Manual*. Published by ACE, San Diego, CA.

American College of Sports Medicine (ACSM) (1991). *Guidelines for Exercise Testing and Prescription*. 4th edition, Lea and Febiger, Philadelphia, PA.

American College of Sports Medicine Position Stand (1990). The Recommended Quantity and Quality of Exercise for Developing and Maintaining Cardiorespiratory and Muscular Fitness in Healthy Adults. *Medicine and Science in Sports and Exercise*, Volume 22, No. 2, April, pp. 265-274.

Baechle, Tom, and Groves, Barney (1992). *Weight Training - Steps To Success*. Human Kinetics Publishers, Champaign, IL. (800) 747-4457

Barnard, R.J., et al. (1973). Cardiovascular responses to sudden strenuous exercise: heart rate, blood pressure, and ECG. *Journal Applied Physiology*, 34:883.

Barnard, R.J., et al. (1973). Ischemic response to sudden strenuous exercise in healthy men. *Circulation*, 48:936.

Basmajian, John, and DeLuca, Carlo (1979). *Muscles Alive - Their Functions Revealed By Electromyography*. 4th edition, Williams and Wilkins, Baltimore, MD. (800) 638-0672

Bernardot, Dan, editor (1993). *Sports Nutrition—A Guide For The Professional Working With Active People*. The American Dietetic Association.

Bompa, T. (1983). *Theory and methodology of training*. Dubuque, IL: Kendall- Hunt.

Brooks, Douglas (1990). *Going Solo—The Art of Personal Training*. 2nd edition, Moves International Publishing, Mammoth Lakes, CA (619) 934-0312

Brooks, Douglas et al. (1995). *Resist-A-Ball: Programming Guide For Fitness Professionals*. Moves International Publishing, Mammoth Lakes, CA (619) 934-0312

Brooks, Douglas et al. (1995). *Reebok Interval Program Manual*. Reebok International, Ltd: Stoughton, MA.

Brooks, Douglas (1995). *Planning Your Strength Program*. IDEA Today: San Diego, CA, September.

Brooks, Douglas (1995). *Shaping the Shoulder*. IDEA Today: San Diego, CA, October.

Brooks, Douglas (1995). *Training the Upper Back*. IDEA Today: San Diego, CA, November/ December.

Brooks, Douglas (1996). *Sculpting the Chest*. IDEA Today: San Diego, CA, January.

Brooks, Douglas (1996). *Strengthening the Upper Arms*. IDEA Today: San Diego, CA, March.

Brooks, Douglas, and Copeland-Brooks, Candice (1993). Uncovering the Myths of Abdominal Exercise, *IDEA Today*, April, pp. 42-49.

Videos with Douglas Brooks:

Brooks, Douglas (1995). *The Best Strength Training Exercises: Upper Body.* Moves International: Mammoth Lakes, CA (619) 934-0312.

Brooks, Douglas (1995). *The Best Strength Training Exercises: Lower Body.* Moves International: Mammoth Lakes, CA (619) 934-0312.

Brooks, Douglas (1995). *The Best Strength Training Exercises: Trunk.* Moves International: Mammoth Lakes, CA (619) 934-0312.

Brooks, Douglas (1995). *One on One: Strength Training Workouts for Everyone.* Moves International: Mammoth Lakes, CA (619) 934-0312.

Written References Continued:

Bruner, R., et al. (1992). *Soviet training and recovery methods.* Pleasant Hill, CA: Sport Focus Publishing.

Byrne, Kevin (1991). *Understanding and Managing Cholesterol.* Human Kinetics Books, Champaign, IL. (800) 747-4457

Cailliet, R. (1988). *Low Back Pain Syndrome.* 4th edition, F.A. Davis Company, Philadelphia, PA.

Carter Center (1988). *Healthier People: Health Risk Appraisal Program,* The Carter Center of Emory University, Atlanta, GA, July.

Cohen, Sharon (1993). The 20-Minute Myth, *SHAPE Magazine,* November.

Council For Responsible Nutrition (CRN) (1993). *Benefits of Nutritional Supplements.* Published by Council For Responsible Nutrition, (202) 872-1488

Council For Responsible Nutrition (1991). *The Safety of Vitamins and Minerals: A Summary of the Findings of Key Reviews.*

Couzens, Gerald (1992). Personal Trainers: A Formula for Fitness? *The Physician and Sportsmedicine,* Vol. 20, No. 11, November 1992

Dickinson, Annette, editor (1993). *Benefits of Nutritional Supplements.* Washington, D.C., The Council for Responsible Nutrition.

Dickinson, Annette, editor (1991). *Safety of Vitamins and Minerals: A Summary of the Findings of Key Reviews.* Washington, D.C., The Council for Responsible Nutrition, June.

Dimsdale, J.E., et al. (1987). Post exercise peril: plasma catecholamines and exercise. *JAMA,* 251:630.

Dishman, Rod K., (1994). Prescribing exercise intensity for healthy adults using perceived exertion. *Medicine and Science in Sports and Exercise.* Vol. 26, No. 9, pp. 1087-94.

Dishman, R.K., Farquhar, R.P., and Cureton, K.J. (1994). Responses to preferred intensities of exertion in men differing in activity levels. *Medicine and Science in Sports and Exercise,* Vol. 26, No. 9, pp. 783-90.

Ebelling, C.B., Ward, A., and Rippe, J.M. (1991). Comparison between palpated heart rates and heart rates observed using the Polar Favor heart rate monitor during an aerobics exercise class. *Exercise Physiology and Nutrition Laboratory,* University of Massachusetts Medical School, Worcester, MA.

Ellison, Deborah (1993). *Advanced Exercise Design For Lower Body*. 2nd edition, Movement That Matters, Vista, CA (619) 599-9366

Evans, William, and Rosenberg, Irwin (1991). *Biomarkers.* Simon and Schuster, New York, NY.

Fair, Erik (1992). Fitness Software. *IDEA Today*, San Diego, CA. June, pg. 27.

Fisher, Garth, and Jensen, Clayne (1990). *Scientific Basis of Athletic Conditioning.* 3rd edition, Lea and Febiger, Philadelphia, PA.

Fleck, Steven and Kraemer, William (1987). *Designing Resistance Training Programs.* Human Kinetics Publishers, Champaign, IL.

Francis, Peter, et al. (1994). *The effectiveness of elastic resistance in strength overload.* Pilot study, San Diego State University.

Francis, Peter, and Francis, Lorna (1988). *If It Hurts, Don't Do It.* Prima Publishing, Rocklin, CA. (916) 624-5718

Gesing, Bernard F. (1990). All for One: Client/Trainer/Physician. *IDEA Today*, November/December.

Giese, M. (1988). Organization of an exercise session. In *American College of Sports Medicine Resource Manual,* for guidelines for exercise testing and prescription., pp. 244-247, Philadelphia: Lea and Febiger.

Golding, Lawrence, et al. (1989). *The Y's Way to Physical Fitness.* Human Kinetics Publishers, Champaign, IL. (800) 747-4457

Gordon, Neil (1993). *Diabetes: Your Complete Exercise Guide.* Human Kinetics Publishers, Champaign, IL.

Graves, James, and Pollock, Michael (1993). *Understanding The Physiological Basis Of Muscular Fitness.* Published in, Stairmaster Fitness Handbook, Masters Press, Indianapolis, IN.

Haas, Elson (1992). *Staying Healthy with Nutrition.* Berkeley, CA: Celestial Art Publishing.

Harper, Deby: Information on *Personal Fitness System (PFS)* is available through The Fitness Company, 7127 E. Becker Lane, Suite 168, Scottsdale, AZ, 85254 or contact Deby Harper at (602) 951-8149.

Hendler, Sheldon (1990). *The Doctors Vitamin and Mineral Encyclopedia.* New York: Simon and Schuster.

Heyward, Vivian (1991). *Advanced Fitness Assessment and Exercise Prescription.* 2nd edition, Human Kinetics Books, Champaign, IL.

Hickson, R.C., et al. (1985). Reduced training intensities and loss of aerobic power, endurance, and cardiac growth. *Journal of Applied Physiology,* 58:492-99.

Jackson, Andrew S., and Pollock, Michael L. (1985) Practical Assessment of Body Composition, *The Physician and Sports Medicine;* Vol. 13, No. 5, May 1985, pp. 76-90

Jacobson, Michael, editor (1987). The Right Dose. *Nutrition Action Health Letter*, Washington, D.C., Center for Science in the Public Interest (CSPI).

Kendall, Florence, et al. (1993). *Muscles - Testing and Function.* 4th edition, Williams and Wilkins, Baltimore, MD. (800) 638-0672

Komi, P.V., editor (1992). **Strength and Power in Sport**. *Distributed by Human Kinetics Publishers, Champaign, IL. (800) 747-4457*

Kraemer, William, and Fleck, Steven (1993). **Strength Training For Young Athletes**. *Human Kinetics Publishers, Champaign, IL.*

Leger, L., and Thiveragte L. (1998). *Heart Rate Monitors: Validity, Stability and Functionality.* **Physician and Sports Medicine**, *Vol. 16, No. 5, pp. 153-161.*

Lifeline International: *A* **resource for elastic resistance** *(tubing, bands etc.) and other associated resistance training systems. (800) 553-6633*

Lohman, Timothy, et al. (1988). **Anthropometric Standardization Reference Manual**. *Human Kinetics Books, Champaign, IL.*

Mahan, Kathleen, and Arlin, Marian (1992). **Krause's Food, Nutrition and Diet Therapy**. *Philadelphia, PA: W. B. Saunders, 8th edition.*

Margen, Sheldon, et al. editors (1994). Nutrition. **The University of California at Berkeley, Wellness Reports.**

Marmot, M. G. (1986). *Epidemiology and the Art of the Soluble.* **Lancet:** *i: 897-900.*

McArdle, William, et al. (1991). **Exercise Physiology - Energy, Nutrition and Human Performance**. *3rd edition, Lea and Febiger, Philadelphia, PA.*

McDonagh, M.J.N., and Davies, C.T.M. (1984). *Adaptive response of mammalian skeletal muscle to exercise with high loads.* **European Journal of Applied Physiology**, *52, 139-155.*

Metveyev, L. (1981). **Fundamental of sports training**. *Moscow: Progress Publishers.*

Miller, S.A., and Stephenson, M.G. (1985). **Scientific and Public Health Rationale for the Dietary Guidelines for Americans**. *Vol. 42:739-745.*

Ornish, Dean, et al. (1990). *Can Lifestyle Changes Reverse Coronary Heart Disease?* **The Lancet,** *336, pps. 129-133.*

Ozolin, N. (1971). **The athlete's training system for competition**. *Moscow: Fizkultura i Sport Publication.*

Pate, R., et al. (1995). *Physical Activity and Public Health: A Recommendation From the Centers for Disease Control and Prevention and The American College of Sports Medicine.* **Journal of the American Medical Association**, *273, pps. 402-7.*

Plowman, Sharon (1992). *Physical Activity, Physical Fitness, and Low Back Pain.* **Exercise and Sport Sciences Reviews,** *Volume 20, pp. 221-242.*

Polar Electro Inc., **Heart rate monitors,** *99 Seaview Blvd., Port Washington, N.Y. (800) 227-1314*

Pollock, Michael, and Wilmore, Jack (1990). **Exercise In Health and Disease**. *2nd edition, W.B. Saunders, Philadelphia, PA.*

Purvis, Tom (1994). **Trainer's Video Lecture And Hands-On Series**. *Focus On Fitness: Oklahoma City, Oklahoma. (405) 755-3082*

Roberts, Scott, editor (1996). **The Business of Personal Training**. *Champaign, IL: Human Kinetics Publishers.*

Rockport Walking Institute, *P.O. Box 480, Marlboro, MA 01752, (508) 485-2090*

Safran, M.R., et al. (1988). *The role of warm-up in muscular injury prevention.* **American Journal Sports Medicine**, 16:123.

Schardt, David (1993). *These Feet Were Made For Walking.* **Nutrition Action Health Letter, Center for Science in the Public Interest,** Vol. 20, No. 10, December.

Sharkey, Brian (1991). **New Dimensions In Aerobic Fitness.** Human Kinetics Publishers, Champaign, IL.

Sharkey, Brian (1990). **Physiology of Fitness.** 3rd edition, Human Kinetics Publishers, Champaign, IL.

Sheehan, George (1991). **The Physician And Sports Medicine.** Health Risk Appraisals, Vol. 19, No. 5, pg. 41.

Sherman, Carl (1994). *Reversing Heart Disease: Are Lifestyle Changes Enough?* **The Physician And Sportsmedicine,** Vol. 22, No. 1, January, pps. 91-94.

Siff, Mel, et al. (1993). **Super Training: Special Strength Training For Sporting Excellence.** South Africa: School of Mechanical Engineering, University of Witwatersrand.

Skinner, James (1993). **Understanding The Physiological Basis Of Cardiorespiratory Fitness.** Published in, Stairmaster Fitness Handbook, Masters Press, Indianapolis, IN.

Sleamaker, Rob (1989). **Serious Training for Serious Athletes.** Leisure Press—A Division of Human Kinetics Books, Champaign, IL.

Smith, Bob (1993). **Advanced Fitness Teacher's Manual.** Ludoe Publications: Loughborough University, England.

SPRI: **A resource for elastic resistance** (tubing, bands etc.), other associated resistance training systems and personal training products. (800) 222-7774

Stone, Michael, and O'Bryant, Harold (1987). **Weight Training - A Scientific Approach.** Burgess International Group, Minneapolis, MN.

Thompson, Clem (1989). **Manual of Structural Kinesiology.** 11th edition, Times Mirror/Mosby, St. Louis, MO. (314) 872-8370

Townsend, Hal, et al. (1991). *Electromyographic analysis of the glenohumeral muscles during a baseball rehabilitation program.* **The American Journal of Sports Medicine,** Vol. 19, No. 3.

Vorobyev, A. (1978). **A textbook on weight lifting.** Budapest: International Weightlifting Federation.

Westcott, Wayne (1991). **Strength Fitness.** 3rd edition, Wm. C. Brown Publishers, Dubuque, IA. (319) 588-1451

Wichmann, Susan, and Martin, D.R. (1992). *Heart Disease: Not For Men Only.* **The Physician And Sports Medicine,** Vol. 20, No. 8, August, pps. 138-48.

Wilmore, Jack (1991). *Resistance Training For Health: A Renewed Interest.* **Sports Medicine Digest,** June, pg. 6.

Wilmore, Jack, and Costill, David (1994). **Physiology of Sport and Exercise.** Human Kinetics Publishers, Champaign, IL. (800) 747-4457

Wilmore, Jack, and Costill, David (1988). **Training for Sport and Activity: The Physiological Basis of the Conditioning Process.** 3rd edition, William Brown Publishers, Dubuque, IA.

Van der Beek, et al. (1988). *Thiamin, Riboflavin and Vitamin B6, and C: Impact of Combined Restricted Intake on Functional Performance in Man.* **American Journal of Clinical Nutrition**, 48: 601.

Yessis, M. (1987). **The secret of soviet sports fitness and training.** Published: Arbor House.

Index

ABOUT THE AUTHOR

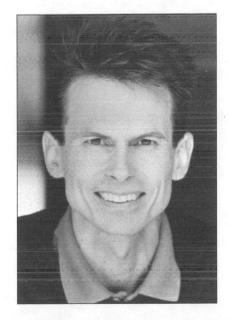

Douglas Brooks, MS, has successfully bridged his academic background, program design and communication skills to become one of the country's premier personal trainers. While his career has expanded as an author and lecturer, video and television educator, Douglas remains a "trainer's trainer" because he practices what he teaches. He writes articles and lectures to trainers internationally on exercise science, strength training and personal training. Douglas also incorporates his experience as a marathon runner, triathlete and skier. He lives near the top of a mountain in Mammoth Lakes, California with his wife and two sons, and cross-trains with all the toys according to the season.

Other books and videos by Douglas Brooks, MS

Going Solo—The Art of Personal Training (book)
Best Strength Exercises—Upper Body (video)
Best Strength Exercises—Lower Body (video)
Best Strength Exercises—Trunk (video)
Stability Ball Training (video)

You'll find
other outstanding
Fitness Instruction resources a

www.humankinetics.com

In the U.S. call

1-800-747-4457

Australia	....	(08) 8277-155
Canada	....	(800) 465-730
Europe	....	+44 (0) 113-278-1708
New Zealand	....	(09) 309-189

HUMAN KINETICS
The Information Leader in Physical Activity
P.O. Box 5076 • Champaign, IL 61825-5076 USA